I0072136

Traumatic Brain Injury:
Assessment and Management

Traumatic Brain Injury: Assessment and Management

Edited by Chris Garcia

hayle
medical

New York

Hayle Medical,
750 Third Avenue, 9th Floor,
New York, NY 10017, USA

Visit us on the World Wide Web at:
www.haylemedical.com

© Hayle Medical, 2019

This book contains information obtained from authentic and highly regarded sources. Copyright for all individual chapters remain with the respective authors as indicated. All chapters are published with permission under the Creative Commons Attribution License or equivalent. A wide variety of references are listed. Permission and sources are indicated; for detailed attributions, please refer to the permissions page and list of contributors. Reasonable efforts have been made to publish reliable data and information, but the authors, editors and publisher cannot assume any responsibility for the validity of all materials or the consequences of their use.

ISBN: 978-1-63241-683-4

Trademark Notice: Registered trademark of products or corporate names are used only for explanation and identification without intent to infringe.

Cataloging-in-Publication Data

Traumatic brain injury : assessment and management / edited by Chris Garcia.
    p. cm.
Includes bibliographical references and index.
ISBN 978-1-63241-683-4
1. Brain--Wounds and injuries. 2. Brain--Wounds and injuries--Treatment.
3. Brain damage. I. Garcia, Chris.
RC387.5 .T73 2019
617.481 044--dc23

Table of Contents

Preface

Traumatic brain injury (TBI), also referred to as intracranial injury, occurs due to trauma to the brain. It can cause a range of physical, cognitive, behavioral, social and emotional symptoms. Its outcome can vary from complete recovery to permanent disability or death. TBI can occur due to an accident, physical violence or a fall. Its diagnosis involves the use of techniques like magnetic resonance imaging (MRI) and computed tomography. Depending on the extent of the injury, confirmed through a diagnosis, treatment can be minimal or extensive involving medications, surgery and rehabilitation therapies. This book discusses the fundamental as well as modern approaches in the assessment and management of traumatic brain injury. The topics included in this book are of utmost significance and bound to provide incredible insights to readers. It will prove to be immensely beneficial to students and researchers in this domain.

Various studies have approached the subject by analyzing it with a single perspective, but the present book provides diverse methodologies and techniques to address this field. This book contains theories and applications needed for understanding the subject from different perspectives. The aim is to keep the readers informed about the progresses in the field; therefore, the contributions were carefully examined to compile novel researches by specialists from across the globe.

Indeed, the job of the editor is the most crucial and challenging in compiling all chapters into a single book. In the end, I would extend my sincere thanks to the chapter authors for their profound work. I am also thankful for the support provided by my family and colleagues during the compilation of this book.

Editor

Targeted Temperature Management in Traumatic Brain Injury

Sombat Muengtaweepongsa and
Pornchai Yodwisithsak

Abstract

Traumatic brain injury (TBI) remains an important health problem worldwide. Pathophysiology of TBI has been intensively investigated. Many novel theories related with pathophysiology of TBI have been regularly proposed. Targeted temperature management (TTM), previously known as therapeutic hypothermia, has a well-established benefit for application as neuroprotective therapy and intracranial pressure (ICP) control. With the novel automatic feedback machine, application of TTM in clinical practice becomes much feasible and safe. Many pre-clinical trials of TTM in models with TBI demonstrated usefulness in multiple aspects. The successful story of TTM in patients with restore of spontaneous circulation (ROSC) after cardiac arrest is a good example for bench to bedside. In the past decade, many clinical trials of TTM in patients with TBI have been conducted with the hope to be another successful study.

Keywords: targeted temperature management, traumatic brain injury, intracranial pressure, surface cooling, endovascular cooling, shivering, skin counter warming

1. Introduction

Therapeutic hypothermia provides neuroprotective effects against acute brain injury with hypoxic ischemic encephalopathy in patients with post-cardiac arrest [1, 2]. However, since the meeting of five major professional physician societies, the term "therapeutic hypothermia" has been substituted with "targeted temperature management (TTM)" [3]. TTM is characterized as a kind of therapy that patient's core temperature is reduced until a therapeutic target with the rationale in salvaging or relieving damaged brain [4]. TTM is accepted as an established treatment in patients with restored spontaneous circulation following cardiac arrest [5]. Pertaining to standard guidelines for resuscitation, TTM is a class I recommendation in the post-cardiac arrest care section [6–10].

Traumatic brain injury is a catastrophic health problem with high morbidity and mortality rate throughout the world [11]. One of the most important characteristics of TBI is its heterogeneity [12]. The heterogeneous nature of TBI leads to broad spectrum of clinical features, variable in outcomes, and unpredictable prognosis [13]. These heterogeneities are also related with failure to demonstrate effectiveness of the treatment in many clinical trials leading to the wide gaps of evidence-based treatment for TBI [14]. Among several options of treatments available for TBI, TTM is one of the potentially effective treatments in patients with TBI.

2. Pathophysiology of traumatic brain injury (TBI)

The primary pathological damage of brain in TBI derives from two important mechanisms. The first mechanism is mechanical insult or direct brain injury that leads to parenchymal contusion, bruise, laceration, and hemorrhage [15–17]. This direct brain injury leads to autoregulation break down and then impairment of cerebral blood flow (CBF) [15]. This so-called "neurometabolic cascade" mechanism resembles the ischemic-mimic pathophysiology [18]. In this cascade, brain tissue switches the energy resource to anaerobic metabolism, leading to the collection of lactate and sodium-potassium pump failure [19]. Cells become depolarized after the pump failure before calcium gets influx [20]. Accumulation of intracellular calcium leads to uncontrolled release of excitotoxic proteins [21]. Mitochondrial dysfunction and cell membrane disruption produce necrotic cells and then programmed cell death by apoptosis. Excitotoxic proteins and other toxic chemicals, including free oxidative radicals, reactive oxygen species, endonucleases, phospholipases, and ATPases, are released into the surrounding by these death cells [22]. These insults further harm adjacent cells. Immunoinflammatory cells come in to eat up death cells and liberate many mediators and cytokines [23]. Blood-brain barrier (BBB) is destroyed by this immunoinflammatory process before leakage of large protein molecules from disrupted BBB especially albumins lead to cerebral edema causing pressure effect and further destruction to environmental brain tissue [24–26]. The inducible nitric oxide syntase (iNOS), which is related to severity of TBI, is significantly expressed during day 3–7 after onset of TBI [27]. Autophagy, previously known as autophagocytosis, is a housekeeping mechanism to remove cellular degradation [28]. Autophagy plays a major role in eliminating debris after TBI [29]. Dysfunction of autophagic activities leads to neuronal cell death in animal models with TBI. Autophagy has neuroprotective properties against TBI [30].

Another primary damage is indirect brain injury related with acceleration or deceleration of the brain. This indirect insult leads to widespread axonal injury and then generalized brain edema. Clinical manifestations of these primary insults begin right at the initiation of TBI. The secondary injury subsequently comes after the primary damage. Therefore, the clinical presentations of this secondary injury, including elevated intracranial pressure (ICP) and brain ischemia, come a bit late [31]. Once the primary damage occurs, it is almost impossible to be salvageable. Any treatments seem to be not effective to relieve the primary pathological damage [32]. The secondary insults may show responsiveness to the treatments [15, 16].

3. Pathophysiology of intracranial pressure (ICP)

Alexander Monro was the first scientist who presented the theory about intracranial pressure during eighteenth century before George Kellie presented his article confirmed Monro's theory 40 years later, known as Monro-Kellie doctrine [33, 34]. This doctrine describes that due to the brain which is surrounded by rigid meninges and skull with constant volume, increment in the quantity of the intracranial compartments will have an effect on intracranial pressure (ICP) [35]. The intracranial compartments, which are actually persistent, consist of brain tissue, cerebrospinal fluid (CSF), and blood. An expansion in either compartment or growth of a space-occupying lesion is going to raise intracranial pressure and may need a reduction in other compartments so as to maintain the constant intracranial volume [36]. A further volume expansion can firstly push CSF and venous blood away from the skull to avoid ICP elevation. However, the ability for ICP protection from volume expansion has significant restriction. If the expansion still goes on until beyond capacity of compensation, ICP finally becomes elevated [37]. ICP elevation produces cerebral herniation [38]. Cerebral perfusion pressure (CPP), which is calculated by mean arterial pressure (MAP) minus ICP, is lower when ICP is elevated. Then, depressed CCP leads to diminution of cerebral blood flow (CBF) [39].

The neurometabolic cascade from primary brain damage leads to cerebral edema and then elevated ICP as mentioned above. This secondary damage by ICP elevation is due to depressed CPP and declined CBF [40]. When CPP or CPF is declined, there is no enough blood to deliver nutrients for the cells [41]. Elevated ICP, particularly which of more than 20 cm of water, in patients with TBI is associated with unfavorable outcomes and increased mortality [42, 43]. The level of CPP in patients with severe TBI should be kept above 60 mm of mercury to achieve favorable outcomes [44].

4. Mechanisms of TTM actions on TBI

The defensive properties of TTM on neurometabolic cascade of TBI are considered to be numerous mechanisms of actions [45]. The best known effect of TTM is the protective function against hypoxic/ischemic encephalopathy [46]. Similar protective actions of TTM against ischemic cascade, for example, reduction of oxygen free radical, inhibition of excitatory amino acid release, prevention of calcium influx, and reduction of cytokines and mediator release are all protective effect against neurometabolic cascade [6, 45, 47]. TTM also relieves TBI via its alternative actions including brain metabolism reduction, prevention of cortical spreading depolarizations, mitochondrial protection, and preventive effect on cell membrane disruption [40, 47]. These effects can delay the neurons and the glials to deteriorate into apoptosis [48].

TTM suppresses iNOS expression leading to outcomes improvement in animal models with TBI [49]. Protective effect on blood-brain barrier disruption is another well-known action of TTM, which helps to reduce brain swelling and lower ICP [48, 50]. Effectiveness of ICP reduction by TTM in various models with TBI has been demonstrated in many clinical and experimental studies [51–53]. However, the benefit of ICP control by TTM in various clinical entities needs to be proven in large-scale trials [54].

5. The course of TTM in clinical practice

The process of TTM is ideally separated into three stages including induction, sustainment, and rewarming [45, 51]. The induction is the initial stage of TTM. The core temperature is rapidly declined to the target during induction stage [55, 56]. The rate of temperature reduction usually depends on the performance of available methods in the center [45]. With effective methods of cooling, core temperature can be brought down with the rate of 2–4°C/h [51]. The target temperature then is smoothly maintained during sustainment stage. Good methods should not allow more than 0.5°C fluctuation of temperature [4]. After the target temperature is sustained until the setting duration, it is slowly elevated back to normal destination during rewarming stage [46]. The rate of temperature rising depends on the indication of TTM. The usual recommended rate of rewarming is 0.2–0.5°C/h. The rapid increasing temperature is associated with rebound rising of ICP and higher risk of infection [57].

6. Methods of TTM

Effective methods are the key of success to achieve excellent process of TTM. Although there are several methods available to use, some of them are not quite popular and no longer in use as a solitary method in clinical practice [46]. According to some pilot studies, the selective brain TTM with cooling helmet or cap may be safe and feasible; however, this method is not accepted to use as a principle method for TTM in patients with TBI [58–61]. The antipyretic drugs alone or combination with other conventional methods may be useful for fever control; however, they are not effective enough to be used as solitary method for TTM [62–64]. The intravenous 4°C normal saline may be advantageous to launch TTM in the absence of energy condition such as pre-hospital setting [65–67]. However, huge volume of saline infusion requirement to lower temperature is usually associated with complications and becomes a major disadvantage to its use as a principle method for TTM [62]. The endovascular cooling technique is somehow invasive but very effective and reliable to use as a principle method for TTM [68, 69]. The surface cooling technique is the most popular method for TTM due to its feasibility, noninvasiveness, and effectiveness [70].

6.1. Invasive endovascular methods

A central venous heat exchange catheter connected with extracorporeal cooling machine is an important characteristic of invasive endovascular techniques [4]. This intravenous catheter is able to insert through femoral, subclavian, or jugular vein [68, 71]. The auto-response temperature modulated system is integrated with the extracorporeal cooling machine [71]. The advantage of invasive endovascular method is efficient accomplishment including fast temperature lowering to the destination, smoothly maintenance during sustainment stage and rewarming with reliably controlled rate [72, 73]. Shivering is a common physiological reaction in patients treated with TTM [74]. Shivering control is an important step during the course of TTM [46]. Anti-shivering therapy includes pharmacologic treatment with many kinds of sedative drugs and nonpharmacologic treatment with skin-counter warming [51, 75]. Sedative effects from pharmacologic anti-shivering therapy may lead to impairment of consciousness and associated complications in patients undergoing TTM [75]. These complications are associated with unfavorable outcome in patients treated with TTM [76]. Skin counter warming can help to avoid many complications by lessen use of pharmacologic anti-shivering therapy [77]. As compared with surface technique, application of skin counter warming as nonpharmacologic anti-shivering therapy is much more possible during treatment with endovascular technique [78]. Due to lacking of drowsiness effect from pharmacologic anti-shivering therapy, skin counter warming can be applied in patients treated with TTM without need of intubation [79]. For this reason, endovascular technique is the most recommended method for patients with conditions that basically do not need intubation and require neurological observation such as patients with acute ischemic stroke [78, 80, 81]. However, not only technical difficulties in venous access but also complications associated with catheter are disadvantage concerns for endovascular technique [82, 83].

6.2. Noninvasive surface methods

The easiest technique for surface method is application of ordinary ice packs to neck, axilla, and groin. Before the era of automatic feedback machine, this simple ice pack was the most popular technique recommended in clinical practice [1, 2, 84]. However, the care team usually becomes exhausted after ice pack application because the team needs to give a very strenuous care and monitoring during the procedure [85]. Other than that, limitations of ice packs include its clumsiness, difficulty in temperature management, and high rate of adverse reactions [86]. The novel machine with automatic feedback temperature modulated system offers favorable temperature control, effortlessness of application, and rapid initiation [87]. This system facilitates its use in clinical practice [57]. This TTM machine is connected with circulating cold water blankets/pads or cold air-blow blankets [88, 89]. Core temperature measurement is mandatory for automatic feedback system. Temperature probe straight connected to the machine provides input data for automatic feedback system [90, 91]. The temperature of fluid or air within the pads or blankets is automatically modulated by the system dependent on the setting of target temperature and input data from the temperature probe [92]. The effectiveness of this system helps to achieve the ideal process of TTM including rapid lowering the temperature to the target, smooth maintenance of the target temperature, and slow rewarming back to the normal setting [46].

There is a surface cooling technique which is designed to use under the circumstance of lacking electrical source. EMCOOLS® HypoCarbon pads consist of graphite elements. This graphite has prominent heat conductivity. The pads are able to apply directly to the superficial skin. Before application, these pads must become frozen up in regular freezer. Electrical supply is not necessary during application. For this reason, HypoCarbon pads are feasible to apply for TTM induction in pre-hospital setting [93–96].

6.3. The novel cooling method

RhinoChill intra-nasal cooling system is a portable device for selective brain cooling. It has a nasal tube to disperse evaporating coolant liquid in nasal cavity [97]. The coolant does not need to be frozen up, and the device is battery-based operation. This system should be feasible for pre-hospital setting [98, 99]. An observational study enrolled 17 patients with out-of-hospital cardiac arrest showed that the intra-nasal cooling device was safe and feasible to apply in pre-hospital setting. Two events of nonfatal adverse reactions included epistaxis and white nose were reported [100]. Rising blood pressure during treatment by this device in patients with acute ischemic stroke was concerned in another observational study [101]. Moreover, there was a case report of a serious adverse event with fatal pneumocephalus. The authors postulated that the air from nasal tube penetrated cribriform plate of ethmoidal sinus leading to pneumocephalus [102]. This serious adverse effect raises concerns to apply the intra-nasal device in patients with traumatic brain injury.

The novel esophageal cooling device helps to achieve rapid induction in patients with post-cardiac arrest [103]. According to its noninvasive property, it is also feasible for fever control in intensive care unit [104]. The device has been approved by The United States Food and Drug Administration (USFDA) and clinical trial [105].

7. Shivering and common physiologic response

When temperature starts to decline, the early physiologic response, such as peripheral vaso-constriction, occurs [57]. Behavioral compensations are the next response. When temperature continues to go down below the threshold, shivering inevitably develops [4, 75]. Shivering is the last resort of the defensive mechanisms against hypothermia, which occurs when vaso-constriction and behavioral compensations are not enough to prevent hypothermia [75]. Heat production increases two-fold to five-fold with shivering [106]. Appearance of shivering may indicate unimpaired neurophysiologic response and should be related with favorable neuro-logic outcomes [107]. Shivering management is a milestone in the course of TTM and should be integrated in the protocol of TTM [77, 108]. Bedside shivering assessment score (BSAS) is helpful for measuring degree of shivering (**Table 1**) [76].

0	No shivering
1	Mild: shivering confines to cervical and/or thorax only
2	Moderate: shivering extends to whole movement of upper limbs
3	Severe: shivering spreads to overall movement of trunk, upper limbs, and lower limbs

Table 1. Bedside shivering assessment score (BSAS) [76].

Increased peripheral arterial resistance during induction stage of TTM is common but usually temporary and does no harm to systemic blood pressure [51]. Sinus bradycardia is also commonly presented during sustainment stage. Heart rate usually lowers less than 50 beats per minute without any effect to hemodynamic status, therefore, requires no treatment [109]. However, this bradycardia should represent intact autonomic function and indicate favorable outcomes [110]. In the experimental animal model with hypothermia, prolonged coagulation and diminution of platelets function are common [111]. However, in the real world practice, clinical bleeding associated with hypothermia is not quite common [112]. During sustainment stage, kidneys are influent by hypothermia to excrete more water leading to volume contraction [113]. Serum potassium is significantly declined during sustainment stage [114]. The most likely mechanisms of hypokalemia are hypothermia induced both intracellular shifting and renal loss of potassium [115]. However, serum potassium is anticipated to become elevated when temperature gets raised during rewarming stage [116]. It is safe and practical to keep serum potassium above 3.0 milli-equivalents per liter during sustainment stage to avoid both related fatal arrhythmia during sustainment stage and overt hyperkalemia during rewarming stage [114, 116]. Raised serum amylase is also common during sustainment stage; nonetheless, this elevated serum amylase is not related with clinical pancreatitis any more [117]. Sustained hyperglycemia (serum glucose > 8 mmol/L for at least 4 hours duration) is common during the course of TTM and may be associated with unfavorable outcomes [118]. Multiple mechanisms associated with hypothermia-induced hyperglycemia are postulated including decreased sugar utilization, reduced endogenous insulin production, and elevated resistance to exogenous insulin [119]. However, supplementary insulin during sustainment stage may shift potassium into cells then worsen the pre-existing hypokalemia [120]. Infection, particularly pneumonia and sepsis, is the most unwanted adverse event in patients treated with TTM, however only uncontrolled infection that should lead to unfavorable outcomes [57, 121].

8. Application of TTM in traumatic brain injury (TBI)

8.1. TTM in animal model with TBI

Benefits of TTM in animal experimental models with TBI have been demonstrated in several studies. Protective effects of TTM against neurometabolic cascade of TBI were proved with many studies in animal models. These protective effects were also histopathologically demonstrated in rats with a liquid percussion TBI. Overall number of necrotic neurons in both CA3 and CA4 layer of hippocampus and thalamus was reduced with hypothermia [122]. Post-traumatic hypothermia is able to suppress both glutamate release and hydroxyl radical elevations in rat models with induced TBI [123]. As mentioned above, disruption of BBB is one of the important steps in neurometabolic cascade leading to cerebral edema. The leakage of endogenous vascular proteins from the disrupted BBB was reduced with hypothermia in rats with the acute hypertensive response after TBI [124]. In the developing brain, TBI may also cause neonatal seizures and epilepsy due to the hyperexcitability of neurons and neural circuits, resulting in long-term functional impairments. Hypothermia improved functional recovery after TBI in developing brain of neonatal rats [125]. As mentioned above, autophagy plays a major role in eliminating function after TBI and has neuroprotective effects. Hypothermia enhances autophagy resulting in improved behavioral outcomes in rats with lateral fluid percussion TBI [126].

Most of studies, animal models demonstrated protective effects of TTM against catastrophic cascade of TBI in many aspects. However, confirmation of its benefit in clinical trials is necessary before application in routine practice.

8.2. Clinical trials of TTM in patients with TBI

Pertaining to very promising outcome of TTM for TBI in pre-clinical trials, many clinical trials have been conducted to prove its benefit in human. Earlier, small scale, single-center, clinical trials demonstrated benefit of TTM in patients with TBI. In 1997, Marion et al. reported a landmark clinical trial of TTM in patients with severe TBI. This study recruited 82 patients with Glasgow Coma Score 5–7 which was relatively small sample size. The favorable outcomes were demonstrated in 3–6 months after treatment with TTM, but no benefit was presented when following up at 12 months [127]. The similar benefit was again supported by later single-center trials. Two clinical trials in patients with severe TBI from China demonstrated good effect of TTM on ICP control with favorable outcomes after 6 months to 1 year [128, 129]. However, the National Acute Brain Injury Study Hypothermia (NABISH), the multi-center landmark trial, reported not only lack of benefit but also potentially harmful of TTM in patients with TBI [130]. Moreover, the following systematic review and meta-analysis, which includes clinical trials before 2003, reveal no benefit of TTM in patients with TBI [131–133]. The inter-center variance in NABISH, which could confound the outcomes of the study, was reported thereafter [134]. This leads to conduct the National Acute Brain Injury Study Hypothermia II (NABISH II) many years later. Unfortunately, as well as the initial one, the NABISH II proved no benefit of TTM in patients with TBI [135]. The negative results in the NABISH I and II were confirmed by the Brain-Hypothermia (B-HYPO) Study from Japan. The B-HYPO showed that TTM with target temperature between 32 and 34°C did not provide any benefit as compared with fever control in patients with TBI [136].

As mentioned above, elevated ICP is a common secondary insult in patients with TBI and associated with unfavorable outcomes [137, 138]. Most of the previous clinical trials of TTM in patients with TBI start rewarming when the peak of ICP is approaching at around 48 h after the onset of TBI, leading to augmentation of ICP [139]. This phenomenon is presumed to be one of the important reasons of negative results in previous clinical trials of TTM in patients with TBI [54]. As mentioned above, ICP reduction is one of the well-known properties of TTM. ICP reduction with TTM should provide some benefit to the specific group of patients with elevated ICP in TBI [52]. Clinical trial of TTM pertaining to level of ICP in patients with TBI was then conducted [140]. A small-scale, single-center, prospective clinical trial demonstrated improvements of survivals and neurological outcomes with TTM in patients with TBI plus refractory intracranial hypertension [141]. Unfortunately, the large scale, multi-center, clinical trial of TTM in patients with TBI pertaining to elevated ICP more than 20 mm Hg (Eurotherm3235 Trial) again reported no clinical benefits [142]. Large scale, multi-center, clinical trial of TTM as second-line treatment for elevated ICP in patients with TBI has still been ongoing [143].

Recent systematic review and meta-analysis of TTM versus normothermia in adult patients with TBI reveals not only no clinical benefit of TTM as compared with normothermia but also increased risk of developing pneumonia and cardiovascular complications associated with TTM [144]. At this moment, application of TTM as routine practice in adult patients with TBI without enrolment into clinical trial is not recommended [145].

As well as in adult, similar results of clinical trials for TTM in children with severe TBI revealed no benefit. Clinical trial of TTM in children with severe TBI conducted by Hutchison et al. reported not only no evidence of a benefit with respect to any short-term or long-term outcomes but also potential complications related with TTM particularly critical hypotension [146]. Several confounding factors in Hutchison's trial such as late treatment initiation, too short treatment duration, and rapid rewarming were reported. However, without all these confounding factors, the Cool Kid Trial reported no benefit of TTM in children with severe TBI [147]. Moreover, preliminary report of early initiation of TTM in children with severe TBI revealed infeasibility with low rate of recruitment [148]. The recent systematic review and meta-analysis confirmed no benefit of TTM in both adults and children with TBI [149].

9. Conclusions

Neurometabolic cascade is a key of primary pathologic damage in traumatic brain injury (TBI). Elevated intracranial pressure (ICP) is a well-known secondary damage related to unfavorable outcomes in patients with TBI. Targeted temperature management (TTM), previously known as therapeutic hypothermia, has many well-established protective effects against catastrophic cascade in TBI. TTM is also a good option for ICP reductive treatment. However, how to transfer from bench to bedside is still controversial for TTM in patients with TBI. The available methods for TTM are feasible and effective to apply in patients with TBI. The course of TTM is easy to achieve under the novel automatic feedback machine. The physiologic response and related complications with TTM are able to be controlled and treated. Routine use of TTM in patients with TBI outside clinical trial is still not recommended.

Author details

Sombat Muengtaweepongsa[1]* and Pornchai Yodwisithsak[2]

*Address all correspondence to: sombatm@hotmail.com

1 Division of Neurology, Department of Medicine, Thammasat University, Pathum Thani, Thailand

2 Division of Neurosurgery, Department of Surgery, Thammasat University, Pathum Thani, Thailand

References

[1] Hypothermia after Cardiac Arrest Study G. Mild therapeutic hypothermia to improve the neurologic outcome after cardiac arrest. New England Journal of Medicine. 2002;**346**(8):549-556

[2] Bernard SA, Gray TW, Buist MD, Jones BM, Silvester W, Gutteridge G, et al. Treatment of comatose survivors of out-of-hospital cardiac arrest with induced hypothermia. New England Journal of Medicine. 2002;**346**(8):557-563

[3] Nunnally ME, Jaeschke R, Bellingan GJ, Lacroix J, Mourvillier B, Rodriguez-Vega GM, et al. Targeted temperature management in critical care: A report and recommendations from five professional societies. Critical Care Medicine. 2011;**39**(5):1113-1125

[4] Mayer SA, Sessler DI, editors. Therapeutic hypothermia. New York: Marcel Dekker; 2005

[5] Arrich J, Holzer M, Havel C, Mullner M, Herkner H. Hypothermia for neuroprotection in adults after cardiopulmonary resuscitation. Cochrane Database of Systematic Reviews. 2016;**2**:CD004128

[6] Nolan JP, Morley PT, Vanden Hoek TL, Hickey RW, Kloeck WG, Billi J, et al. Therapeutic hypothermia after cardiac arrest: An advisory statement by the advanced life support task force of the International Liaison Committee on Resuscitation. Circulation. 2003;**108**(1):118-121

[7] Peberdy MA, Callaway CW, Neumar RW, Geocadin RG, Zimmerman JL, Donnino M, et al. Part 9: Post-cardiac arrest care: 2010 American Heart Association Guidelines for Cardiopulmonary Resuscitation and Emergency Cardiovascular Care. Circulation. 2010;**122**(18 Suppl 3):S768-S786

[8] Callaway CW, Donnino MW, Fink EL, Geocadin RG, Golan E, Kern KB, et al. Part 8: Post-cardiac arrest care: 2015 American Heart Association Guidelines Update for Cardiopulmonary Resuscitation and Emergency Cardiovascular Care. Circulation. 2015;**132**(18 Suppl 2):S465-S482

[9] Nolan JP, Soar J, Cariou A, Cronberg T, Moulaert VR, Deakin CD, et al. European Resuscitation Council and European Society of Intensive Care Medicine Guidelines for Post-resuscitation Care 2015: Section 5 of the European Resuscitation Council Guidelines for Resuscitation 2015. Resuscitation. 2015;**95**:202-22

[10] Hazinski MF, Nolan JP, Aickin R, Bhanji F, Billi JE, Callaway CW, et al. Part 1: Executive summary: 2015 international consensus on cardiopulmonary resuscitation and emergency cardiovascular care science with treatment recommendations. Circulation. 2015;**132**(16 Suppl 1):S2-S39

[11] Maas AIR, Stocchetti N, Bullock R. Moderate and severe traumatic brain injury in adults. The Lancet Neurology. 2008;**7**(8):728-741

[12] Lingsma HF, Roozenbeek B, Steyerberg EW, Murray GD, Maas AIR. Early prognosis in traumatic brain injury: From prophecies to predictions. The Lancet Neurology. 2010;**9**(5):543-554

[13] Saatman KE, Duhaime AC, Bullock R, Maas AI, Valadka A, Manley GT. Classification of traumatic brain injury for targeted therapies. Journal of Neurotrauma. 2008;**25**(7):719-738

[14] Carney N, Totten AM, O'Reilly C, Ullman JS, Hawryluk GW, Bell MJ, et al. Guidelines for the management of severe traumatic brain injury, fourth edition. Neurosurgery. 2017;**80**(1):6-15

[15] Werner C, Engelhard K. Pathophysiology of traumatic brain injury. British Journal of Anaesthesia. 2007;**99**(1):4-9

[16] Graham DI, McIntosh TK, Maxwell WL, Nicoll JAR. Recent advances in neurotrauma. Journal of Neuropathology & Experimental Neurology. 2000;**59**(8):641-651

[17] Wilberger J, Ortega J, Slobounov S. Concussion mechanisms and pathophysiology. In: Slobounov S, Sebastianelli W, editors. Foundations of Sport-Related Brain Injuries. Boston, MA: Springer US; 2006. pp. 45-63

[18] Giza CC, Hovda DA. The neurometabolic cascade of concussion. Journal of Athletic Training. 2001;**36**(3):228-235

[19] Xing C, Arai K, Lo EH, Hommel M. Pathophysiologic cascades in ischemic stroke. International Journal of Stroke. 2012;**7**(5):378-385

[20] Stead SM, Daube JR. Basics of Neurophysiology. Clinical Neurophysiology. 2016:3-29

[21] Hinkle JL, Bowman L. Neuroprotection for ischemic stroke. The Journal of Neuroscience Nursing: Journal of the American Association of Neuroscience Nurses. 2003;**35**(2):114-118

[22] Yi J-H, Hazell AS. Excitotoxic mechanisms and the role of astrocytic glutamate transporters in traumatic brain injury. Neurochemistry International. 2006;**48**(5):394-403

[23] Kadhim HJ, Duchateau J, Sébire G. Cytokines and brain injury: Invited review. Journal of Intensive Care Medicine. 2008;**23**(4):236-249

[24] Strbian D, Durukan A, Pitkonen M, Marinkovic I, Tatlisumak E, Pedrono E, et al. The blood-brain barrier is continuously open for several weeks following transient focal cerebral ischemia. Neuroscience. 2008;**153**(1):175-181

[25] Xi G, Keep RF, Hoff JT. Pathophysiology of brain edema formation. Neurosurgery Clinics of North America. 2002;**13**(3):371-383

[26] Shlosberg D, Benifla M, Kaufer D, Friedman A. Blood-brain barrier breakdown as a therapeutic target in traumatic brain injury. Nature Reviews Neurology. 2010;**6**(7):393-403

[27] Wada K, Chatzipanteli K, Kraydieh S, Busto R, Dietrich WD. Inducible nitric oxide synthase expression after traumatic brain injury and neuroprotection with aminoguanidine treatment in rats. Neurosurgery. 1998;**43**(6):1427-1436

[28] Glick D, Barth S, Macleod KF. Autophagy: Cellular and molecular mechanisms. The Journal of Pathology. 2010;**221**(1):3-12

[29] Zhang Y-B, Li S-X, Chen X-P, Yang L, Zhang Y-G, Liu R, et al. Autophagy is activated and might protect neurons from degeneration after traumatic brain injury. Neuroscience Bulletin. 2008;**24**(3):143-149

[30] Lipinski MM, Wu J, Faden AI, Sarkar C. Function and mechanisms of autophagy in brain and spinal cord trauma. Antioxidants and Redox Signaling. 2015;23(6):565-577

[31] Finfer SR, Cohen J. Severe traumatic brain injury. Resuscitation. 2001;48(1):77-90

[32] Reilly P, Bullock R. Head Injury : Pathophysiology & Management. 2005:444

[33] Kim DJ, Czosnyka Z, Kasprowicz M, Smieleweski P, Baledent O, Guerguerian AM, et al. Continuous Monitoring of the Monro-Kellie Doctrine: Is It Possible? J Neurotrauma. 2012;29(7):1354-63

[34] Kellie G. Appearances observed in the dissection of two individuals; death from cold and congestion of the brain. Trans Med-Chir Soc Edinburgh. 1824;1:84

[35] Neff S, Subramaniam RP. Monro-Kellie doctrine. Journal of Neurosurgery. 1996;85(6):1195

[36] Mokri B. The Monro-Kellie hypothesis: Applications in CSF volume depletion. Neurology. 2001;56(12):1746-1748

[37] Kincaid MS, Lam AM. Monitoring and managing intracranial pressure. Continuum. 2006;12(1):16

[38] Sheth K, McCullough M, Kazmi S, Lazaridis C, O'Phelan K, Shepherd SA, et al. Cerebral Herniation Syndromes and Intracranial Hypertension. Rutgers University Press; 2016

[39] Villa F, Citerio G. Intracranial pressure monitoring. Oxford Textbook of Neurocritical Care. 2016:107

[40] Germans MR, Boogaarts HD, Macdonald RL. Neuroprotection in Critical Care Neurology. Seminars in Neurology. 2016;36(6):642-648

[41] Greve MW, Zink BJ. Pathophysiology of traumatic brain injury. Mount Sinai Journal of Medicine: A Journal of Translational and Personalized Medicine. 2009;76(2):97-104

[42] Marmarou A, Anderson RL, Ward JD. Impact of ICP instability and hypotension on outcome in patients with severe head trauma. Journal of Neurosurgery. 1991;75:S59-S66

[43] Karamanos E, Teixeira PG, Sivrikoz E, Varga S, Chouliaras K, Okoye O, et al. Intracranial pressure versus cerebral perfusion pressure as a marker of outcomes in severe head injury: A prospective evaluation. The American Journal of Surgery. 2014;208(3):363-371

[44] Juul N, Morris GF, Marshall SB, Trial tECotIS, Marshall LF. Intracranial hypertension and cerebral perfusion pressure: Influence on neurological deterioration and outcome in severe head injury. Journal of Neurosurgery. 2000;92(1):1-6

[45] Polderman KH. Mechanisms of action, physiological effects, and complications of hypothermia. Critical Care Medicine. 2009;37(Suppl):S186-S202

[46] Muengtaweepongsa S. Methods and clinical applications of targeted temperature management. Neurology Asia. 2015;20(4):325-333

[47] Polderman KH. Application of therapeutic hypothermia in the ICU: Opportunities and pitfalls of a promising treatment modality. Part 1: Indications and evidence. Intensive Care Medicine. 2004;30(4):556-575

[48] Gonzalez-Ibarra F, Varon J, Lopez-Meza E. Therapeutic Hypothermia: Critical Review of the Molecular Mechanisms of Action. Frontiers in Neurology. 2011;**2**(4)

[49] Chatzipanteli K, Wada K, Busto R, Dietrich WD. Effects of moderate hypothermia on constitutive and inducible nitric oxide synthase activities after traumatic brain injury in the rat. Journal of Neurochemistry. 1999;**72**(5):2047-2052

[50] Chi OZ, Liu X, Weiss HR. Effects of mild hypothermia on blood-brain barrier disruption during isoflurane or pentobarbital anesthesia. Anesthesiology. 2001;**95**(4):933-938

[51] Choi HA, Badjatia N, Mayer SA. Hypothermia for acute brain injury—Mechanisms and practical aspects. Nature Reviews Neurology. 2012;**8**(4):214-222

[52] Sadaka F, Veremakis C. Therapeutic hypothermia for the management of intracranial hypertension in severe traumatic brain injury: A systematic review. Brain Injury. 2012;**26**(7-8):899-908

[53] Farid S, Ashok P, Christopher V, Rekha L. Therapeutic Hypothermia in Traumatic Brain Injury. Rijeka, Croatia: INTECH Open Access Publisher; 2013

[54] Sinclair HL, Andrews P. Bench-to-bedside review: Hypothermia in traumatic brain injury. Critical Care. 2010;**14**(1):204

[55] Suwannakin A, Muengtaweepongsa S. Initial experience of therapeutic hypothermia after cardiac arrest with surface cooling method in Thammasat Chalerm Prakiat Hospital: Two cases report. Journal of the Medical Association of Thialand. 2011;**94**(Suppl. 7):S190-S192

[56] Pinichjindasup A, Homvises B, Muengtaweepongsa S. Therapeutic hypothermia with extracorporeal membrane oxygenation (ECMO) and surface cooling in post-cardiac arrest patients: 4 case reports. Journal of the Medical Association of Thailand. 2014;**97**(8):223

[57] Polderman KH. Application of therapeutic hypothermia in the intensive care unit. Opportunities and pitfalls of a promising treatment modality—Part 2: Practical aspects and side effects. Intensive Care Medicine. 2004;**30**(5):757-769

[58] Hachimi-Idrissi S, Corne L, Ebinger G, Michotte Y, Huyghens L. Mild hypothermia induced by a helmet device: A clinical feasibility study. Resuscitation. 2001;**51**(3):275-281

[59] Wang H, Olivero W, Lanzino G, Elkins W, Rose J, Honings D, et al. Rapid and selective cerebral hypothermia achieved using a cooling helmet. Journal of Neurosurgery. 2004;**100**(2):272-277

[60] Qiu W, Shen H, Zhang Y, Wang W, Liu W, Jiang Q, et al. Noninvasive selective brain cooling by head and neck cooling is protective in severe traumatic brain injury. Journal of Clinical Neurosciences. 2006;**13**(10):995-1000

[61] Liu W, Qiu W, Zhang Y, Wang W, Lu F, Yang X. Effects of selective brain cooling in patients with severe traumatic brain injury: A preliminary study. Journal of International Medical Research. 2006;**34**(1):58-64

[62] Polderman KH, Herold I. Therapeutic hypothermia and controlled normothermia in the intensive care unit: Practical considerations, side effects, and cooling methods*. Critical Care Medicine. 2009;**37**(3):1101-1120

[63] Zhang Z. Antipyretic therapy in critically ill patients with established sepsis: A trial sequential analysis. PLoS One. 2015;**10**(2):e0117279

[64] Zhang Z, Chen L, Ni H. Antipyretic therapy in critically ill patients with sepsis: An interaction with body temperature. PLoS One. 2015;**10**(3):e0121919

[65] Polderman KH, Rijnsburger ER, Peerdeman SM, Girbes ARJ. Induction of hypothermia in patients with various types of neurologic injury with use of large volumes of ice-cold intravenous fluid*. Critical Care Medicine. 2005;**33**(12):2744-2751 10.1097/01. CCM.0000190427.88735.19

[66] Bernard S, Buist M, Monteiro O, Smith K. Induced hypothermia using large volume, ice-cold intravenous fluid in comatose survivors of out-of-hospital cardiac arrest: A preliminary report. Resuscitation. 2003;**56**(1):9-13

[67] Kim F, Olsufka M, Carlbom D, Deem S, Longstreth WT, Jr., Hanrahan M, et al. Pilot study of rapid infusion of 2 L of 4 degrees C normal saline for induction of mild hypothermia in hospitalized, comatose survivors of out-of-hospital cardiac arrest. Circulation. 2005;**112**(5):715-719

[68] Keller E, Imhof H-G, Gasser S, Terzic A, Yonekawa Y. Endovascular cooling with heat exchange catheters: A new method to induce and maintain hypothermia. Intensive Care Medicine. 2003;**29**(6):939-943

[69] Pittl U, Schratter A, Desch S, Diosteanu R, Lehmann D, Demmin K, et al. Invasive versus non-invasive cooling after in- and out-of-hospital cardiac arrest: a randomized trial. Clin Res Cardiol. 2013;**102**(8):607-614

[70] Fukuda T. Targeted temperature management for adult out-of-hospital cardiac arrest: Current concepts and clinical applications. Journal of Intensive Care. 2016;**4**(1):30

[71] Georgiadis D, Schwarz S, Kollmar R, Schwab S. Endovascular cooling for moderate hypothermia in patients with acute stroke: First results of a novel approach. Stroke. 2001;**32**(11):2550-2553

[72] Al-Senani FM, Graffagnino C, Grotta JC, Saiki R, Wood D, Chung W, et al. A prospective, multicenter pilot study to evaluate the feasibility and safety of using the CoolGard (TM) System and Icy (TM) catheter following cardiac arrest. Resuscitation. 2004;**62**(2):143-150

[73] Lyden PD, Allgren RL, Ng K, Akins P, Meyer B, Al-Sanani F, et al. Intravascular cooling in the treatment of stroke (ICTuS): Early clinical experience. Journal of Stroke and Cerebrovascular Diseases. 2005;**14**(3):107-114

[74] Karnatovskaia LV, Wartenberg KE, Freeman WD. Therapeutic hypothermia for neuroprotection: History, mechanisms, risks, and clinical applications. The Neurohospitalist. 2014;**4**(3):153-163

[75] Mahmood MA, Zweifler RM. Progress in shivering control. Journal of Neurological Sciences. 2007;**261**(1-2):47-54

[76] Logan A, Sangkachand P, Funk M. Optimal management of shivering during therapeutic hypothermia after cardiac arrest. Critical Care Nurse. 2011;**31**(6):e18-e30

[77] Choi HA, Ko S-B, Presciutti M, Fernandez L, Carpenter AM, Lesch C, et al. Prevention of shivering during therapeutic temperature modulation: The Columbia anti-shivering protocol. Neurocritical Care. 2011;**14**(3):389-394

[78] Lyden PD, Hemmen TM, Grotta J, Rapp K, Raman R. Endovascular therapeutic hypothermia for acute ischemic stroke: ICTuS 2/3 protocol. International Journal of Stroke. 2014;**9**(1):117-125

[79] De Georgia MA, Krieger DW, Abou-Chebl A, Devlin TG, Jauss M, Davis SM, et al. Cooling for acute ischemic brain damage (COOL AID): A feasibility trial of endovascular cooling. Neurology. 2004;**63**(2):312-317

[80] Worp HB, Macleod MR, Bath PM, Demotes J, Durand-Zaleski I, Gebhardt B, et al. EuroHYP-1: European multicenter, randomized, phase III clinical trial of therapeutic hypothermia plus best medical treatment vs. best medical treatment alone for acute ischemic stroke. International Journal of Stroke. 2014

[81] Krieger DW, De Georgia MA, Abou-Chebl A, Andrefsky JC, Sila CA, Katzan IL, et al. Cooling for acute ischemic brain damage (cool aid): An open pilot study of induced hypothermia in acute ischemic stroke. Stroke. 2001;**32**(8):1847-1854

[82] Fischer M, Lackner P, Beer R, Helbok R, Pfausler B, Schneider D, et al. Cooling Activity is Associated with Neurological Outcome in Patients with Severe Cerebrovascular Disease Undergoing Endovascular Temperature Control. Neurocrit Care. 2015;**23**(2):205-209

[83] Oh SH, Oh JS, Kim YM, Park KN, Choi SP, Kim GW, et al. An observational study of surface versus endovascular cooling techniques in cardiac arrest patients: A propensity-matched analysis. Critical Care. 2015;**19**:85

[84] Larsson I-M, Wallin E, Rubertsson S. Cold saline infusion and ice packs alone are effective in inducing and maintaining therapeutic hypothermia after cardiac arrest. Resuscitation. 2010;**81**(1):15-19

[85] Seder DB, Van der Kloot TE. Methods of cooling: Practical aspects of therapeutic temperature management. Critical Care Medicine. 2009;**37**(7 Suppl):S211-S222

[86] Merchant RM, Abella BS, Peberdy MA, Soar J, Ong MEH, Schmidt GA, et al. Therapeutic hypothermia after cardiac arrest: Unintentional overcooling is common using ice packs and conventional cooling blankets. Critical Care Medicine. 2006;**34**(12):S490-S494

[87] Vaity C, Al-Subaie N, Cecconi M. Cooling techniques for targeted temperature management post-cardiac arrest. Critical Care. 2015;**19**(1):103

[88] Vargas M, Sutherasan Y, Servillo G, Pelosi P. What is the proper target temperature for out-of-hospital cardiac arrest? Best Practice & Research. Clinical Anaesthesiology. 2015;**29**(4):425-434

[89] Bindra A, Gupta D. Targeted temperature management in neurocritical care: Boon or bust. Journal of Neuroanaesthesiology and Critical Care. 2016;**3**(2):96-109

[90] Holzer M. Devices for rapid induction of hypothermia. European Journal of Anaesthesiology. Supplement. 2008;**42**:31-38

[91] Hall GW, Burnett DR, Seidman D. Method and Apparatus for Inducing Therapeutic Hypothermia. Google Patents; 2010

[92] Glover GW, Thomas RM, Vamvakas G, Al-Subaie N, Cranshaw J, Walden A, et al. Intravascular versus surface cooling for targeted temperature management after out-of-hospital cardiac arrest—An analysis of the TTM trial data. Critical Care. 2016;**20**(1):381

[93] Uray T, Sterz F, Janata A, Wandaller C, Holzer M, Laggner AN, et al. Surface cooling with a new cooling-blanket for rapid induction of mild hypothermia in humans after cardiac arrest: A feasibility trial. Circulation. 2006;**114**(18):1190

[94] Dhaese HL, Martens PR, Muller NH, Casier IM, Mulier JP, Heytens L. The use of emergency medical cooling system pads in the treatment of malignant hyperthermia. European Journal of Anaesthesiology. 2010;**27**(1):83-85

[95] Testori C, Sterz F, Behringer W, Spiel A, Firbas C, Jilma B. Surface cooling for induction of mild hypothermia in conscious healthy volunteers–A feasibility trial. Critical Care. 2011;**15**(5):R248

[96] Uray T, Mayr FB, Stratil P, Aschauer S, Testori C, Sterz F, et al. Prehospital surface cooling is safe and can reduce time to target temperature after cardiac arrest. Resuscitation. 2015;**87**:51-56

[97] Busch HJ, Eichwede F, Fodisch M, Taccone FS, Wobker G, Schwab T, et al. Safety and feasibility of nasopharyngeal evaporative cooling in the emergency department setting in survivors of cardiac arrest. Resuscitation. 2010;81(8):943-949

[98] Castrén M, Nordberg P, Svensson L, Taccone F, Vincent JL, Desruelles D, et al. Intra-arrest transnasal evaporative cooling. A randomized, prehospital, multicenter study (PRINCE: Pre-ROSC IntraNasal Cooling Effectiveness). Circulation. 2010;**122**(7):729-736

[99] Nordberg P, Taccone FS, Castren M, Truhlár A, Desruelles D, Forsberg S, et al. Design of the PRINCESS trial: Pre-hospital resuscitation intra-nasal cooling effectiveness survival study (PRINCESS). BMC Emergency Medicine. 2013;**13**(1):21

[100] Grave M-S, Sterz F, Nürnberger A, Fykatas S, Gatterbauer M, Stättermayer AF, et al. Safety and feasibility of the RhinoChill immediate transnasal evaporative cooling device during out-of-hospital cardiopulmonary resuscitation: A single-center, observational study. Medicine. 2016;**95**(34):e4692

[101] Poli S, Purrucker J, Priglinger M, Sykora M, Diedler J, Rupp A, et al. Safety evaluation of nasopharyngeal cooling (RhinoChill®) in stroke patients: An observational study. Neurocritical Care. 2014;**20**(1):98-105

[102] Harris S, Bansbach J, Dietrich I, Kalbhenn J, Schmutz A. RhinoChill((R))-more than an "ice-cream headache (1)" serious adverse event related to transnasal evaporative cooling. Resuscitation. 2016;**103**:e5-e6

[103] Markota A, Fluher J, Kit B, Balažič P, Sinkovič A. The introduction of an esophageal heat transfer device into a therapeutic hypothermia protocol: A prospective evaluation. The American Journal of Emergency Medicine. 2016;**34**(4):741-745

[104] Hegazy A, Lapierre D, Althenayan E. Targeted temperature management after cardiac arrest and fever control with an esophageal cooling device. Critical Care. 2015;**19**(Suppl 1):P424

[105] CritiCool Specification M, (Rehovot, Israel). 510K for CritiCool system http://www.accessdata.fda.gov/scripts/cdrh/cfdocs/cfpmn/denovo.cfm?ID=DEN140018 [updated 01/23/2017]. Available from: http://www.accessdata.fda.gov/scripts/cdrh/cfdocs/cfpmn/denovo.cfm?ID=DEN140018

[106] Giesbrecht GG, Sessler DI, Mekjavic IB, Schroeder M, Bristow GK. Treatment of mild immersion hypothermia by direct body-to-body contact. Journal of Applied Physiology (1985). 1994;**76**(6):2373-2379

[107] Nair SU, Lundbye JB. The occurrence of shivering in cardiac arrest survivors undergoing therapeutic hypothermia is associated with a good neurologic outcome. Resuscitation. 2013;**84**(5):626-629

[108] Presciutti M, Bader MK, Hepburn M. Shivering management during therapeutic temperature modulation: Nurses' perspective. Critical Care Nurse. 2012;**32**(1):33-42

[109] Thomsen JH, Hassager C, Bro-Jeppesen J, Soholm H, Nielsen N, Wanscher M, et al. Sinus bradycardia during hypothermia in comatose survivors of out-of-hospital cardiac arrest—A new early marker of favorable outcome? Resuscitation. 2015;**89**:36-42

[110] Muengtaweepongsa S, Jantanukul A, Suwanprasert K. Should the heart rate including the heart rate variability be important prognostigators in cardiac arrest? Resuscitation. 2016;**98**:E15-E

[111] Wolberg AS, Meng ZH, Monroe DMI, Hoffman M. A systematic evaluation of the effect of temperature on coagulation enzyme activity and platelet function. Journal of Trauma and Acute Care Surgery. 2004;**56**(6):1221-1228

[112] Srivilaithon W, Muengtaweepongsa S. The Outcomes of Targeted Temperature Management After Cardiac Arrest at Emergency Department: A Real-World Experience in a Developing Country. Therapeutic hypothermia and temperature management. 2017;**7**(1):24-29

[113] Varon J, Acosta P. Therapeutic hypothermia: Past, present, and future. Chest. 2008;**133**(5): 1267-1274

[114] Mirzoyev SA, McLeod CJ, Bunch TJ, Bell MR, White RD. Hypokalemia during the cooling phase of therapeutic hypothermia and its impact on arrhythmogenesis. Resuscitation. 2010;**81**(12):1632-1636

[115] Sprung J, Cheng EY, Gamulin S, Kampine JP, Bosnjak ZJ. The effect of acute hypothermia and serum potassium concentration on potassium cardiotoxicity in anesthetized rats. Acta Anaesthesiologica Scandinavica. 1992;**36**(8):825-830

[116] Soeholm H, Kirkegaard H. Serum potassium changes during therapeutic hypothermia after out-of-hospital cardiac arrest-should it be treated? Therapeutic Hypothermia and Temperature Management. 2012;**2**(1):30-36

[117] Bernard SA, Buist M. Induced hypothermia in critical care medicine: A review. Critical Care Medicine. 2003;**31**(7):2041-2051

[118] Nielsen N, Sunde K, Hovdenes J, Riker RR, Rubertsson S, Stammet P, et al. Adverse events and their relation to mortality in out-of-hospital cardiac arrest patients treated with therapeutic hypothermia*. Critical Care Medicine. 2011;**39**(1):57-64

[119] Cueni-Villoz N, Devigili A, Delodder F, Cianferoni S, Feihl F, Rossetti AO, et al. Increased blood glucose variability during therapeutic hypothermia and outcome after cardiac arrest*. Critical Care Medicine. 2011;**39**(10):2225-2231

[120] Lehot JJ, Piriz H, Villard J, Cohen R, Guidollet J. Glucose homeostasis. Comparison between hypothermic and normothermic cardiopulmonary bypass. Chest. 1992;**102**(1): 106-111

[121] Gagnon DJ, Nielsen N, Fraser GL, Riker RR, Dziodzio J, Sunde K, et al. Prophylactic antibiotics are associated with a lower incidence of pneumonia in cardiac arrest survivors treated with targeted temperature management. Resuscitation. 2015;**92**:154-159

[122] Dietrich W, Alonso O, Busto R, Globus M, Ginsberg M. Post-traumatic brain hypothermia reduces histopathological damage following concussive brain injury in the rat. Acta Neuropathologica. 1994;**87**:250-258

[123] Globus MY, Alonso O, Dietrich WD, Busto R, Ginsberg MD. Glutamate release and free radical production following brain injury: Effects of posttraumatic hypothermia. Journal of Neurochemistry. 1995;**65**(4):1704-1711

[124] Jiang JY, Lyeth BG, Kapasi M, Jenkins L, Povlishock J. Moderate hypothermia reduces blood-brain barrier disruption following traumatic brain injury in the rat. Acta Neuropathologica. 1992;**84**(5):495-500

[125] Gu X, Wei ZZ, Espinera A, Lee JH, Ji X, Wei L, et al. Pharmacologically induced hypothermia attenuates traumatic brain injury in neonatal rats. Experimental Neurology. 2015;**267**:135-142

[126] Jin Y, Lei J, Lin Y, Gao GY, Jiang JY. Autophagy inhibitor 3-MA weakens neuroprotective effects of posttraumatic brain injury moderate hypothermia. World Neurosurgery. 2016;**88**:433-446

[127] Marion DW, Penrod LE, Kelsey SF, Obrist WD, Kochanek PM, Palmer AM, et al. Treatment of traumatic brain injury with moderate hypothermia. New England Journal of Medicine. 1997;**336**(8):540-546

[128] Zhi D, Zhang S, Lin X. Study on therapeutic mechanism and clinical effect of mild hypothermia in patients with severe head injury. Surgical Neurology. 2003;**59**(5):381-385

[129] Jiang J, Yu M, Zhu C. Effect of long-term mild hypothermia therapy in patients with severe traumatic brain injury: 1 year follow up review of 87 cases. Journal of Neurosurgery. 2000;**93**:546-549

[130] Clifton GL, Miller ER, Choi SC, Levin HS, McCauley S, Smith KR, Jr., et al. Lack of effect of induction of hypothermia after acute brain injury. New England Journal of Medicine. 2001;**344**(8):556-563

[131] Henderson W, Dhingra V, Chittock D, Fenwick J, Ronco J. Hypothermia in the management of traumatic brain injury: A systematic review and meta-analysis. Intensive Care Medicine. 2003;**29**:1637-1644

[132] Peterson K, Carson S, Cairney N. Hypothermia treatment for traumatic brain injury: A systematic review and meta-analysis. Journal of Neurotrauma. 2008;**25**:62-71

[133] McIntyre L, Fergusson D, Hebert P, Moher D, Hutchison J. Prolonged therapeutic hypothermia after traumatic brain injury in adults: A systematic review. JAMA. 2003;**289**:2992-2999

[134] Clifton GL, Choi SC, Miller ER, Levin HS, Smith KR, Jr., Muizelaar JP, et al. Intercenter variance in clinical trials of head trauma—Experience of the National Acute Brain Injury Study: Hypothermia. Journal of Neurosurgery. 2001;**95**(5):751-755

[135] Clifton GL, Valadka A, Zygun D, Coffey CS, Drever P, Fourwinds S, et al. Very early hypothermia induction in patients with severe brain injury (the National Acute Brain Injury Study: Hypothermia II): A randomised trial. Lancet Neurology. 2011;**10**(2):131-139

[136] Maekawa T, Yamashita S, Nagao S, Hayashi N, Ohashi Y. Prolonged mild therapeutic hypothermia versus fever control with tight hemodynamic monitoring and slow rewarming in patients with severe traumatic brain injury: A randomized controlled trial. Journal of Neurotrauma. 2015;**32**(7):422-429

[137] Ghajar J. Traumatic brain injury. Lancet. 2000;**356**(9233):923-929

[138] Ducrocq S, Meyer P, Orliaguet G, Blanot S, Laurent-Vannier A, Renier D, et al. Epidemiology and early predictive factors of mortality and outcome in children with traumatic severe brain injury: Experience of a French pediatric trauma center. Pediatric Critical Care Medicine. 2006;**7**:461-467

[139] Wijayatilake DS, Shepherd SJ, Sherren PB. Updates in the management of intra-cranial pressure in traumatic brain injury. Current Opinion in Anaesthesiology. 2012;**25**(5):540-547

[140] Lei J, Gao G, Mao Q, Feng J, Wang L, You W, et al. Rationale, methodology, and implementation of a nationwide multicenter randomized controlled trial of long-term mild hypothermia for severe traumatic brain injury (the LTH-1 trial). Contemporary Clinical Trials. 2015;**40**:9-14

[141] Polderman KH, Tjong Tjin Joe R, Peerdeman SM, Vandertop WP, Girbes AR. Effects of therapeutic hypothermia on intracranial pressure and outcome in patients with severe head injury. Intensive Care Medicine. 2002;**28**(11):1563-1573

[142] Andrews PJ, Sinclair HL, Rodriguez A, Harris BA, Battison CG, Rhodes JK, et al. Hypothermia for intracranial hypertension after traumatic brain injury. New England Journal of Medicine. 2015;**373**(25):2403-2412

[143] Ahmad FU, Starke RM, Komotar RJ, Connolly ES. A randomized clinical trial of hypothermia as a preferred second-line treatment for elevated intracranial pressure after traumatic brain injury. Neurosurgery. 2016;**78**(2):N10-N11

[144] Zhu Y, Yin H, Zhang R, Ye X, Wei J. Therapeutic hypothermia versus normothermia in adult patients with traumatic brain injury: A meta-analysis. SpringerPlus. 2016;**5**(1):801

[145] Yokobori S, Yokota H. Targeted temperature management in traumatic brain injury. Journal of Intensive Care. 2016;**4**(1):28

[146] Hutchison JS, Ward RE, Lacroix J, Hebert PC, Barnes MA, Bohn DJ, et al. Hypothermia therapy after traumatic brain injury in children. New England Journal of Medicine. 2008;**358**(23):2447-2456

[147] Adelson PD, Wisniewski SR, Beca J, Brown SD, Bell M, Muizelaar JP, et al. Comparison of hypothermia and normothermia after severe traumatic brain injury in children (Cool Kids): A phase 3, randomised controlled trial. The Lancet Neurology. 2013;**12**(6):546-553

[148] Beca J, McSharry B, Erickson S, Yung M, Schibler A, Slater A, et al. Hypothermia for traumatic brain injury in children–A phase II randomized controlled trial. Critical Care Medicine. 2015;**43**(7):1458-1466

[149] Sandestig A, Romner B, Grande PO. Therapeutic hypothermia in children and adults with severe traumatic brain injury. Therapeutic Hypothermia and Temperature Management. 2014;**4**(1):10-20

2

Diffuse Axonal Injury: A Devastating Pathology

Christ Ordookhanian, Katherine Tsai,
Sean W. Kaloostian and Paul E. Kaloostian

Abstract

Traumatic brain injury (TBI) also known as intracranial injury is the result of a lesion within the brain due to an external force. Common forms of TBI result from falls, violence, and/or vehicle crashes; the classification of this pathology is dependent on the severity of the lesion as well as the mechanism of trauma to the head. One of the most common onsets of traumatic brain injuries result from mild to severe lesions to the white matter tracts of the brain called diffuse axonal injury (DAI); however, additional forms of TBI's can present in non-penetrating forms. Penetrating forms of TBI's such as trauma to the head via a foreign object do also contribute to the many millions of TBI cases per year, but we will not discuss these traumatic injuries as in depth within this chapter. The onset of diffuse axonal injury will vary on a per-patient basis from mild to severe, based on a standardized neurological examination rated on the Glasgow Coma Scale (GCS), which indicates the severity of brain damage present. While there is a spectrum of severity for DAI patients, a concussion is typically observed within a larger majority of patients in addition to other overwhelming trauma.

Keywords: trauma, diffuse, axonal, injury, intracranial

1. Introduction

In this chapter, we will discuss in depth the pathology of diffuse axonal injury (DAI) touching upon clinical presentation/keynote characteristics, medical diagnosis, radiological imaging, treatment, prognosis, historical outcomes, and quality of life aftercare [1]. While diffuse axonal injury is included within the broader category of intracranial injury, it is essential to note the physiological severity it plays on the life of the patient. Trauma to any region of the head should prompt immediate concern and medical attention. While DAI is one of the worst forms of lesions to the brain, we would like to approach this topic with a sense of urgency as it is frequently seen in medical centers worldwide [2].

2. Diffuse axonal injury: a devastating pathology

2.1. Keynote characteristics

Alongside the many forms of intracranial injuries, the differential key characteristics of DAI are the lesions which occur within the white matter. White matter is composed of several bundles of myelinated axons which connects gray matter together. Gray matter houses the neuronal cell bodies within the brain and is highly regulated in regard to transmission of neuronal impulses [3–5]. Lesions of white matter can vary in size greatly, as they typically present as 1–18 mm wide in trauma and affect the frontal and temporal lobes mostly. However, it is not limited to that region entirely as regions of the brainstem and corpus callosum have also been affected quite frequently according to literature [6, 7]. Axonal injury to the brain is at times an irreversible trauma, which results in loss of consciousness and even death. Forces of greater magnitude striking the head almost immediately disconnect axons within the site of impact. Secondary axon disconnections also develop resulting in severe brain injury [8, 9]. Human physiological symptoms as a result of trauma also set in, such as swelling and degeneration of nerves. The bodily response places the brain under the extreme amount of pressure and is often exposed to irreversible damage [10, 11]. While it was once assumed that sheer force is the responsible factor for the disconnection of axons, it is indeed false to assume that. It is the biochemical response to the impact stimuli which causes that largest impact on axons. However, impact does in fact cause some lesions but not comparable to the damage done by biochemical cascades which follow the impact [12, 13]. Biochemical pathways within our bodies are greatly responsible for the axonal disconnect which occurs secondary to the traumatic impact. The biochemical response is due to the physical stress and stretching caused by the force of impact. The impact disrupts the proteolytic metabolism and degradation of cytoskeleton; sodium channels open within the axolemma causing a strong wave of neuronal depolarization. To balance the influx of cationic sodium, calcium channels also open allowing the stronger cation metal to leave the neuron and into the cell to depolarize the neuron. The excess of calcium ions within the extracellular cavity activates a cascade of enzymes, leading to the activation of phospholipases and other enzymes that act on the cytoskeleton and cause severe damage. This biochemical pathway ends with axonal separation and cell death [14]. Axonal stretching and disconnect occur 1–6 hours after initial trauma. While irreversible brain damage has already occurred, severe damage is yet to come. While the axonal network is compromised, the axonal transport still continues and is halted at any point where the neuronal network is cleaved or compromised. At the site of axon disconnect, transport products and cell debris begin to build up, causing local swelling and severe compression [15–17].

In **Figure 1**, take note of the leading causes of diffuse axonal injury, their severity, and chance of recovery.

2.2. Clinical presentation

Many patients that have sustained a traumatic brain injury (TBI) to a certain degree suffer from diffuse axonal injury (DAI). Many patients presenting to emergency and trauma centers with DAI are unconscious and have strikingly poor neurological examination results. The Glasgow Coma Scale (GCS) (**Figures 2** and **3**) is a neurological scale which establishes an objective way to rate the state of consciousness of patients. The sum of the three categories will allow for the determination of the GCS score and patient consciousness [18]. Patients presenting with DAI are often reflecting vivid signs of functional impairment of the brainstem and impairment of the reticular activating system as many of the physiological vital signs are maintained through external sources (e.g., life support) [19]. While alertness and responsiveness may develop slowly over a longer course of time with intensive rehabilitation, the rate of mortality with patients presenting with DAI is extremely high, as high as 50% in severe cases. In patients whom consciousness can be restored, cognitive and memory impairments persist through the remainder of the patient's life [20, 21].

Cause	Severity	Chance of Recovery
1. Automobile Accidents	Extreme	Mild
2. Sport Related Accidents	Extreme	Mild
3. Violence	Extreme	Low to Mild
4. Accidental Falls in Elderly	Extreme	Low
5. Child Abuse (Shaken Baby)	Extreme	Minimal to None
6. Intoxicated Related Falls	Extreme	Mild

Figure 1. Most common causes of diffuse axonal injury. Listed from the highest to the lowest occurrence.

	1	2	3	4	5	6
Visual	Eyes closed	Eyes open to sharp stimuli	Eyes open to sounds	Eyes open without induced stimuli		
Motor	No movement	Movement to sharp stimuli	Muscle flexion to sharp stimuli	Muscle flexion and bodily movement	Able to localize touch	Appears to have normal movement
Verbal	No sounds	Slow intensity sounds	Incoherent words	Understandable words spoken	Normal conversation	

Figure 2. The Glasgow Coma Scale.

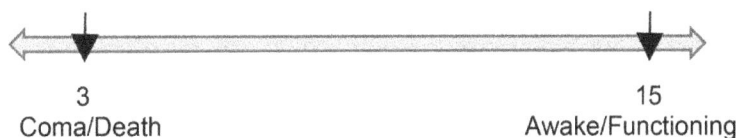

3
Coma/Death

15
Awake/Functioning

Figure 3. The Glasgow Coma Scale range.

The GCS ranges from 3 to 15, three being coma/death and 15 being a fully functioning and awake person. These scores can be the summation of the visual, motor, and verbal scores.

2.3. Medical diagnosis

Due to the fact that there are no distinctive clinical symptoms that patients present with that allow medical professionals to immediately diagnose DAI, physicians must rely on neurological examinations and radiographic imaging to diagnose patients and predict their prognosis. Magnetic resonance imaging (MRI) is the preferred examination for DAI, accompanied with computed topography (CT) scans [22]. A key indicator for the onset of DAI is the minimal yet visible bleeding within the region of the corpus callosum and/or the cerebral cortex. It is essential to note that while trauma may cause axonal disconnect, the vast majority of axonal damage occurs through secondary biochemical degradation. Thus, patients may first appear to be in a functional state, but over 1–6 hours, a patient's condition may drastically change [23, 24].

2.4. Use of DTI to diagnose DAI

Newer radiographic studies such as diffusion tensor imaging (DTI) is an MRI technique, which enables radiologists to measure the diffusion of water in the tissue to then create neural tract images. This method provides pertinent structural information and can even do so for cardiac muscles and prostate muscles [25]. In cases where MRI may demonstrate a negative result to DAI, DTI has been able to show a degree of injury to the white matter fiber tract [26].

2.5. Use of evoked potential to diagnose DAI

Sensory-evoked potential examination studies the electrical activity within the brain and its responsiveness to stimulations such as light, sound, and touch. Neuronal impulses travel via chemical and electrical pathways; these studies detect electrical potentials within the cerebral neuronal network. When patients present to medical centers already in a state of a coma, medical teams must perform a series of neurological examinations which may be challenging when patients are unconscious. A neurological examination conducted typically by neurosurgeons is to test all the 12 cranial nerves and observe appropriate reflexes; a positive result indicates the level of intactness of the central nervous system [27]. Visual-evoked response (VER) test can be used to test and diagnose nerves that affect sight; these are called optic nerves. Electrodes placed along the patient's scalp can detect and record electrical signals as the patient's eyes are exposed to light stimuli [28]. Brainstem auditory-evoked response (BAER) test examines one's hearing ability and the neuronal network involved in the detection of sound. Results that signify a compromised neuronal network can be indicative of brainstem damage or the presence of a tumor within the brainstem; for the sake of this chapter, we will assume that head trauma was the result of brainstem damage. Once again, through electrodes placed on the patients scalp and earlobes, auditory stimuli are presented to the patient, and the patient's reactions are recorded. Auditory stimuli must vary in frequency and tone to establish a complete understanding of the patient's responses [29]. Lastly, somatosensory-evoked response (SSER) examinations can be utilized to detect issues within the spinal cord often seen clinically with patients presenting with numbness of the arms and legs. In patients presenting with TBI, verbal communication is limited or unsustainable; thus SSER can be utilized to detect any neurological issues present within the spine [30]. Mild electrical stimuli will be presented to the patients scalp via electrodes; nerves will then transfer the electrical signal to the brain through which reading can be visualized on a medical recorder device. The duration of time which it takes for electrical signals to travel can indicate the presence of spinal trauma or compromise [31]. These examinations are utilized quite commonly throughout medical practice especially when neurological compromise is suspected; through the detection of electrical impulses through the scalp, medical personnel can gain an understanding of the patient's neurological state, especially in suspected DAI patients where an unconscious state is commonly presented with.

2.6. Use of electroencephalogram to diagnose DAI

Traumatic brain trauma is indicative of patients with suspected DAI; electroencephalograms provide medical teams a sufficient amount of information regarding a patient's state of consciousness and cognitive processing. DAI patients have experienced a traumatic injury, which is accompanied with impaired consciousness and cognitive function as well as impaired motor functions with severe cases posing with damage to vital neuronal structures such as the brainstem [32, 33]. Essentially, the severity of the traumatic impact on the brain may alter or completely change the prognosis and outcome of rehabilitation efforts [34]. Within the chronic stage of diffuse axonal injury, it has been observed that the mean frequency of the brain alpha wave activity was dramatically low and remained low over the mean of all the wave peaks. Brain waves are monitored via electroencephalogram, and low alpha waves do indicate an abnormal brain function. In addition, brain spindle activation in normal patients appears to have similar activity and strengths; in patients presenting with DAI, activation spindle activity varies across the brain and greatly varies among slow to fast spindle fibers. Despite the low alpha waves observed in patients presenting with a coma, delta and theta waves are also diminished; thus, sleep cycles are dysregulated and abnormal adding to the uphill climb during the rehabilitation process [35–37]. While electroencephalograms carry a stigma that they present no meaningful results which a diagnosis can be based off of, we would like to emphasize the impactful contribution electroencephalograms have on medical diagnosis as well as their daily use in medical centers worldwide.

2.7. Radiological findings: computed topography (CT)

As we have discussed previously, diffuse axonal injury (DAI) is characterized through lesions within the white matter of one's brain; severe case lesions are present within the corpus callosum and brainstem. Thus far, we have discussed many of the electro-neuromonitoring techniques utilized within medical centers, but to obtain a clear diagnosis, radiographic imaging techniques are coupled with electro-neuromonitoring practices and physician neurological exams to yield a confirmed DAI diagnosis. Within this section we discuss in depth the radiological examinations conducted to confirm DAI diagnosis. Computed topography (CT) scans is typically utilized first, while CT scans are not entirely as sensitive to visualize subtle DAI; a slight abnormality observed in a CT scan can spark the interest for further investigation by MRI. A non-contrast CT scan of the brain with head injury is a routine and can allow visualization of lesions which are overtly hemorrhagic. A hemorrhagic lesion within the brain will appear hyperdense and present as a few millimeters in diameter [38].

While lesions may be apparent on CT imaging following trauma, the highest visibility will be observed a few days after the trauma, followed by a significant amount of cerebral swelling, compression, and intracranial pressure [39, 40]. While computed topography is not recommended for the sole diagnosis of TBI, coupling with additional diagnostic data allows CT scans to add to the holistic diagnosis. CT scans have been shown to identify TBI in only 19% of nonhemorrhagic lesions; however, when utilizing T2-weighted imaging (T2WI), identification rate rises to 92% accurate diagnosis [41]. T2-weighted imaging (T2WI) is the basic pulse sequence within an MRI; weighting highlights the variability between T2 relaxation times. When lesions are of hemorrhagic entity, CT scans are sensitive enough to visualize lesions quite well; only for nonhemorrhagic lesions do CT scans have difficulty visualizing with appropriate detail. A general rule of thumb is that if small lesions are visible in CT scans, then the overall damage is greater than expected and often classified as severe trauma.

As we mentioned above, a significant amount of damage results after the initial traumatic impact; **Figure 4** illustrates the CT scan of a patient's head for whom was diagnosed with DAI.

2.8. Radiological findings: magnetic resonance imaging (MRI)

While computed topography (CT) scans provide valuable information to the medical care team, the use of magnetic resonance imaging (MRI) is by far the modality of choice when a DAI is suspected [43]. If a CT scan shows a normal pathology, an MRI will be performed to validate those results. There are specific series of MRI's that can be completed to assess for the presence of a DAI. In this section, we will discuss two forms of MRI. The first form is gradient-recalled echo (GRE) sequence imaging, and the second is susceptibility-weighted

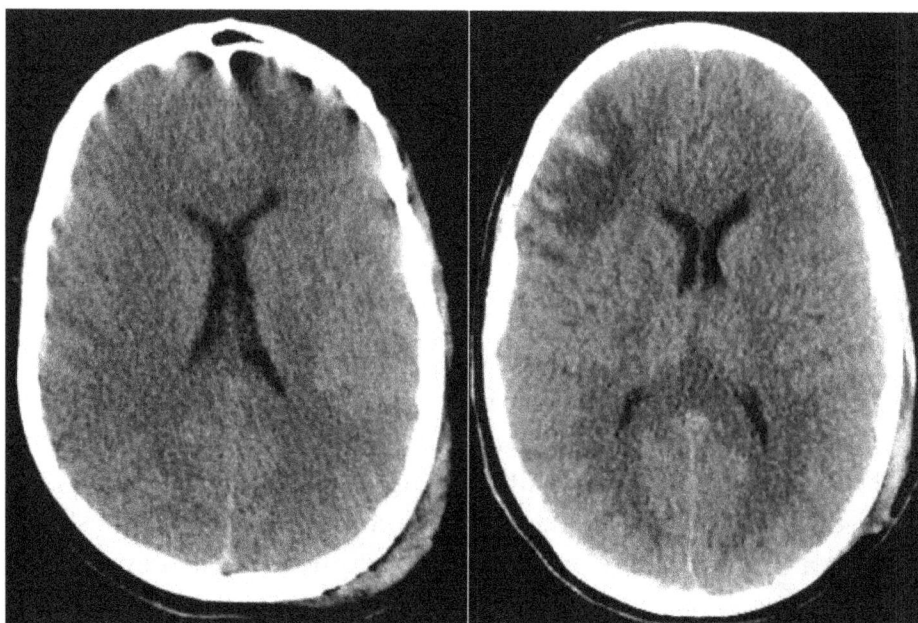

Figure 4. Computed topography scan of patient diagnosed with DAI [42]. From left to right, CT scan of day 1 vs. 11.

imaging (SWI) [44]. GRE imaging methods utilize gradient fields to produce transverse magnetism and flip angles that are less than 90°. SWI is an MRI sequence, which is particularly sensitive to substances which disturb the magnetic field; this method of MRI is extremely useful in detecting blood [45–47]. The use of SWI and GRE is paramount in analyzing the severity of lesions that occur in TBI and suspected DAI. As the junction point of white-gray brain matter is most susceptible to lesions, the use of MRI, specifically GRE and SWI, is crucial in obtaining a diagnosis and severity of DAI [48]. As lesions can be both hemorrhagic and nonhemorrhagic, the use of MRI with increasing fluid-attenuated inversion recovery (FLAIR) signal can be utilized to study lesions that are completely nonhemorrhagic [49]. A FLAIR is fluid attenuation inversion recovery, which utilizes a long inversion time (TI) of the pulse sequence such that at equilibrium there is no net-transverse magnetism of the fluid and thus is visualized. The use of FLAIR is quite common in evaluation of the central nervous system (CNS), especially for head injuries [50, 51]. While MRI technologies are among the most accurate in the field of medicine and modern technology has opened the door to even more precise medical diagnosis, just because the MRI does not show a problematic pathology for the diagnosis of DAI, it does not mean the patient is clear of that diagnosis.

In **Figure 5** through **Figures 6–8**, we can see the MRI scans of patients who were diagnosed with DAI using the GRE and SWI technologies we discussed earlier, as well as the T2 W1 and FLAIR methodologies.

2.9. Treatment options for DAI

While there are many events that may bring on DAI, the treatment is very much similar to that of any head trauma. DAI-suspected patients present to medical centers worldwide with

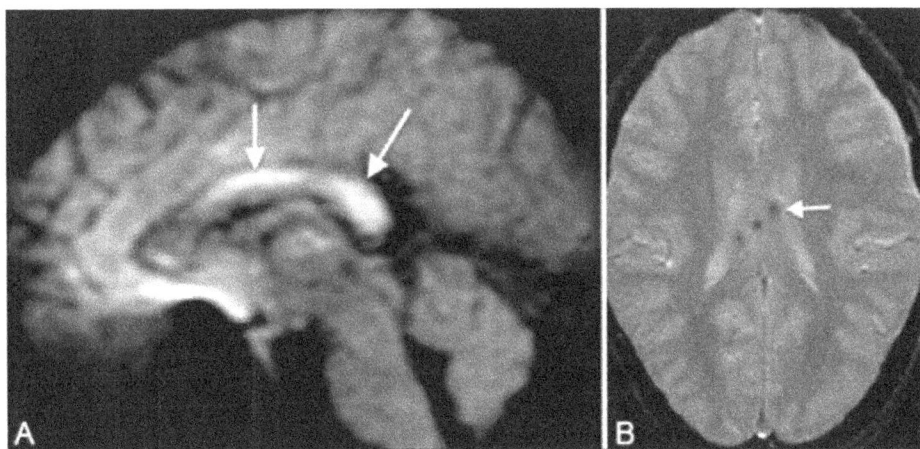

Figure 5. (A) MRI-GRE image of a 30-year-old male patient presenting with head trauma. (B) Image depicting hemorrhagic DAI [52]. Magnetic resonance imaging (MRI) of a 30-year-old patient which presented to medical professionals in an unconscious state of mind with a severe brain injury. (A) Arrows pointing to high-signal foci within the corpus callosum, a structure responsible for cerebral cortex communication between paralleled structures on the two hemispheres. Arrows indicate a restricted diffusion, technically known as abnormally low ADC (apparent diffusion coefficient) values. (B) Appearance of "blooming," indicated by the arrow, apparent in a gradient-recalled echo (GRE) sequence, much similar to a spin-echo MRI. Blooming is an artifact of radiological images which exaggerates the presence of lesions which is extremely useful in the detection of small lesions. Blooming may be seen when certain elements/compounds are present during imaging such as hemosiderin or metals (calcium).

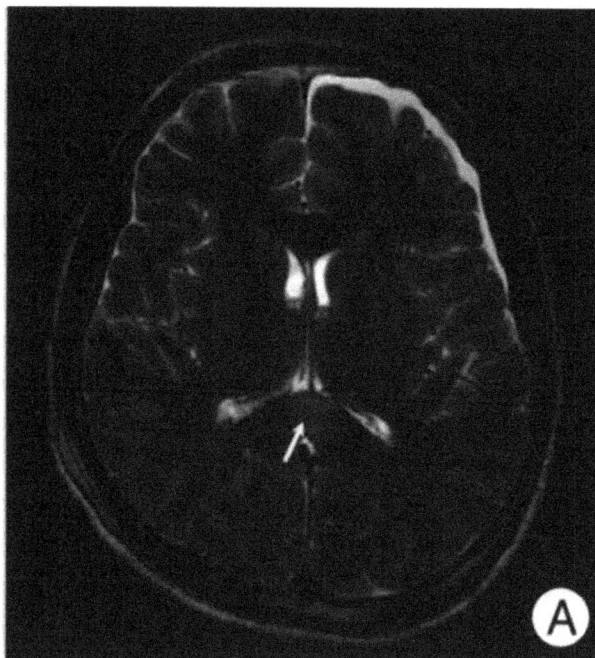

Figure 6. A 21-year-old patient presenting to ER following traumatic bicycle accident. Glasgow coma scale score of 6 (see **Figures 2–3**). Patient presents with nonhemorrhagic lesions visualized through high signal intensity at T2 W1, discussed above. This image is shown under high signal intensity at T2W1 indicating lesions within the corpus callosum of a 21-year-old patient following a traumatic brain injury resultant of a bicycle injury. The arrow is indicative of a nonhemorrhagic lesion at the splenium (posterior end) of the corpus callosum [53].

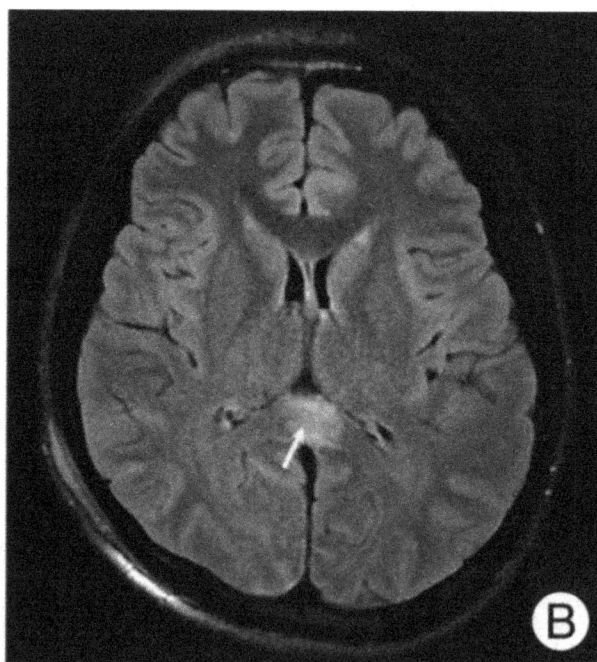

Figure 7. Additional imaging of the 21-year-old bicycle accident patient described above. Image captured using the FLAIR methodology also discussed above. Same patient as above (21-year-old bicycle accident patient) presenting with traumatic brain injury and nonhemorrhagic lesions of the splenium of the corpus callosum. This image is obtained using the fluid-attenuated inversion recovery MRI sequence, often called FLAIR sequence. This form of imaging is useful in suppressing the cerebrospinal fluid (CSF) effects on radiological imaging allowing the higher-intensity appearance of lesions. In this image, the FLAIR imaging also confirms the initial diagnosis [53].

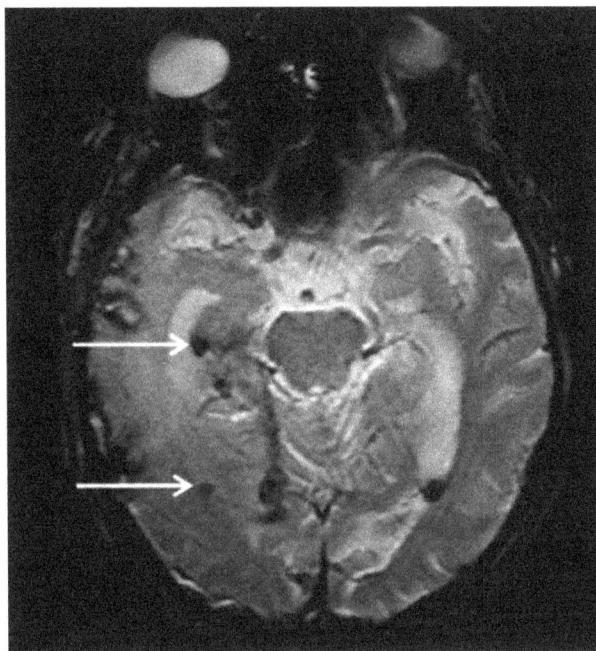

Figure 8. Hemorrhagic DAI [54]. An 83-year-old female patient presenting to the clinic post-fall. The image above is an axial gradient-recalled echo (GRE) image, which indicates and draws focus to the right temporal lobe which, indicated by the white arrows, shows the resulting injury of a hemorrhagic diffuse axonal injury.

symptoms of being unconsciousness and/or in a severe coma to which the patient has sustain mild to severe brain damage often of the irreversible form. In the event that a patient regains consciousness and makes a near-full recovery through the management of brain swelling, hemorrhage, and neurological network status, there are a multitude of therapeutic modalities that can be pursued to maximize the chance of a near-full recovery. This plan entails a variety of medical professional care for the patient each in a specific regard [55]. Upon discharge from trauma and emergency centers, patients enter a long and intensive program for multiple forms of therapeutic care consisting of the following modalities: speech therapy, physical therapy, occupational therapy, recreational therapy, adaptive equipment training, and counseling [56]. Deficits resulting from TBI include impairments in movement, balance, and coordination, accompanied by sensory deficits, behavioral changes, cognitive defects, and communicative defects. In our efforts to restore quality of life back to the patient's life, we will discuss the several modalities of therapy and their application to patients recovering from DAI.

Speech therapy, conducted by a licensed speech and language therapist, first completes a formal evaluation of patients cognitive and communication skills as well as their swallowing skills. An oral examination is also conducted to ensure the strength and coordination of the muscles involved in producing speech. Following the assessment, therapists will engage in a series of short conversations to gage the patient's ability to form understandable and coherent speech; patients are often presented with a series of questions relating to their life and daily tasks prior to the traumatic accident. In the event that a patient presents difficulty utilizing muscles involved in speech or forming speech in itself, therapists will then evaluate the patient's ability to swallow or gag in the presence of a gag stimulus. Concluding the series of examination, the therapist conduct is a developed plan that highlights the focus areas for a patient, often separated into primary, secondary, and tertiary goals. Primary goals are to get the patients general responses to sensory stimuli to appropriate levels, followed by education of the patient's family and friends on proper interactions with a person going through speech therapy. Secondary goals are to build cognitive skills such as attention and reduce any confusion a patient may have. Gaining a sense of balance while sitting and standing is also a secondary goal of therapists, allowing the patient to reestablish the necessary muscle memory and neuronal demands balance has on a human body. Later on, through the process of recovery, tertiary goals include the patient reestablishing cognitive maps and problem-solving skills. Often hard to accomplish even for the first time, therapists work on these skills as well as social skills for life outside of the medical center. While the title of speech therapy seems limited to the physical act of producing speech, it is actually a major component of not only speech-forming techniques but also techniques that must be remastered in areas such as cognition and basic physical skills such as balance [57–60]. The process of relearning task one learned earlier in life, involves the reconstruction of neuronal networks, is an example of the many neuronal networks and pathways within a human mind [61].

In addition to speech therapy, patients also go through extensive physical therapy to restore the patient's life as close to their pre-trauma life as possible. Physical therapists work closely with both the patient and their family to develop goals and an individualized treatment plan pertaining to the symptoms displayed by the patient. Depending on the severity of damage the brain has sustained and the patient's level of consciousness, a series of daily task-specific trainings will be conducted. A patient who is said to be in a "vegetative state" has retained basic brain function but is unaware of their surroundings and requires assistance with body positioning. Additionally, patients who are said to be in "minimally conscious state" show beginning signs of inconsistent awareness; however, they require assistance with almost all physical movement. A vast majority of patients presenting to physical therapists are in a form of a vegetative state following a mild to severe head trauma, specifically when a DAI is diagnosed [62]. The primary goals for physical therapy are to aid the patient in regaining a sense of alertness, the understanding of physical movement, and the ability to follow commands. Secondary goals include movement, muscle strength, and flexibility. Additionally, movement around common daily objects such as beds is also a secondary concern for physical therapists. The activities conducted within physical therapy sessions include a tremendous amount of both mental and physical learning, balance and coordination, as well as strength and energy [63–65].

While physical therapy focuses on movement, strength, and balance as a whole, occupational therapy takes a more targeted approach in dealing with day-to-day activities such as walking down stairs, brushing one's teeth, and opening a door, to name a few. Occupational therapists, just like any other therapist, begin therapy by assessing the severity of the patient's physical disability. Often, the Canadian Occupational Performance Measure (COPM) is used to assess the patient's performance and life satisfaction [66]. Additionally, patient questionnaires are utilized to gain a psychological baseline as the school of thought behind occupational therapy strongly believes in the patient's psychological motivation. The Community Integration Questionnaire (CIQ) and the Satisfaction with Life Scale (SWLS) both assess a patient's social interaction, productivity, and cognitive judgments. With these metrics, occupational therapists are able to design personal goals for the patient to first improve self-awareness, then improve physical activity which related to daily life, and lastly to restore as much as memory recall as possible [67, 68]. Occupational therapy is not as structured as speech or physical therapy; this form of therapy truly evaluates a patient's quality of life and psychological state prior to beginning any form of therapy which involves movement. **Figure 9** illustrates the many factors of occupational therapy in a primary care setting, highly correlative to what is seen in post-trauma care [69].

While patients receive a tremendous amount of in-hospital care, they also receive a unique and more social form of treatment called recreational therapy. This form of therapy involves the therapist designing activities to improve and enhance the patient's self-esteem and social skills while also practicing balance, coordination, strength, and additional motor skills. These therapists aim to design social outings for the patient and their friends/families to allow the patient to not only feel loved and supported but to also reintroduce key life skills such as team building and social interaction. Within this form of therapy, highly trained canines may be utilized as well as more hobby-like activities such as gardening, recreational sports, and even holiday functions, such as decorating or baking [70, 71]. While this form of therapy is less aggressive and directed, data has continuously shown the remarkable outcomes that recreational therapy has not only on the patient's physical abilities but also on the overall happiness of the patient and their quality of life, a truly life-changing treatment in the posttraumatic realm [72].

For many patients that have suffered from a severe form of DAI, adaptive assistive technologies will be essential to restoring the quality of life back for the patient. Adaptive assistive technologies are medical devices that are used to aid the patient in completing daily living activities such as bathing, walking, and eating [73]. These forms of medical devices are crucial for the treatment of DAI in that they provide patients who otherwise would be confined to a bed the ability to be mobile again. Common forms of these devices include wheelchairs, crutches, prosthetics, and orthotics. Despite the mobility, these devices can also assist with sensory such as hearing and touch, as well as safety with devices that alert the patient when an alarm may sound or a door bell may ring. For many of us, we take these devices for granted and do not understand their true lifesaving powers, especially for DAI patients who have experienced a great deal of trauma and require these devices in order to live a quality of life [74, 75]. Engineers today are working on the development of novel assistive technologies, such as the intelligent power wheelchair seen in **Figure 10**, which will allow

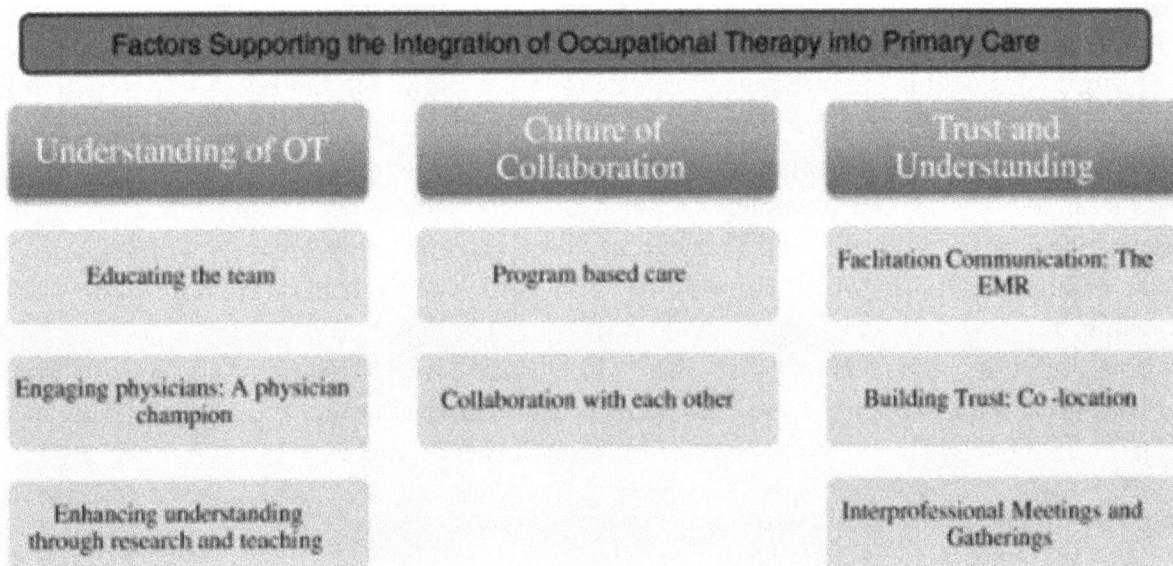

Figure 9. Factors involved in occupation therapy [69].

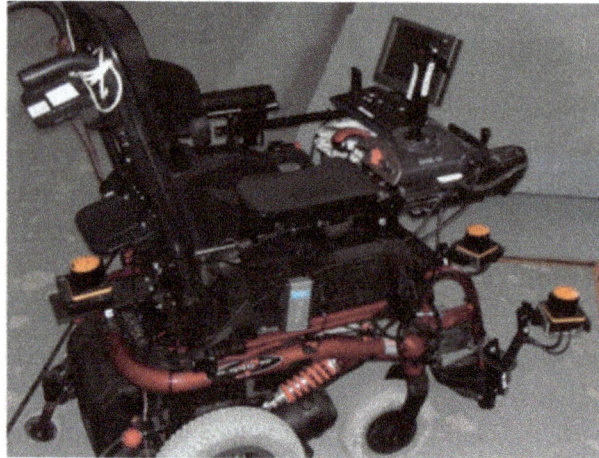

Figure 10. Assistive technology: Intelligent power wheelchair prototype for clinical applications.

many DAI patients who may never have the ability to walk again to be able to venture the world and be more independent. Many posttraumatic DAI patients buffer from immobility and are confined to the limits of a wheelchair; with technological advances such as these, we expect to see a tremendous gain in patient's quality of life [76].

We have currently discussed the many forms of treatment available to patients who have sustained a TBI, specifically DAI; however, despite all form of treatment to restore mental and physical quality of life, counseling is also just as an important characteristic. Any injury to the brain is catastrophic and especially for the patient and their family. One of the most highly utilized forms of treatment is counseling, often for patients that present with a sense of worthlessness, loneliness, and frustration over their predicament [77, 78]. Counseling sets out to answer a series of questions regarding the patient's life; these questions tend to deal with first, identifying the problem and then understanding the severity of the problem. Through every second of counseling, it is important that the patient feels that counseling will be the solution to many of their problems as well as that patient's privacy will be upheld to the maximum extent [79].

Through the many different modalities of therapy, the treatment for DAI is one that can span over the year with no real guarantee that progress will be made. The diagnosis of DAI is life-changing at best and is often the result of severe brain trauma. In the event that a patient is successful in the battle to regain consciousness and expelled out of their coma, the uphill battle to restore a quality of life begins [80]. Through the many forms of DAI treatment available to patients today, slight improvements are possible, and faith in the various treatment methods is at an all-time high [81, 82]. The primary form of counseling patients receives frankly a conversation regularly with therapists focusing on reducing frustration and anxiety and resorting the sense of self-worth. At the end of the day, the patient must come to term with their new situation and establish a new life; while this is easier to be said than done, counseling has successfully completed this task multiple times. To patients climbing the uphill battle of DAI treatment, we wish you the best of luck and a speedy recovery.

2.10. The history behind DAI

In 1956, Sabina Strich, the scientist known to have first identified and described the diffuse degeneration of white matter and white-gray matter lesions, published the first ever study focused on the matter seen within the cerebral region of five patients that had sustained closed-head injuries of severe form [83]. A case study of five patients set the landmark for pathological investigations into brain damage and traumatic head injuries, specifically diffuse axonal injury [84]. While in 1956, the human brain was not entirely understood as well as technology was not at the level it is today to have been able to radiographically or investigatingly screen for the presence of head trauma, thus the rate of mortality was strikingly high. Of the five subjects Strich was investigating, all patients succumbed to their brain injuries weeks to months after the initial trauma. While there was no striking evidence for the presence of DAI, Strich came to the realization that extended degeneration of axons over a time period after the trauma was responsible for the high rate of mortality. The pathologic term DAI was established after Strich published her findings; later, it was agreed that DAI was a multipart pathology in that not only does the initial trauma cause severe damage, but also secondary factors such as biochemical cascades, edema, and hypoxia also contribute to the pathology as a whole [85, 86]. It was in the early 1980s where the official term, DAI, was introduced and accepted worldwide as a pathology which played a key integral role in the posttraumatic development of the patient [87].

2.11. Neuroinflammation: a novel understanding

Inflammatory response within the brain resulting after a traumatic brain injury, specifically a DAI, is mediated by microglia. Oehmichen et al. conducted an experiment in which microglia were immunohistochemically labeled to enable their ability to track areas of axonal injury by observing infiltration [88–90]. Microglia will localize to the region of trauma and become activated such that they are able to isolate compromised structures and locate injured axons. Infiltration mentioned briefly above will become evident after 24 hours in young patients or 48 hours in elder patients and can last for as long as 2 weeks or even a month for particular cases [91]. Cytokines are the key factor involved in inflammation; interleukin (IL) families 1, 6, and 10 also play a role as mediators of inflammation, accompanied by TNF, a tumor necrosis factor which is a cell signaling protein utilized by the body during inflammation. Within a rat model, traumatic brain injury is correlated with a rapid increase in cortical IL-1 alpha and beta sub-factors of the IL-1 family. These interleukins were demonstrated to rapidly increase the rate of inflammation within the rat model [92]. Additionally, interleukin-6 (IL-6) family has also been shown to increase in expression 1–6 hours after the traumatic brain injury. The highest levels of IL-6 mRNA transcription and IL-6 cytokine expression occurred in regions where diffuse axonal damage was the greatest [93]. Within the body, interleukin (IL)-6 plays a key role in the homeostatic control of inflammation-activating cofactors such as granulocytes, lymphocytes, and NK, which rapidly diffuse within the blood in the event of a traumatic injury [94, 95]. The inflammatory response while deadly if not controlled actually increases the likely hood of neuronal damage recovery; however, due to the constant volume of the given region and risk of cerebral compression, inflammation must be controlled to minimize any risks of mortality or compression-induced damage.

2.12. Conclusion

In this chapter, we have discussed in detail the pathology of diffuse axonal injury (DAI) as a result of traumatic brain injury (TBI). Although this pathology represents a mild to severe disease which complicates or often deprives patients from a normal life, implementation of effective therapy and rehabilitation treatment, along with the adaptation of novel therapy

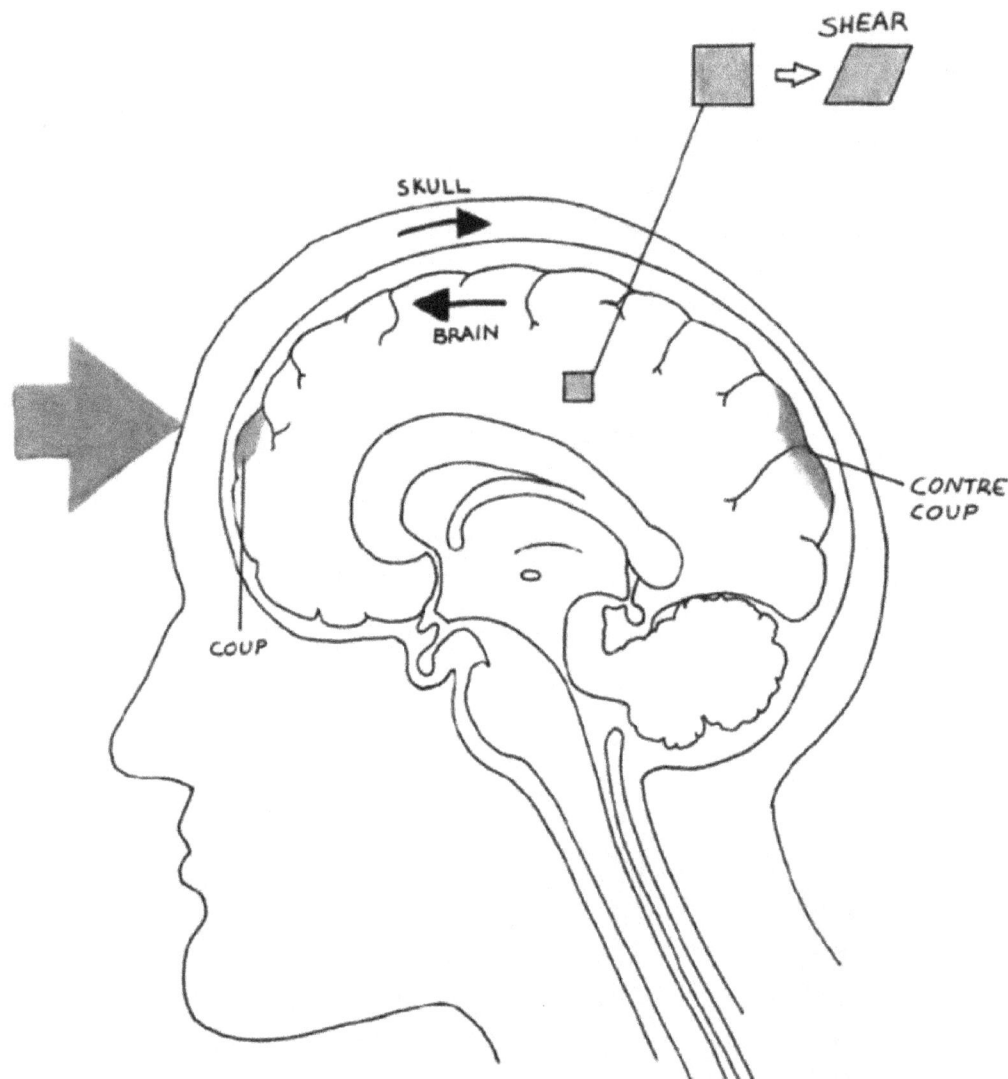

Figure 11. Demonstration of the most common form of DAI impact injury [96].

methodologies, patient course and prognosis may be substantially improved, mitigating traumatic sequelae and long-term posttraumatic outcomes. We hope that you have learned a great deal in regard to DAI, its pathology, and biochemical characteristics. In **Figure 11**, we hope to visualize the most common physical action that results in DAI. Axonal injury is typically resulting from an external force that is acted upon the brain causing a rotational force to be acted upon the axon along with a severe impact of the brain along the skull. Stay safe!

Disclosure

All figures displayed within this manuscript were obtained through the Open Access Biomedical Image Search Engine, with the image owners receiving appropriate citation for the contributions. In accordance to the terms of the Creative Commons Attribution License, the reproduction and distribution of each figure used in this manuscript are accompanied by the citation of the original author(s) or licensors. Original publication within their respected journals is also cited. Our intended uses of these figures are in good and accepted academic practice.

Author details

Christ Ordookhanian[1], Katherine Tsai[1], Sean W. Kaloostian[2] and Paul E. Kaloostian[1]*

*Address all correspondence to: paulkaloostian@hotmail.com

1 Riverside School of Medicine, University of California, Riverside, CA, USA

2 Irvine Medical Center, University of California, Irvine, CA, USA

References

[1] Kokkoz C et al. Diagnosis of delayed diffuse axonal injury. The American Journal of Emergency Medicine. 2017

[2] Lahner D, Fritsch G. Pathophysiology of intracranial injuries. Unfallchirurg. 2017

[3] Leenders KL et al. Cerebral blood flow, blood volume and oxygen utilization. Normal values and effect of age. Brain. 1990;**113**(Pt 1):27-47

[4] Marner L et al. Marked loss of myelinated nerve fibers in the human brain with age. The Journal of Comparative Neurology. 2003;**462**(2):144-152

[5] Sowell ER et al. Mapping cortical change across the human life span. Nature Neuroscience. 2003;**6**(3):309-315

[6] Sindelar B, Bailes JE. Neurosurgical emergencies in sport. Neurologic Clinics. 2017;**35**(3): 451-472

[7] Sanchez EJ et al. Evaluation of head and brain injury risk functions using sub-injurious human volunteer data. Journal of Neurotrauma. 2017;**34**(16):2410-2424

[8] Johnson VE, Stewart W, Smith DH. Axonal pathology in traumatic brain injury. Experimental Neurology. 2013;**246**:35-43

[9] Ng LJ et al. A mechanistic end-to-end concussion model that translates head kinematics to neurologic injury. Frontiers in Neurology. 2017;**8**:269

[10] Paterakis K et al. Outcome of patients with diffuse axonal injury: The significance and prognostic value of MRI in the acute phase. The Journal of Trauma. 2000;**49**(6):1071-1075

[11] Tang-Schomer MD et al. Mechanical breaking of microtubules in axons during dynamic stretch injury underlies delayed elasticity, microtubule disassembly, and axon degeneration. The FASEB Journal. 2010;**24**(5):1401-1410

[12] Vascak M et al. Mild traumatic brain injury evokes pyramidal neuron axon initial segment plasticity and diffuse presynaptic inhibitory terminal loss. Frontiers in Cellular Neuroscience. 2017;**11**:157

[13] Iwata A et al. Traumatic axonal injury induces proteolytic cleavage of the voltage-gated sodium channels modulated by tetrodotoxin and protease inhibitors. The Journal of Neuroscience. 2004;**24**(19):4605-4613

[14] Arundine M et al. Vulnerability of central neurons to secondary insults after in vitro mechanical stretch. The Journal of Neuroscience. 2004;**24**(37):8106-8123

[15] Staal JA et al. Cyclosporin-a treatment attenuates delayed cytoskeletal alterations and secondary axotomy following mild axonal stretch injury. Developmental Neurobiology. 2007;**67**(14):1831-1842

[16] Staal JA et al. Initial calcium release from intracellular stores followed by calcium dys-regulation is linked to secondary axotomy following transient axonal stretch injury. Journal of Neurochemistry. 2010;**112**(5):1147-1155

[17] Chung RS et al. Mild axonal stretch injury in vitro induces a progressive series of neurofilament alterations ultimately leading to delayed axotomy. Journal of Neurotrauma. 2005;**22**(10):1081-1091

[18] Vieira RC et al. Diffuse axonal injury: Epidemiology, outcome and associated risk factors. Frontiers in Neurology. 2016;**7**:178

[19] Su E, Bell M. Diffuse axonal injury. Laskowitz D, Grant G, eds. In: Translational Research in Traumatic Brain Injury. 2016: Boca Raton (FL)

[20] Hutchinson EB et al. Diffusion MRI and the detection of alterations following traumatic brain injury. Journal of Neuroscience Research. 2017

[21] Scott G et al. Amyloid pathology and axonal injury after brain trauma. Neurology. 2016;**86**(9):821-828

[22] Cicuendez M et al. Magnetic resonance in traumatic brain injury: A comparative study of the different conventional magnetic resonance imaging sequences and their diagnostic value in diffuse axonal injury. Neurocirugía (Asturias, Spain). 2017

[23] Crooks CY, Zumsteg JM, Bell KR. Traumatic brain injury: A review of practice management and recent advances. Physical Medicine and Rehabilitation Clinics of North America. 2007;**18**(4):681-710 vi

[24] Maas AI, Stocchetti N, Bullock R. Moderate and severe traumatic brain injury in adults. Lancet Neurology. 2008;**7**(8):728-741

[25] Manenti G et al. Diffusion tensor magnetic resonance imaging of prostate cancer. Investigative Radiology. 2007;**42**(6):412-419

[26] Corbo J, Tripathi P. Delayed presentation of diffuse axonal injury: A case report. Annals of Emergency Medicine. 2004;**44**(1):57-60

[27] Sleigh JW et al. Somatosensory evoked potentials in severe traumatic brain injury: A blinded study. Journal of Neurosurgery. 1999;**91**(4):577-580

[28] Papathanasopoulos P et al. Pattern reversal visual evoked potentials in minor head injury. European Neurology. 1994;**34**(5):268-271

[29] Thomas JG. An analysis of the human brain stem auditory evoked response yielding new criteria for defining its abnormality. Journal of the Neurological Sciences. 1984;**63**(2):207-228

[30] Azad TD et al. Diagnostic utility of intraoperative neurophysiological monitoring for intramedullary spinal cord Tumors: Systematic review and meta-analysis. Clinical Spine Surgery. 2017

[31] Fukuda S. Somatosensory evoked potential. Masui. 2006;**55**(3):280-293

[32] Light GA et al. Electroencephalography (EEG) and event-related potentials (ERPs) with human participants, Chapter 6: P. Current Protocols in Neuroscience, Unitas. 2010;**6**(25):1-24

[33] Malver LP et al. Electroencephalography and analgesics. British Journal of Clinical Pharmacology. 2014;**77**(1):72-95

[34] Binnie CD, Prior PF. Electroencephalography. Journal of Neurology, Neurosurgery, and Psychiatry. 1994;**57**(11):1308-1319

[35] Wittebole X et al. Electrocardiographic changes after head trauma. Journal of Electro-cardiology. 2005;**38**(1):77-81

[36] Molteni E et al. Combined behavioral and EEG power analysis in DAI improve accu-racy in the assessment of sustained attention deficit. Annals of Biomedical Engineering. 2008;**36**(7):1216-1227

[37] Kane NM et al. Quantitative electroencephalographic evaluation of non-fatal and fatal traumatic coma. Electroencephalography and Clinical Neurophysiology. 1998;**106**(3): 244-250

[38] Gentry LR et al. Prospective comparative study of intermediate-field MR and CT in the evaluation of closed head trauma. AJR. American Journal of Roentgenology. 1988;**150**(3):673-682

[39] Lee B, Newberg A. Neuroimaging in traumatic brain imaging. NeuroRx. 2005;**2**(2):372-383

[40] Sharif-Alhoseini M et al. Indications for brain computed tomography scan after minor head injury. Journal of Emergencies, Trauma and Shock. 2011;**4**(4):472-476

[41] Davis PC, Expert Panel I. On neurologic, head trauma. AJNR. American Journal of Neuroradiology. 2007;**28**(8):1619-1621

[42] Hocker SE, Fogelson J, Rabinstein AA. Refractory intracranial hypertension due to fen-tanyl administration following closed head injury. Frontiers in Neurology. 2013;**4**:3

[43] Ezaki Y et al. Role of diffusion-weighted magnetic resonance imaging in diffuse axonal injury. Acta Radiologica. 2006;**47**(7):733-740

[44] Boyle GE, et al. An interactive taxonomy of MR imaging sequences. Radiographics. 2006;**26**(6):p. e24; quiz e24

[45] Schweser F et al. Differentiation between diamagnetic and paramagnetic cerebral lesions based on magnetic susceptibility mapping. Medical Physics. 2010;**37**(10):5165-5178

[46] Tong KA et al. Susceptibility-weighted MR imaging: A review of clinical applications in children. AJNR. American Journal of Neuroradiology. 2008;**29**(1):9-17

[47] Wu Z et al. Identification of calcification with MRI using susceptibility-weighted imaging: A case study. Journal of Magnetic Resonance Imaging. 2009;**29**(1):177-182

[48] Yuh EL et al. Magnetic resonance imaging improves 3-month outcome prediction in mild traumatic brain injury. Annals of Neurology. 2013;**73**(2):224-235

[49] Okuda T et al. Brain lesions: When should fluid-attenuated inversion-recovery sequences be used in MR evaluation? Radiology. 1999;**212**(3):793-798

[50] Bakshi R et al. Fluid-attenuated inversion recovery magnetic resonance imaging detects cortical and juxtacortical multiple sclerosis lesions. Archives of Neurology. 2001;**58**(5): 742-748

[51] Bangerter NK et al. Fluid-attenuated inversion-recovery SSFP imaging. Journal of Magnetic Resonance Imaging. 2006;**24**(6):1426-1431

[52] Kazi AZ et al. MRI evaluation of pathologies affecting the corpus callosum: A pictorial essay. Indian Journal of Radiology Imaging. 2013;**23**(4):321-332

[53] Chung SW et al. Locations and clinical significance of non-hemorrhagic brain lesions in diffuse axonal injuries. Journal of Korean Neurosurgical Association. 2012;**52**(4):377-383

[54] Mehan WA Jr et al. Optimal brain MRI protocol for new neurological complaint. PLoS One. 2014;**9**(10):e110803

[55] Smith DH, Hicks R, Povlishock JT. Therapy development for diffuse axonal injury. Journal of Neurotrauma. 2013;**30**(5):307-323

[56] Yang JY et al. Diagnosis and treatment of diffuse axonal injury in 169 patients. Chinese Journal of Traumatology. 2005;**8**(6):345-348

[57] Beaulieu CL et al. Occupational, physical, and speech therapy treatment activities during inpatient rehabilitation for traumatic brain injury. Archives of Physical Medicine and Rehabilitation. 2015;**96**(8 Suppl):S222-S234 e17

[58] Duff MC, Proctor A, Haley K. Mild traumatic brain injury (MTBI): Assessment and treatment procedures used by speech-language pathologists (SLPs). Brain Injury. 2002;**16**(9):773-787

[59] Stierwalt JA, Murray LL. Attention impairment following traumatic brain injury. Seminars in Speech and Language. 2002;**23**(2):129-138

[60] Seel RT et al. Patient effort in traumatic brain injury inpatient rehabilitation: Course and associations with age, brain injury severity, and time Postinjury. Archives of Physical Medicine and Rehabilitation. 2015;**96**(8 Suppl):S235-S244

[61] Wu CC et al. On the crucial cerebellar wound healing-related pathways and their crosstalks after traumatic brain injury in Danio Rerio. PLoS One. 2014;**9**(6):e97902

[62] Lendraitiene E, Krisciunas A. Physical therapy for persons with traumatic brain injury. Medicina (Kaunas, Lithuania). 2010;**46**(10):712-719

[63] Chantsoulis M et al. Neuropsychological rehabilitation for traumatic brain injury patients. Annals of Agricultural and Environmental Medicine. 2015;**22**(2):368-379

[64] Hellweg S, Johannes S. Physiotherapy after traumatic brain injury: A systematic review of the literature. Brain Injury. 2008;**22**(5):365-373

[65] Hugentobler JA et al. Physical therapy intervention strategies for patients with prolonged mild traumatic brain injury symptoms: A case series. International Journal of Sports Physical Therapy. 2015;**10**(5):676-689

[66] Wheeler S et al. Occupational therapy interventions for adults with traumatic brain injury. American Journal of Occupational Therapy. 2017;**71**(3):7103395010p1-7103395010p3

[67] Radomski MV et al. Effectiveness of Interventions to Address Cognitive Impairments and Improve Occupational Performance After Traumatic Brain Injury: A Systematic Review. Am J Occup Ther. 2016;**70**(3);7003180050p1-9

[68] Vargo MM et al. Interdisciplinary rehabilitation referrals in a concussion clinic cohort: An exploratory analysis. PM & R. 2016;**8**(3):241-248

[69] Donnelly C et al. The integration of occupational therapy into primary care: A multiple case study design. BMC Family Practice. 2013;**14**:60

[70] Hodges JS, Luken K, Zook B. Recreational therapy can help adult brain injury survivors get back into the community. North Carolina Medical Journal. 2001;**62**(6):355-358

[71] Sorensen B, Luken K. Improving functional outcomes with recreational therapy. The Case Manager. 1999;**10**(5):48-52 quiz 53

[72] Hammond FM et al. Group therapy use and its impact on the outcomes of inpatient rehabilitation after traumatic brain injury: Data from traumatic brain injury-practice based evidence project. Archives of Physical Medicine and Rehabilitation. 2015;**96**(8 Suppl):S282-S292 e5

[73] Lane AK, Benoit D. Driving, brain injury and assistive technology. NeuroRehabilitation. 2011;**28**(3):221-229

[74] Carver MD. Adaptive equipment to assist with one-handed intermittent self-catheterization: A case study of a patient with multiple brain injuries. The American Journal of Occupational Therapy. 2009;**63**(3):333-336

[75] Flanagan SR, Cantor JB, Ashman TA. Traumatic brain injury: Future assessment tools and treatment prospects. Neuropsychiatric Disease and Treatment. 2008;**4**(5):877-892

[76] Boucher P et al. Design and validation of an intelligent wheelchair towards a clinically-functional outcome. Journal of Neuroengineering and Rehabilitation. 2013;**10**(1):58

[77] Cooper Z et al. Withdrawal of life-sustaining therapy in injured patients: Variations between trauma centers and nontrauma centers. The Journal of Trauma. 2009;**66**(5):1327-1335

[78] Santana Carlos VM. Importance of communication in counselling the spinal cord injury patient. Paraplegia. 1978;**16**(2):206-211

[79] Dorf E et al. Therapy after injury to the hand. The Journal of the American Academy of Orthopaedic Surgeons. 2010;**18**(8):464-473

[80] Brooks N et al. The five year outcome of severe blunt head injury: A relative's view. Journal of Neurology, Neurosurgery, and Psychiatry. 1986;**49**(7):764-770

[81] Bovet C, Carlson M, Taylor M. Quality of life, unmet needs, and iatrogenic injuries in rehabilitation of patients with Ehlers-Danlos syndrome hypermobility type/joint hypermobility syndrome. American Journal of Medical Genetics. Part A. 2016;**170**(8):2044-2051

[82] Fann JR, Hart T, Schomer KG. Treatment for depression after traumatic brain injury: A systematic review. Journal of Neurotrauma. 2009;**26**(12):2383-2402

[83] Howe FA et al. Magnetic resonance neurography. Magnetic Resonance in Medicine. 1992;**28**(2):328-338

[84] Strich SJ. Diffuse degeneration of the cerebral white matter in severe dementia following head injury. Journal of Neurology, Neurosurgery, and Psychiatry. 1956;**19**(3):163-185

[85] Esiri M. Obituary for Dr Sabina Strich. Neuropathology and Applied Neurobiology. 2016;**42**(2):210-211

[86] Czeiter E et al. Traumatic axonal injury in the spinal cord evoked by traumatic brain injury. Journal of Neurotrauma. 2008;**25**(3):205-213

[87] Mesfin FB, Dulebohn SC. Diffuse Axonal Injury (DAI), in StatPearls. 2017: Treasure Island (FL)

[88] Oehmichen M, Theuerkauf I, Meissner C. Is traumatic axonal injury (AI) associated with an early microglial activation? Application of a double-labeling technique for simultaneous detection of microglia and AI. Acta Neuropathologica. 1999;**97**(5):491-494

[89] GrandPre T, Li S, Strittmatter SM. Nogo-66 receptor antagonist peptide promotes axonal regeneration. Nature. 2002;**417**(6888):547-551

[90] Wofford KL et al. Rapid neuroinflammatory response localized to injured neurons after diffuse traumatic brain injury in swine. Experimental Neurology. 2017;**290**:85-94

[91] Lin Y, Wen L. Inflammatory response following diffuse axonal injury. International Journal of Medical Sciences. 2013;**10**(5):515-521

[92] Lu KT et al. Extracellular signal-regulated kinase-mediated IL-1-induced cortical neuron damage during traumatic brain injury. Neuroscience Letters. 2005;**386**(1):40-45

[93] Nwachuku EL et al. Time course of cerebrospinal fluid inflammatory biomarkers and relationship to 6-month neurologic outcome in adult severe traumatic brain injury. Clinical Neurology and Neurosurgery. 2016;**149**:1-5

[94] Yu Y et al. Regulatory T cells exhibit neuroprotective effect in a mouse model of traumatic brain injury. Molecular Medicine Reports. 2016;**14**(6):5556-5566

[95] Zhang Z, Fauser U, Schluesener HJ. Early attenuation of lesional interleukin-16 up-regulation by dexamethasone and FTY720 in experimental traumatic brain injury. Neuropathology and Applied Neurobiology. 2008;**34**(3):330-339

[96] Kleiven S. Why most traumatic brain injuries are not caused by linear acceleration but skull fractures are. Frontiers in Bioengineering and Biotechnology. 2013;**1**:15

Traumatic Axonal Injury in Patients with Mild Traumatic Brain Injury

Sung Ho Jang

Abstract

Mild traumatic brain injury (TBI) is a subtype of TBI that is classified by the severity of head trauma, whereas traumatic axonal injury (TAI) is a diagnostic term with a pathological meaning. In this chapter, TAI in patients with mild TBI is described in terms of definition, history, and diagnostic approach. The presence of TAI in patients with mild TBI has been demonstrated by autopsy studies since the 1960s. However, because conventional brain CT or MRI are not powered with contrast resolution to determine TAI in mild TBI, diagnosis of TAI in live patients with mild TBI was impossible. Since the introduction of diffusion tensor imaging, hundreds of studies have demonstrated TAI in live patients with mild TBI in the 2000s. The precise diagnosis of TAI in patients with mild TBI is clinically important for proper management and prognosis prediction following mild TBI. Several requirements are necessary for diagnosis of TAI in mild TBI: first, head trauma history; second, development of new clinical symptoms and signs after head trauma; third, evidence of TAI of the neural tracts on diffusion tensor imaging or diffusion tensor tractography; and fourth, coincidence of the newly developed clinical features and the function of injured neural tracts.

Keywords: diffusion tensor imaging, diffusion tensor tractography, mild traumatic brain injury, traumatic axonal injury, concussion

1. Introduction

Traumatic brain injury (TBI) is a major cause of disability in adults, and is classified as mild, moderate, and severe according to the severity of head trauma [1]. Mild TBI poses a significant public health problem: it composes 70–90% of all TBI [1–4]. The incidence of hospital-treated patients with mild TBI is 100–300/100,000 population although the true population-based rate including mild TBI not treated in hospitals is estimated above 600/100,000 [1–4]. Mild TBI

Pathoanatomy			
Diffuse		**Focal**	
Concussion		Contusion	
Traumatic axonal injury/diffuse axonal injury		Penetrating	
Blast		Hematoma	
Abusive head trauma		- Epidural	
		- Subarachnoid	
		- Subdural	
		- Intraventricular	
		- Intracerebral	
Severity of head trauma	**Loss of consciousness**	**Post-traumatic amnesia**	**Glasgow Coma Scale**
Mild	≤30 min	≤24 hours	13–15
Moderate	>30 min, ≤24 hours	>24 hours, ≤7 days	9–12
Severe	> 24 hours	>7 days	3–8

Table 1. Traumatic brain injury subtypes.

and concussion (a transient disorder of brain function without long-term sequelae) have been used interchangeably, although the two terms have different definitions and belong to different subtypes of TBI (**Table 1**) [5–7].

Since the 1980s, the term "traumatic axonal injury (TAI)" that describes impaired axoplasmic transports, axonal swelling and disconnection after the head trauma, including mild TBI, has been used in pathological studies using animal brain [8–11]. Since the 1960s, pathological studies using autopsy reported axonal injury in patients with mild TBI or concussion [12–14]. However, because conventional brain CT or MRI are not powered with contrast resolution to determine TAI in mild TBI, diagnosis of TAI in live patients with mild TBI was impossible for a long time. Since the development of diffusion tensor imaging (DTI) in the 2000s, many researchers demonstrated TAI in live patients with mild TBI [15–85]. Because mild TBI and TAI are different TBI subtypes, the precise diagnosis of TAI in patients with mild TBI is clinically important for proper management and prognosis prediction (**Table 1**) [6, 7].

In this chapter, TAI in patients with mild TBI is described in terms of definition, history, and diagnostic approach.

2. Traumatic axonal injury in patients with mild traumatic axonal injury

2.1. Definition and problem of the term "mild traumatic brain injury"

The American Congress of Rehabilitation Medicine in 1993 defined mild TBI as a traumatically induced physiological disruption of brain function resulting from the head being struck or striking an object, or an acceleration and deceleration movement of the brain, as manifested by at least one of the following: any period of loss of consciousness up to 30 min, post-traumatic amnesia not exceeding 24 hours, and an initial Glasgow Coma Scale score of 13–15 [86–89]. Blast may also cause mild TBI [90].

Opinions critical of the use of the term "mild TBI," as indicating a benign condition, have been expressed [5, 91, 92]. In 2012, Rapp et al. insisted that mild TBI is a category mistake because of the heterogeneity of the clinical population and features, and the complex idiosyncratic time course of the appearance of these deficits in patients with mild TBI [92]. Subsequently, McMahon et al. reported that the term "mild TBI" is a misnomer because some of the patients with mild TBI show severe neurological sequelae [91]. In 2015, Sharp and Jenkins insisted that mild TBI is not always a benign condition as its name implies and patients with mild TBI sometimes fail to recover [5]. These critical opinions appear to stem from the observations of concurrent TAI in patients with mild TBI that cannot be detected on conventional brain CT or MRI. Such lesions have been described by hundreds of DTI studies since the 2000s [15–85].

2.2. Definition and diagnostic history of traumatic axonal injury in mild TBI

Neural axons in the white matter are particularly vulnerable to diffuse head trauma due to mechanical loading of the brain during TBI [8, 93]. TAI, a pathological term, is defined as tearing of axons due to indirect shearing forces during acceleration, deceleration, and rotation of the brain, or direct head trauma [6, 9, 10, 15–23, 94, 95].

Since the 1980s, many researchers, including Povlishock, have used the term "TAI" in their pathological studies using animal brain [8–11]. In the human brain, several studies have demonstrated trauma-related axonal injury in pathological autopsy studies of patients who died of other causes following TBI, including concussion or mild TBI, since the middle of the last century [12–14, 96]. However, due to insensitivity of conventional brain MRI for detection of TAI in mild TBI, diagnosis of TAI in live patients with mild TBI was impossible for a long time. In the 1990s, the development of DTI opened a new era for diagnosis of the subcortical white matter pathology in the live human brain. Because DTI provides invaluable information about subcortical white matter that cannot be obtained by conventional MRI, DTI was initially used to detect white matter pathology undetectable by conventional CT or MRI in brain pathologies such as cerebral palsy, hypoxic-ischemic brain injury, and congenital brain disease [97–99]. Since Arfanakis's study in 2002, TAI has been demonstrated in hundreds of DTI studies in mild TBI [15–85]. As a result, DTI become an important diagnostic tool for TAI in patients with mild TBI, particularly in patients whose conventional brain CT or MRI is negative.

The history of the use of term TAI with regard to the term "diffuse axonal injury (DAI)" has given rise to some confusion [6]. Adams et al. began to use the term "DAI" by defining DAI as the presence of microscopic axonal injury in the white matter of the cerebral hemisphere, corpus callosum, and brainstem caused by mechanical forces during head injury [100–102]. After that, instead of DAI, "TAI" or "diffuse TAI" was used to correct the mistaken term "diffuse" (because the distribution of the lesions of axonal injury is not diffuse but multifocal), and to include the meaning of trauma in terms of the etiology of axonal injury [6–8, 93]. Generally, the traditional definition of DAI indicates patients in profound and prolonged coma at the onset of head trauma, and who suffer a poor outcome [6–8, 93, 102, 103]. Because more restricted patterns of axonal injury than the traditional DAI were detected in milder TBI with the development of DTI, the term "TAI" is used for these more limited injuries: in practice, TAI indicates milder injury than DAI [6–8, 93, 98, 103].

2.3. Comparison of diffusion tensor imaging and diffusion tensor tractography in detecting TAI in mild TBI

The left corticospinal tract shows partial tearing (arrow) at the subcortical white matter. When a researcher measures diffusion tensor imaging parameters using the region of interest (ROI) method, if the ROI is placed in the partially torn area (B), traumatic axonal injury of the left corticospinal tract can be detected, whereas if the ROI is placed in the normal-appearing area (D), traumatic axonal injury of the left corticospinal tract cannot be detected.

Two methods are used to detect TAI in mild TBI: (1) region of interest (ROI) method: measurement of DTI parameters in a certain ROI of the brain, and (2) diffusion tensor tractography (DTT) for the neural tracts (**Figure 1**). DTT allows for visualization and estimation of the neural tracts three dimensionally by reconstruction from DTI data: measurement of DTT parameters and configurational analysis of the reconstructed neural tracts [19, 20, 24–56, 61, 72, 98]. Many more studies have used the ROI method than DTT; however, this method can yield false results for the following reasons. First, high individual variability of the anatomical location of the neural tracts in the human brain can lead to measurement of DTI parameters in a false location for the target neural tract, especially in compact areas such as the corona radiata, posterior limb of the internal capsule, or brainstem [104]. In addition, the results can differ depending on whether a ROI is placed in a TAI lesion (for example, a partially torn area) or normal-appearing area. For example, when a neural tract was partially torn by TAI following mild TBI, if the ROI was placed in the normal-appearing area, TAI cannot be detected using the ROI method although this patient had TAI following mild TBI (**Figure 1**). Second, high interanalyzer variability of the ROI method can lead to false results [105].

By contrast, DTT for reconstruction of the neural tracts usually employs a combined ROI method that reconstructs only neural fibers passing more than two ROI areas. The ROI areas and reconstruction conditions for the neural tracts are well defined for each neural tract [6, 50, 106–113]. High repeatability and reliability of DTT method for the neural tracts have been demonstrated in many studies [6, 24, 50, 106–111, 113]. Therefore, experienced analyzers can reconstruct the neural tracts without significant inter- and intra-analyzer variation. The main advantage of DTT over DTI is that the entire neural tract can be evaluated in terms of DTT parameters, including fractional anisotropy, mean diffusivity and tract volume, and configurational analysis. Fractional anisotropy value indicates the degree of directionality of microstructures, such as axons, myelin, and microtubules, while mean diffusivity value suggests the magnitude of water diffusion [114]. Tract volume is determined by counting the number of voxels contained within a neural tract [114]. Therefore, a significant decrement of fractional anisotropy or tract volume, or increment of mean diffusivity compared with normal subjects, indicates injury of a neural tract. In addition, on configuration analysis of the

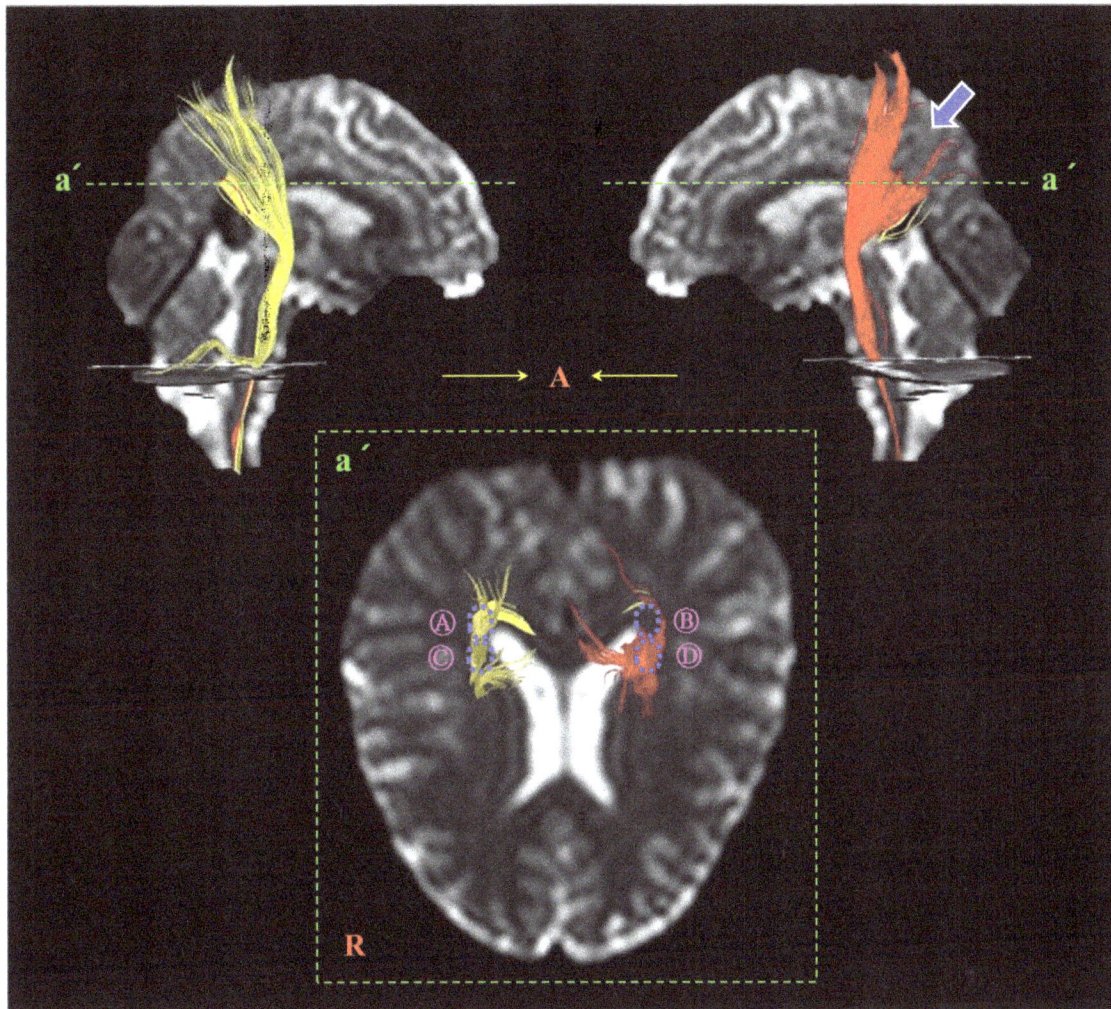

Figure 1. Possible false measurement of diffusion tensor imaging parameters in a partially torn corticospinal tract in a patient with mild traumatic brain injury.

reconstructed neural tracts, abnormal findings including tearing, narrowing, or discontinuation have been used to detect TAI of the neural tracts in patients with mild TBI (**Figure 2**) [19, 20, 24, 26–37, 39–56]. As a result, DTT would be better than DTI to detect TAI in a neural tract in an individual patient. More than 30 papers have demonstrated TAI in individual patients with mild TBI in the corticospinal tract, corticoreticulospinal tract, spinothalamic tract, fornix, cingulum, optic radiation, ascending reticular activating system, papez circuit, pre-fronto-thalamic tracts, inferior cerebellar peduncle, corticofugal tracts form the secondary motor area, arcuate fasciculus, corticobulbar tract, and dentatorubrothalamic tract [19, 20, 24, 26–37, 39–56]. However, DTT may underestimate the neural tracts due to regions of fiber complexity and crossing that can prevent full reflection of the underlying fiber architecture [105, 115, 116]. In addition, TAI on DTT often cannot be discriminated from abnormalities by previous head trauma, other concurrent neurological diseases, aging, or immaturity, although some findings suggest characteristic features of TAI in several neural tracts [26, 28, 29, 39, 48, 51–54].

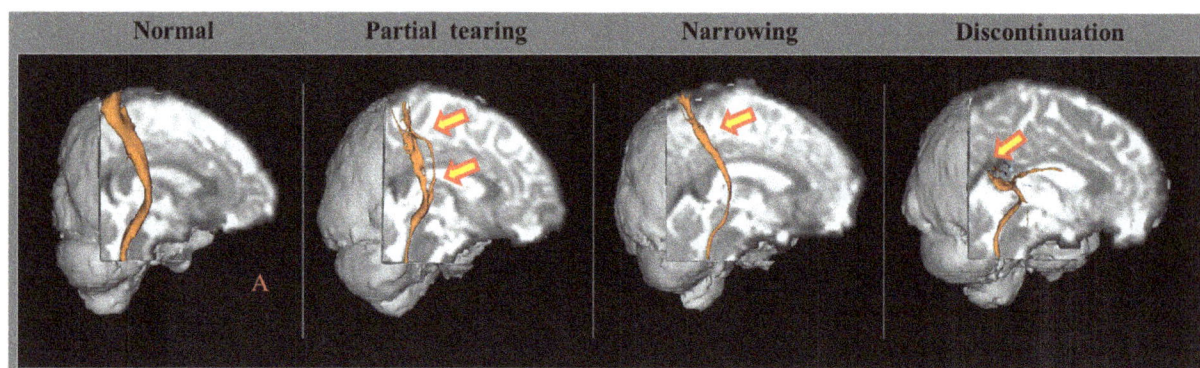

Figure 2. Configurational analysis of the spinothalamic tract in patients with mild traumatic brain injury.

2.4. Diagnostic approach of traumatic axonal injury in patients with mild TBI

TAI is a diagnostic term with a pathological meaning; therefore, pathological study by brain biopsy is required to confirm TAI of a neural tract in patients with mild TBI. However, performing brain biopsy for an injured neural tract in patients with mild TBI is impossible because mild TBI is not a life-threatening disease like, for example, brain tumor. The sensitivity and specificity of DTT for diagnosis of TAI of a neural tract in patients with mild TBI can be calculated only through direct comparison of DTT findings of an injured tract with the pathological results of brain tissue, if we accept the latter as the diagnostic "gold standard." As a result, precise demonstration of sensitivity and specificity of DTT for diagnosis of TAI of an injured neural tract in live patients with mild TBI is impossible. However, in 2007, Mac Donald et al. demonstrated that TAI on pathological and DTI results agree in a mouse model of mild TBI that showed normal findings on conventional MRI [117]. They concluded that DTI is highly sensitive for detection of TAI and conventional MRI is not as sensitive as DTI for axonal injury [117].

There are more than 30 recent papers that reported TAI in individual patients with mild TBI using DTT [19, 20, 24, 26–37, 39–56]. The methods to diagnose TAI of the neural tracts of the above studies can be summarized as follows (**Flow Sheet 1**). First, head trauma history compatible with mild TBI is required. According to the definition of mild TBI from the American Congress of Rehabilitation Medicine, the patient must have a head trauma history with three conditions of mild TBI: loss of consciousness, post-traumatic amnesia, and Glasgow Coma Scale [86]. If a patient did not suffer loss of consciousness, any alteration in mental state (feeling dazed, disoriented, or confused) at the time of the accident is necessary. Second, development of new clinical symptoms and signs after head trauma is required. The patient must show new clinical features after the head trauma, which were never observed before the head trauma. The possibility of delayed onset of the clinical symptom due to secondary axonal injury that refers to a condition in which axons were not damaged at the time of injury, but undergo axonal injury caused by the sequential neural injury process of an injured neural tract, should also be considered [9, 10, 24, 26, 27]. Third, evidence of TAI of a neural tract on DTT is required [19, 20, 24, 26–37, 39–56]. TAI of a neural tract can be detected by configuration (tearing, narrowing, or discontinuation) or DTT parameters (significant decrement of fractional anisotropy or tract volume, or increment of mean diffusivity) on DTT for a neural

Head trauma history compatible with mild TBI

↓

Development of new clinical symptoms and signs after head trauma

↓

Traumatic axonal injury findings on DTT for clinically relevant neural tracts
-Configuration: tearing, narrowing or discontinuation
-Significant change of DTT parameters: decreased fractional anisotropy or
tract volume, or increased mean diffusivity

↓

R/O Previous head trauma, concurrent neurological disease, aging or artifact of DTT

↓

R/O Other pathologies
(peripheral nerve injury, spinal cord injury, and musculoskeletal problems)

↓

Consider response to management for clinical symptoms

↓

Consider other clinical features and DTT findings of other neural tracts,

↓

Diagnosis

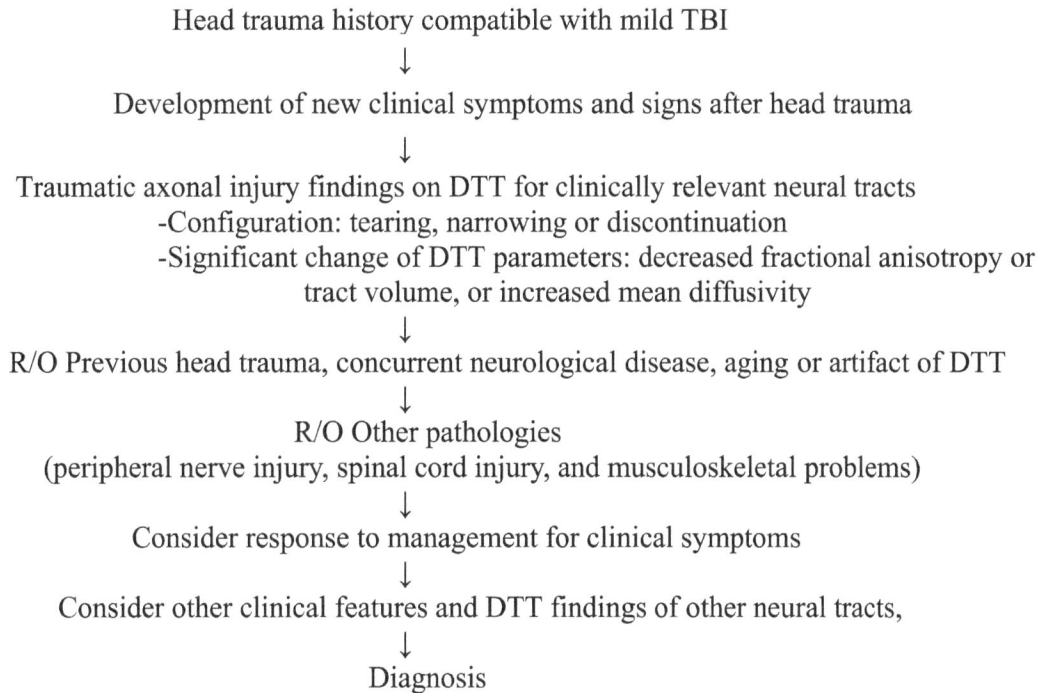

Flow Sheet 1. Diagnostic approach of traumatic axonal injury of a neural tract in patients with mild traumatic brain injury.

tract (**Figure 2**). Fourth, DTT abnormality by previous head trauma, concurrent neurological disease, aging, immaturity, or artifact of DTT should be ruled out. In addition, the newly developed clinical features and the function of the injured neural tracts must coincide. Fifth, other pathologies including peripheral nerve injury, spinal cord injury, and musculoskeletal problems should be ruled out through other studies such as electromyography study, radiological study, or ultrasonography. Additionally, improvement of a clinical symptom with management of an injured neural tract could be an additional evidence for TAI. For example, when a patient develops central pain due to injury of the spinothalamic tract following mild TBI, and if the patient's pain improves with the administration of specific drugs for central pain, it would be an additional evidence for TAI in this patient. In addition, the clinical features and DTT findings of other neural tracts should be considered because TAI usually occurs in multiple neural tracts following diffuse head trauma like mild TBI [29, 30, 34].

For example, a 43-year-old female patient suffered injury from a car accident. She hit her head on the seats with acceleration-deceleration injury while sitting in a passenger seat in a minibus after a collision with a car from behind. She had no head trauma history, and findings were consistent with the three conditions of mild TBI [86, 87]. Since the head trauma, she noticed memory impairment, mild weakness of both hands, and central pain of the entire body. On DTT, the injuries of cingulum (discontinuations of both anterior cingula), the fornix (discontinuation of the left fornical crus), corticospinal tract (partial tearing at the subcortical white matter of both corticospinal tracts), and spinothalamic tract (partial tearing of the left spinothalamic tract) were detected (**Figure 3**). In this patient, TAI by this car accident was confidently diagnosed by the head trauma history, development of new clinical features, and injury evidence of the various neural tracts on DTT. The patient provided written informed consent.

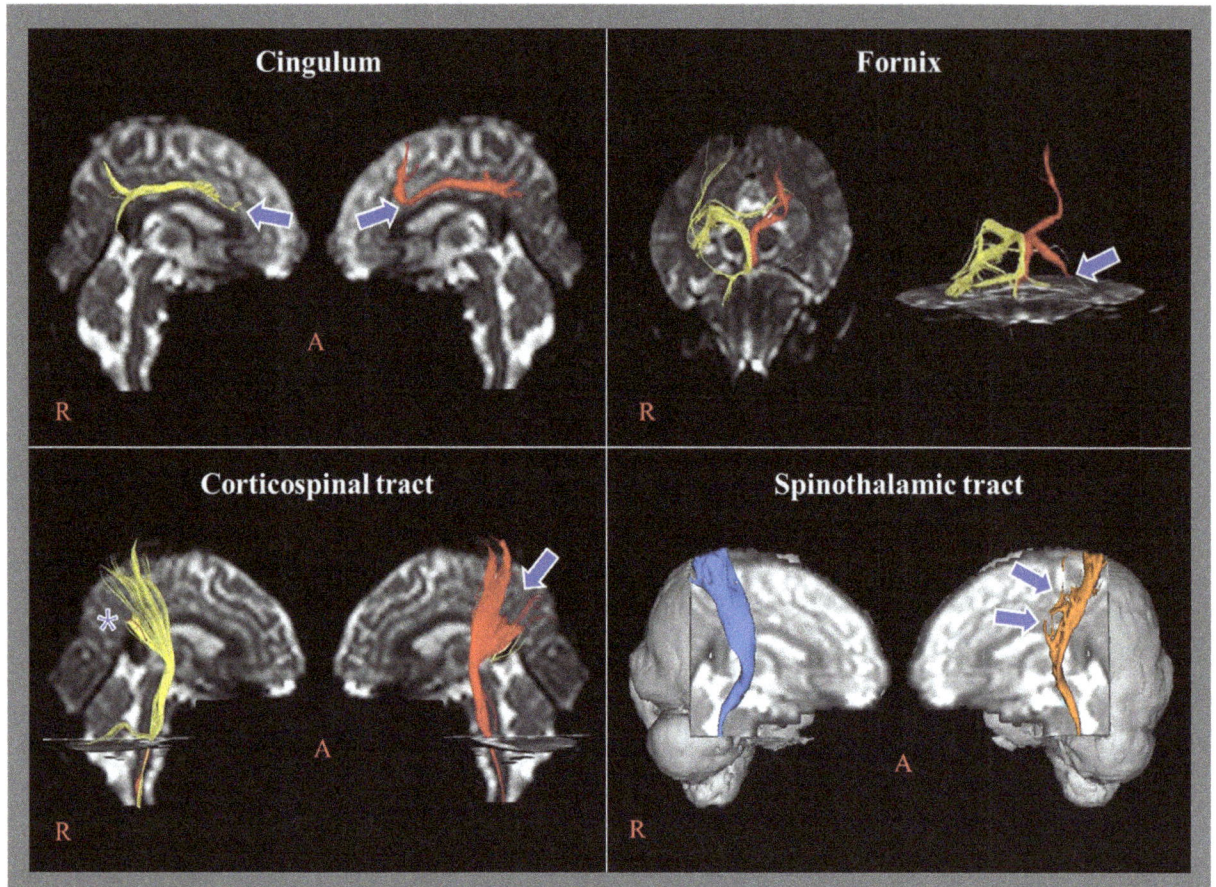

Figure 3. Traumatic axonal injuries of several neural tracts in a patient with mild traumatic brain injury. (->:traumatic axonal injury, *suspicious traumatic axonal injury).

3. Conclusion

In this chapter, TAI in patients with mild TBI is described in terms of definition, history, and diagnostic approach. Precise diagnosis of TAI in patients with mild TBI is clinically important. The introduction of DTI has enabled diagnosis of TAI in the live patients with mild TBI [15–85]. Several requirements are necessary for diagnosis of TAI in patients with mild TBI: head trauma history, development of new clinical symptoms and signs after head trauma, evidence of TAI of the neural tracts on DTI or DTT, and coincidence of the newly developed clinical features and the function of injured neural tracts. DTT seems a better tool than the ROI method on DTI to locate partial injury in a neural tract in an individual patient, because DTT can evaluate the entire neural tract. Limitations of DTT should be considered, although the reconstruction methods of various neural tracts have been well defined, and high repeatability and reliability of these methods have been demonstrated [6, 24, 50, 105–111, 113, 115, 116, 118, 119]. Further studies of the diagnostic criteria for TAI with sensitivity, specificity, and reliability in mild TBI should be encouraged.

Acknowledgements

This work was supported by the National Research Foundation (NRF) of Korea Grant funded by the Korean Government (MSIP) (2015R1A2A2A01004073).

Author details

Sung Ho Jang

Address all correspondence to: strokerehab@hanmail.net

Department of Physical Medicine and Rehabilitation, College of Medicine, Yeungnam University and Daemyungdong, Namku, Taegu, Republic of Korea

References

[1] Decuypere M, Klimo P Jr. Spectrum of traumatic brain injury from mild to severe. The Surgical Clinics of North America. 2012;**92**:939-957. DOI: 10.1016/j.suc.2012.04.005

[2] Kraus JF, Nourjah P. The epidemiology of mild, uncomplicated brain injury. The Journal of Trauma. 1988;**28**:1637-1643. DOI: 10.1097/00005373-198812000-00004

[3] De Kruijk JR, Twijnstra A, Leffers P. Diagnostic criteria and differential diagnosis of mild traumatic brain injury. Brain Injury. 2001;**15**:99-106. DOI: 10.1080/026990501458335

[4] Cassidy JD, Carroll LJ, Peloso PM, Borg J, von Holst H, Holm L, Kraus J, Coronado VG. Incidence, risk factors and prevention of mild traumatic brain injury: Results of the WHO Collaborating Centre Task Force on Mild Traumatic Brain Injury. Journal of Rehabilitation Medicine 2004:28-60. DOI: 10.1080/16501960410023732

[5] Sharp DJ, Jenkins PO. Concussion is confusing us all. Practical Neurology. 2015;**15**:172-186. DOI: 10.1136/practneurol-2015-001087

[6] Jang SH. Dignostic history of traumatic axonal injury in patients with cerebral concussion and mild traumatic brain injury. Brain & Neurorehabil. 2016;**9**:1-8. DOI: 10.12786/bn.2016.9.e1

[7] Saatman KE, Duhaime AC, Bullock R, Maas AI, Valadka A, Manley GT, Workshop Scientific T, Advisory PM. Classification of traumatic brain injury for targeted therapies. Journal of Neurotrauma. 2008;**25**:719-738. DOI: 10.1089/neu.2008.0586

[8] Maxwell WL, Povlishock JT, Graham DL. A mechanistic analysis of nondisruptive axonal injury: A review. Journal of Neurotrauma. 1997;**14**:419-440. DOI: 10.1089/neu.1997.14.419

[9]   Povlishock JT. Traumatically induced axonal injury: Pathogenesis and Pathobiological implications. Brain Pathology. 1992;**2**:1-12

[10] Povlishock JT, Christman CW. The pathobiology of traumatically induced axonal injury in animals and humans: A review of current thoughts. Journal of Neurotrauma. 1995;**12**:555-564. DOI: 10.1089/neu.1995.12.555

[11] Povlishock JT, Becker DP, Cheng CL, Vaughan GW. Axonal change in minor head injury. Journal of Neuropathology and Experimental Neurology. 1983;**42**:225-242. DOI: 10.1097/00005072-198305000-00002

[12] Oppenheimer DR. Microscopic lesions in the brain following head injury. Journal of Neurology, Neurosurgery, and Psychiatry. 1968;**31**:299-306. DOI: 10.1136/jnnp.31.4.299

[13] Blumbergs PC, Scott G, Manavis J, Wainwright H, Simpson DA, McLean AJ. Staining of amyloid precursor protein to study axonal damage in mild head injury. Lancet. 1994;**344**:1055-1056. DOI: 10.1016/s0140-6736(94)91712-4

[14] Bigler ED. Neuropsychological results and neuropathological findings at autopsy in a case of mild traumatic brain injury. Journal of the International Neuropsychological Society. 2004;**10**:794-806. DOI: 10.1017/S1355617704105146

[15] Arfanakis K, Haughton VM, Carew JD, Rogers BP, Dempsey RJ, Meyerand ME. Diffusion tensor MR imaging in diffuse axonal injury. AJNR – American Journal of Neuroradiology. 2002;**23**:794-802

[16] Inglese M, Makani S, Johnson G, Cohen BA, Silver JA, Gonen O, Grossman RI. Diffuse axonal injury in mild traumatic brain injury: A diffusion tensor imaging study. Journal of Neurosurgery. 2005;**103**:298-303. DOI: 10.3171/jns.2005.103.2.0298

[17] Niogi SN, Mukherjee P, Ghajar J, Johnson C, Kolster RA, Sarkar R, Lee H, Meeker M, Zimmerman RD, Manley GT, McCandliss BD. Extent of microstructural white matter injury in postconcussive syndrome correlates with impaired cognitive reaction time: A 3T diffusion tensor imaging study of mild traumatic brain injury. AJNR – American Journal of Neuroradiology. 2008;**29**:967-973. DOI: 10.3174/ajnr.A0970

[18] Shenton ME, Hamoda HM, Schneiderman JS, Bouix S, Pasternak O, Rathi Y, Vu MA, Purohit MP, Helmer K, Koerte I, Lin AP, Westin CF, Kikinis R, Kubicki M, Stern RA, Zafonte R. A review of magnetic resonance imaging and diffusion tensor imaging findings in mild traumatic brain injury. Brain Imaging and Behavior. 2012;**6**:137-192. DOI: 10.1007/s11682-012-9156-5

[19] Jang SH, Kim SY. Injury of the corticospinal tract in patients with mild traumatic brain injury: A diffusion tensor tractography study. Journal of Neurotrauma. 2016;**33**:1790-1795. DOI: 10.1089/neu.2015.4298

[20] Yang DS, Kwon HG, Jang SH. Injury of the thalamocingulate tract in the papez circuit in patients with mild traumatic brain injury. American Journal of Physical Medicine & Rehabilitation. 2016;**95**:E34-E38. DOI: 10.1097/Phm.0000000000000413

[21] Jang SH, Kim TH, Kwon YH, Lee MY, Lee HD. Postural instability in patients with injury of corticoreticular pathway following mild traumatic brain injury. American Journal of Physical Medicine & Rehabilitation. 2016;**95**:580-587. DOI: 10.1097/Phm.0000000000000446

[22] Jang SH, Lee AY, Shin SM. Injury of the arcuate fasciculus in the dominant hemisphere in patients with mild traumatic brain injury a retrospective cross-sectional study. Medicine. 2016;**95**:e3007. DOI: 10.1097/MD.0000000000003007

[23] Jang SH, Kwon HG. Injury of the ascending reticular activating system in patients with fatigue and hypersomnia following mild traumatic brain injury two case reports. Medicine. 2016;**95**:e2628. DOI: 10.1097/md.0000000000002628

[24] Seo JP, Jang SH. Injury of the spinothalamic tract in a patient with mild traumatic brain injury: Diffusion tensor tractography study. Journal of Rehabilitation Medicine. 2014;**46**:374-377. DOI: 10.2340/16501977-1783

[25] Kim JH, Ahn SH, Cho YW, Kim SH, Jang SH. The relation between injury of the spinothalamocortical tract and central pain in chronic patients with mild traumatic brain injury. The Journal of Head Trauma Rehabilitation. 2015;**30**:E40-E46. DOI: 10.1097/Htr.0000000000000121

[26] Jang SH, Kwon HG. Degeneration of an injured spinothalamic tract in a patient with mild traumatic brain injury. Brain Injury. 2016;**30**:1026-1028. DOI: 10.3109/02699052.2016.1146961

[27] Jang SH, Lee HD. Central pain due to spinothalamic tract injury caused by indirect head trauma following a pratfall. Brain Injury. 2016;**30**:933-936. DOI: 10.3109/02699052.2016.1146966

[28] Jang SH, Seo YS. Central pain due to spinothalamic tract injury by head trauma caused by a falling object. Ann Rehabil Med. 2016;**10**:1149-1150. DOI: 10.5535/arm.2016.40.6.1149

[29] Jang SH, Lee HD. Severe and extensive traumatic axonal injury following minor and indirect head trauma. Brain Injury. 2017;**31**:416-419. DOI: 10.1080/02699052.2016.1239274

[30] Jang SH, Ahn SH, Cho YW, Lim JW, Cho IT. Diffusion tensor tractography for detection of concomitant traumatic brain injury in patients with traumatic spinal cord injury. The Journal of Head Trauma Rehabilitation. 2017. DOI: 10.1097/HTR.0000000000000300 [Epub ahead of print]

[31] Jang SH, Kim SH, Seo JP. Spinothalamic tract injury due to primary brainstem injury: A case report. American Journal of Physical Medicine & Rehabilitation. 2016;**95**:E42-E43. DOI: 10.1097/Phm.0000000000000414

[32] Jang SH, Kwon HG. Apathy due to injury of the prefrontocaudate tract following mild traumatic brain injury. American Journal of Physical Medicine & Rehabilitation. 2017;**96**:E130-E133. DOI: 10.1097/Phm.0000000000000630

[33] Jang SH, Kwon HG. Aggravation of excessive daytime sleepiness concurrent with aggravation of an injured ascending reticular activating system in a patient with mild traumatic brain injury: A case report. Medicine (Baltimore). 2017;**96**:e5958. DOI: 10.1097/MD.0000000000005958

[34] Jang SH, Kwon HG. Akinetic mutism in a patient with mild traumatic brain injury: A diffusion tensor tractography study. Brain Injury. 2017:1-5. DOI: 10.1080/02699052.2017.1288265

[35] Jang SH, Kwon HG. Diffuse injury of the papez circuit by focal head trauma: A diffusion tensor tractography study. Acta Neurologica Belgica. 2017;117:389-391. DOI: 10.1007/s13760-016-0665-7

[36] Jang SH, Kwon HG. Injury of the ascending reticular activating system in patients with fatigue and hypersomnia following mild traumatic brain injury: Two case reports. Medicine (Baltimore). 2016;95:e2628. DOI: 10.1097/MD.0000000000002628

[37] Jang SH, Kwon HG. Injury of the dentato-rubro-thalamic tract in a patient with mild traumatic brain injury. Brain Injury. 2015;29:1725-1728. DOI: 10.1097/MD.0000000000007220

[38] Jang SH, Lee AY, Shin SM. Injury of the arcuate fasciculus in the dominant hemisphere in patients with mild traumatic brain injury: A retrospective cross-sectional study. Medicine (Baltimore). 2016;95:e3007. DOI: 10.1097/MD.0000000000003007

[39] Jang SH, Lee HD. Compensatory neural tract from contralesional fornical body to ipsilesional medial temporal lobe in a patient with mild traumatic brain injury: A case report. American Journal of Physical Medicine & Rehabilitation. 2016;95:e14-e17. DOI: 10.1097/PHM.0000000000000390

[40] Jang SH, Lee HD. Weak phonation due to injury of the corticobulbar tract in a patient with mild traumatic brain injury. Neural Regeneration Research. [In press]

[41] Jang SH, Seo JP. Damage to the optic radiation in patients with mild traumatic brain injury. Journal of Neuro-Ophthalmology. 2015;35:270-273. DOI: 10.1097/WNO.0000000000000249

[42] Jang SH, Seo JP. Motor execution problem due to injured corticofugal tracts from the supplementary motor area in a patient with mild traumatic brain injury. American Journal of Physical Medicine & Rehabilitation. 2017. DOI: 10.1097/phm.0000000000000699 [Epub ahead of print]

[43] Jang SH, Seo WS, Kwon HG. Post-traumatic narcolepsy and injury of the ascending reticular activating system. Sleep Medicine. 2016;17:124-125. DOI: 10.1016/j.sleep.2015.09.020

[44] Jang SH, Seo YS. Dysarthria due to injury of the corticobulbar tract in a patient with mild traumatic brain injury. American Journal of Physical Medicine & Rehabilitation. 2016;95:E187-E187. DOI: 10.1097/Phm.0000000000000519

[45] Jang SH, Yi JH, Kwon HG. Injury of the dorsolateral prefronto-thalamic tract in a patient with depression following mild traumatic brain injury: A case report. Medicine. 2016;95:e5009. DOI: 10.1097/MD.0000000000005009

[46] Jang SH, Yi JH, Kwon HG. Injury of the inferior cerebellar peduncle in patients with mild traumatic brain injury: A diffusion tensor tractography study. Brain Injury. 2016;30:1271-1275. DOI: 10.1080/02699052.2016.1178805

[47]   Jang SH, Kwon HG. Injury of the papez circuit in a patient with traumatic spinal cord injury and concomitant mild traumatic brain injury. Neural Regeneration Research. [In press]

[48]   Kim JW, Lee HD, Jang SH. Severe bilateral anterior cingulum injury in patients with mild traumatic brain injury. Neural Regeneration Research. 2015;**10**:1876-1878. DOI: 10.4103/1673-5374.170321

[49]   Kwon HG, Jang SH. Delayed gait disturbance due to injury of the corticoreticular pathway in a patient with mild traumatic brain injury. Brain Injury. 2014;**28**:511-514. DOI: 10.3109/02699052.2014.887228

[50]   Lee HD, Jang SH. Injury of the corticoreticular pathway in patients with mild traumatic brain injury: A diffusion tensor tractography study. Brain Injury. 2015;**29**:1219-1222. DOI: 10.3109/02699052.2015.1045028

[51]   Lee HD, Jang SH. Changes of an injured fornix in a patient with mild traumatic brain injury: Diffusion tensor tractography follow-up study. Brain Injury. 2014;**28**:1485-1488. DOI: 10.3109/02699052.2014.930178

[52]   Seo JP, Jang SH. Traumatic axonal injury of the corticospinal tract in the subcortical white matter in patients with mild traumatic brain injury. Brain Injury. 2015;**29**:110-114. DOI: 10.3109/02699052.2014.973447

[53]   Jang SH, Lee HD. Abundant unusual neural branches from the fornix in patients with mild traumatic brain injury: A diffusion tensor tractography study. Brain Injury. 2017:1-4. DOI: 10.1080/02699052.2017.1350997

[54]   Yeo SS, Jang SH. Neural reorganization following bilateral injury of the fornix crus in a patient with traumatic brain injury. Journal of Rehabilitation Medicine. 2013;**45**:595-598. DOI: 10.2340/16501977-1145

[55]   Jang SH, Kwon HG. Selective injury of fornical column in a patient with mild traumatic brain injury. American Journal of Physical Medicine & Rehabilitation. 2015;**94**:E86. DOI: 10.1097/Phm.0000000000000317

[56]   Jang SH, Kim SH, Seo JP. Recovery of an injured cingulum concurrent with improvement of short-term memory in a patient with mild traumatic brain injury. Brain Injury. [In press]

[57]   Jang SH, Park SM, Kwon HG. Relation between injury of the periaqueductal gray and central pain in patients with mild traumatic brain injury: Observational study. Medicine. 2016;**95**:e4017. DOI: 10.1097/MD.0000000000004017

[58]   Jang SH, Yi JH, Kim SH, Kwon HG. Relation between injury of the hypothalamus and subjective excessive daytime sleepiness in patients with mild traumatic brain injury. Journal of Neurology, Neurosurgery, and Psychiatry. 2016;**87**:1260-U1134. DOI: 10.1136/jnnp-2016-31309

[59]   Jang SH, Lee HD. Diffusion tensor tractography studies on mechanisms of recovery of injured fornical crus: A mini-review. Neural Regeneration Research. [In press]

[60] Jang SH, Kim TH, Kwon YH, Lee MY. Lee HD postural instability in patients with injury of corticoreticular pathway following mild traumatic brain injury. American Journal of Physical Medicine & Rehabilitation. 2016;**95**:580-587. DOI: 10.1097/PHM.0000 000000000446

[61] MM D'S, Trivedi R, Singh K, Grover H, Choudhury A, Kaur P, Kumar P, Tripathi RP. Traumatic brain injury and the post-concussion syndrome: A diffusion tensor tractography study. Indian J Radiol Imaging. 2015;**25**:404-414. DOI: 10.4103/0971-3026.169445

[62] Khong E, Odenwald N, Hashim E, Cusimano MD. Diffusion tensor imaging findings in post-concussion syndrome patients after mild traumatic brain injury: A systematic review. Frontiers in Neurology. 2016;**7**:156. DOI: 10.3389/fneur.2016.00156

[63] Asken BM, DeKosky ST, Clugston JR, Jaffee MS, Bauer RM. Diffusion tensor imaging (DTI) findings in adult civilian, military, and sport-related mild traumatic brain injury (mTBI): A systematic critical review. Brain Imaging and Behavior. 2017. DOI: 10.1007/s11682-017-9708-9

[64] Alhilali LM, Delic JA, Gumus S, Fakhran S. Evaluation of white matter injury patterns underlying neuropsychiatric symptoms after mild traumatic brain injury. Radiology. 2015;**277**:793-800. DOI: 10.1148/radiol.2015142974

[65] Churchill NW, Caverzasi E, Graham SJ, Hutchison MG, Schweizer TA. White matter microstructure in athletes with a history of concussion: Comparing diffusion tensor imaging (DTI) and neurite orientation dispersion and density imaging (NODDI). Human Brain Mapping. 2017;**38**:4201-4211. DOI: 10.1002/hbm.23658

[66] Delano-Wood L, Bangen KJ, Sorg SF, Clark AL, Schiehser DM, Luc N, Bondi MW, Werhane M, Kim RT, Bigler ED. Brainstem white matter integrity is related to loss of consciousness and postconcussive symptomatology in veterans with chronic mild to moderate traumatic brain injury. Brain Imaging and Behavior. 2015;**9**:500-512. DOI: 10.1007/s11682-015-9432-2

[67] Edlow BL, Copen WA, Izzy S, Bakhadirov K, van der Kouwe A, Glenn MB, Greenberg SM, Greer DM, Wu O. Diffusion tensor imaging in acute-to-subacute traumatic brain injury: A longitudinal analysis. BMC Neurology 2016;**16**:2. DOI: 10.1186/s12883-015-0525-8

[68] Ewing-Cobbs L, Johnson CP, Juranek J, DeMaster D, Prasad M, Duque G, Kramer L, Cox CS, Swank PR. Longitudinal diffusion tensor imaging after pediatric traumatic brain injury: Impact of age at injury and time since injury on pathway integrity. Human Brain Mapping. 2016;**37**:3929-3945. DOI: 10.1089/neu.2016.4584

[69] Genc S, Anderson V, Ryan NP, Malpas CB, Catroppa C, Beauchamp MH, Silk TJ. Recovery of white matter following pediatric traumatic brain injury depends on injury severity. Journal of Neurotrauma. 2017;**34**:798-806. DOI: 10.1089/neu.2016.4584

[70] Hashim E, Caverzasi E, Papinutto N, Lewis CE, Jing RW, Charles O, Zhang SD, Lin A, Graham SJ, Schweizer TA, Bharatha A, Cusimano MD. Investigating microstructural abnormalities and neurocognition in sub-acute and chronic traumatic brain injury patients with normal-appearing white matter: A preliminary diffusion tensor imaging study. Frontiers in Neurology. 2017;**8**:97. DOI: 10.3389/fneur.2017.00097

[71] Hu H, Zhou Y, Wang Q, Su SS, Qiu YM, Ge JW, Wang Z, Xiao ZP. Association of abnormal white matter integrity in the acute phase of motor vehicle accidents with posttraumatic stress disorder. Journal of Affective Disorders. 2016;**190**:714-722. DOI: 10.1016/j.jad.2015.09.044

[72] Kasahara K, Hashimoto K, Abo M, Senoo A. Voxel- and atlas-based analysis of diffusion tensor imaging may reveal focal axonal injuries in mild traumatic brain injury – comparison with diffuse axonal injury. Magnetic Resonance Imaging. 2012;**30**:496-505. DOI: 10.1016/j.mri.2011.12.018

[73] Lancaster MA, Olson DV, McCrea MA, Nelson LD, LaRoche AA, Muftuler LT. Acute white matter changes following sport-related concussion: A serial diffusion tensor and diffusion kurtosis tensor imaging study. Human Brain Mapping. 2016;**37**:3821-3834. DOI: 10.1002/hbm.23278

[74] Leh SE, Schroeder C, Chen JK, Chakravarty MM, Park MTM, Cheung B, Huntgeburth SC, Gosselin N, Hock C, Ptito A, Petrides M. Microstructural integrity of hippocampal subregions is impaired after mild traumatic brain injury. Journal of Neurotrauma. 2017;**34**:1402-1411. DOI: 10.1089/neu.2016.4591

[75] Lopez KC, Leary JB, Pham DL, Chou YY, Dsurney J, Chan L. Brain volume, connectivity, and neuropsychological performance in mild traumatic brain injury: The impact of post-traumatic stress disorder symptoms. Journal of Neurotrauma. 2017;**34**:16-22. DOI: 10.1089/neu.2015.4323

[76] Mayinger MCM-BK, Hufschmidt J, Muehlmann M. Brain volume, connectivity, and neuropsychological performance in mild traumatic brain injury s: A longitudinal diffusion tensor imaging study. Brain Imaging and Behavior. 2017 [Epub ahead of print]

[77] Meier TB, Bergamino M, Bellgowan PSF, Teague TK, Ling JM, Jeromin A, Mayer AR. Longitudinal assessment of white matter abnormalities following sports-related concussion. Human Brain Mapping. 2016;**37**:833-845. DOI: 10.1002/hbm.23072

[78] Messe A, Caplain S, Paradot G, Garrigue D, Mineo JF, Ares GS, Ducreux D, Vignaud F, Rozec G, Desal H, Pelegrini-Issac M, Montreuil M, Benali H, Lehericy S. Diffusion tensor imaging and white matter lesions at the subacute stage in mild traumatic brain injury with persistent neurobehavioral impairment. Human Brain Mapping. 2011;**32**:999-1011. DOI: 10.1002/hbm.21092

[79] Miller DR, Hayes JP, Lafleche G, Salat DH, Verfaellie M. White matter abnormalities are associated with chronic postconcussion symptoms in blast-related mild traumatic brain injury. Human Brain Mapping. 2016;**37**:220-229. DOI: 10.1002/hbm.23022

[80] Miller DRHJ, Lafleche G, Salat DH, Verfaellie M. White matter abnormalities are associated with overall cognitive status in blast-related mTBI. Brain Imaging and Behavior. 2016;**11**:1129-1138. DOI: 10.1007/s11682-016-9593-7

[81] Mu W, Catenaccio E, Lipton ML. Neuroimaging in blast-related mild traumatic brain injury. The Journal of Head Trauma Rehabilitation. 2017;**32**:55-69. DOI: 10.1097/HTR.0000000000000213

[82] Oehr L, Anderson J. Diffusion-tensor imaging findings and cognitive function following hospitalized mixed-mechanism mild traumatic brain injury: A systematic review and meta-analysis. Archives of Physical Medicine and Rehabilitation. 2017. DOI: 10.1016/j. apmr.2017.03.019 [Epub ahead of print]

[83] Strain J, Didehbani N, Cullum CM, Mansinghani S, Conover H, Kraut MA, Hart J, Womack KB. Depressive symptoms and white matter dysfunction in retired NFL players with concussion history. Neurology. 2013;**81**:25-32. DOI: 10.1212/WNL.0b013e318299ccf8

[84] Ware JB, Biester RC, Whipple E, Robinson KM, Ross RJ, Nucifora PG. Combat-related mild traumatic brain injury: Association between baseline diffusion-tensor imaging findings and long-term outcomes. Radiology. 2016;**280**:212-219. DOI: 10.1148/radiol.2016151013

[85] Wilde EA, Li XQ, Hunter JV, Narayana PA, Hasan K, Biekman B, Swank P, Robertson C, Miller E, McCauley SR, Chu ZD, Faber J, McCarthy J, Levin HS. Loss of consciousness is related to white matter injury in mild traumatic brain injury. Journal of Neurotrauma. 2016;**33**:2000-2010. DOI: 10.1089/neu.2015.4212

[86] Mild Traumatic Brain Injury Committee. Definition of mild traumatic brain injury. The Journal of Head Trauma Rehabilitation. 1993;**8**:86-87. DOI: 10.1097/00001199-199309000-00010

[87] Alexander MP. Mild traumatic brain injury: Pathophysiology, natural history, and clinical management. Neurology. 1995;**45**:1253-1260. DOI: 10.1212/wnl.45.7.1253

[88] Carroll LJ, Cassidy JD, Holm L, Kraus J, Coronado VG. Methodological issues and research recommendations for mild traumatic brain injury: The who collaborating centre task force on mild traumatic brain injury. Journal of Rehabilitation Medicine. 2004;**36**:113-125. DOI: 10.1080/16501960410023877

[89] Levin HS, Diaz-Arrastia RR. Diagnosis, prognosis, and clinical management of mild traumatic brain injury. Lancet Neurology. 2015;**14**:506-517. DOI: 10.1016/S1474-4422(15)00002-2

[90] Rosenfeld JV, McFarlane AC, Bragge P, Armonda RA, Grimes JB, Ling GS. Blast-related traumatic brain injury. Lancet Neurology. 2013;**12**:882-893. DOI: 10.1016/S1474-4422(13)70161-3

[91] McMahon P, Hricik A, Yue JK, Puccio AM, Inoue T, Lingsma HF, Beers SR, Gordon WA, Valadka AB, Manley GT, Okonkwo DO. Symptomatology and functional outcome in mild traumatic brain injury: Results from the prospective track-TBI study. Journal of Neurotrauma. 2014;**31**:26-33. DOI: 10.1089/neu.2013.2984

[92] Rapp PE, Curley KC. Is a diagnosis of "mild traumatic brain injury" a category mistake? Journal of Trauma and Acute Care Surgery. 2012;**73**:S13-S23. DOI: 10.1097/TA.0b013e318260604b

[93] Johnson VE, Stewart W, Smith DH. Axonal pathology in traumatic brain injury. Experimental Neurology. 2013;**246**:35-43. DOI: 10.1016/j.expneurol.2012.01.013

[94] Buki A, Povlishock JT. All roads lead to disconnection? Traumatic axonal injury revisited. Acta Neurochirurgica. 2006;**148**:181-193. DOI: 10.1007/s00701-005-0674-4

[95] Parizel PM, Ozsarlak, Van Goethem JW, van den Hauwe L, Dillen C, Verlooy J, Cosyns P, De Schepper AM , Imaging findings in diffuse axonal injury after closed head trauma. European Radiology. 1998;**8**:960-965. DOI: 10.1007/s003300050496

[96] Rand CW, Courville CB. Histologic changes in the brain in cases of fatal injury to the head; alterations in nerve cells. Archives of Neurology and Psychiatry. 1946;**55**:79-110. DOI: 10.1001/archneurpsyc.1946.02300130003001

[97] Basser PJ, Mattiello J, LeBihan D. MR diffusion tensor spectroscopy and imaging. Biophysical Journal. 1994;**66**:259-267. DOI: 10.1016/S0006-3495(94)80775-1

[98] Shenton ME, Hamoda HM, Schneiderman JS, Bouix S, Pasternak O, Rathi Y, Vu MA, Purohit MP, Helmer K, Koerte I, Lin AP, Westin CF, Kikinis R, Kubicki M, Stern RA, Zafonte R. A review of magnetic resonance imaging and diffusion tensor imaging findings in mild traumatic brain injury. Brain Imaging and Behavior. 2012;**6**:137-192. DOI: 10.1007/s11682-012-9156-5

[99] Lee AY, Shin DG, Park JS, Hong GR, Chang PH, Seo JP, Jang SH. Neural tracts injuries in patients with hypoxic ischemic brain injury: Diffusion tensor imaging study. Neuroscience Letters. 2012;**528**:16-21. DOI: 10.1016/j.neulet.2012.08.053

[100] Blumbergs PC. Changing concepts of diffuse axonal injury. Journal of Clinical Neuroscience. 1998;**5**:123-124. DOI: 10.1016/S0967-5868(98)90026-1

[101] Adams JH, Doyle D, Ford I, Gennarelli TA, Graham DI, McLellan DR. Diffuse axonal injury in head injury: Definition, diagnosis and grading. Histopathology. 1989;**15**:49-59. DOI: 10.1111/j.1365-2559.1989.tb03040.x

[102] Adams JH, Graham DI, Murray LS, Scott G. Diffuse axonal injury due to nonmissile head injury in humans. Annals of Neurology. 1982;**12**:557-563. DOI: 10.1002/ana.410120610

[103] Hill CS, Coleman MP, Menon DK. Traumatic axonal injury. Mechanisms and translational opportunities. Trends in Neurosciences. 2016;**39**:311-324. DOI: 10.1016/j.tins.2016.03.002

[104] Jang SH. A review of corticospinal tract location at corona radiata and posterior limb of the internal capsule in human brain. NeuroRehabilitation. 2009;**24**:279-283. DOI: 10.3233/Nre-2009-0479

[105] Lee SK, Kim DI, Kim J. Diffusion-tensor MR imaging and fiber tractography: A new method of describing aberrant fiber connections in developmental CNS anomalies – response. Radiographics. 2005;**25**:53-65. DOI: 10.1148/rg.251045085

[106] Brandstack N, Kurki T, Laalo J, Kauko T, Tenovuo O. Reproducibility of tract-based and region-of-interest DTI analysis of long association tracts. Clinical Neuroradiology. 2016;**26**: 199-208. DOI: 10.1007/s00062-014-0349-8

[107] Wang JY, Abdi N, Bakhadirov K, Diaz-Arrastia R, Devous MD. A comprehensive reliability assessment of quantitative diffusion tensor tractography. NeuroImage. 2012;**60**:1127-1138. DOI: 10.1016/j.neuroimage.2011.12.062

[108] Hasan KM, Kamali A, Abid H, Kramer LA, Fletcher JM, Ewing-Cobbs L. Quantification of the spatiotemporal microstructural organization of the human brain association, projection and commissural pathways across the lifespan using diffusion tensor tractography. Brain Structure & Function. 2010;**214**:361-373. DOI: 10.1007/s00429-009-0238-0

[109] Danielian LE, Iwata NK, Thomasson DM, Floeter MK. Reliability of fiber tracking measurements in diffusion tensor imaging for longitudinal study. NeuroImage. 2010;**49**:1572-1580. DOI: 10.1016/j.neuroimage.2009.08.062

[110] Malykhin N, Concha L, Seres P, Beaulieu C, Coupland NJ. Diffusion tensor imaging tractography and reliability analysis for limbic and paralimbic white matter tracts. Psychiatry Research. 2008;**164**:132-142. DOI: 10.1016/j.pscychresns.2007.11.007

[111] Wakana S, Caprihan A, Panzenboeck MM, Fallon JH, Perry M, Gollub RL, Hua K, Zhang J, Jiang H, Dubey P, Blitz A, van Zijl P, Mori S. Reproducibility of quantitative tractography methods applied to cerebral white matter. NeuroImage 2007;**36**:630-644. DOI: 10.1016/j.neuroimage.2007.02.049

[112] Mori S, Crain BJ, Chacko VP, van Zijl PC. Three-dimensional tracking of axonal projections in the brain by magnetic resonance imaging. Annals of Neurology 1999;**45**:265-269. DOI: 10.1002/1531-8249(199902)45:2<265::aid-ana21>3.0.co;2-3

[113] Danielian LE, Iwata NK, Thomasson DM, Floeter MK. Reliability of fiber tracking measurements in diffusion tensor imaging for longitudinal study. NeuroImage. 2010;**49**:1572-1580. DOI: 10.1016/j.neuroimage.2009.08.062

[114] Basser PJ, Jones DK. Diffusion-tensor MRI: Theory, experimental design and data analysis – A technical review. NMR in Biomedicine. 2002;**15**:456-467. DOI: 10.1002/nbm.783

[115] Yamada K, Sakai K, Akazawa K, Yuen S, Nishimura T. MR tractography: A review of its clinical applications. Magnetic Resonance in Medical Sciences. 2009;**8**:165-174. DOI: 10.2463/mrms.8.165

[116] Parker GJ, Alexander DC. Probabilistic anatomical connectivity derived from the microscopic persistent angular structure of cerebral tissue. Philosophical Transactions of the Royal Society of London. Series B, Biological Sciences. 2005;**360**:893-902. DOI: 10.1098/rstb.2005.1639

[117] Mac Donald CL, Dikranian K, Bayly P, Holtzman D, Brody D. Diffusion tensor imaging reliably detects experimental traumatic axonal injury and indicates approximate time of injury. The Journal of Neuroscience. 2007;**27**:11869-11876. DOI: 10.1523/JNEUROSCI.3647-07.2007

[118] Kwon HG, Choi BY, Kim SH, Chang CH, Jung YJ, Lee HD, Jang SH. Injury of the cingulum in patients with putaminal hemorrhage: A diffusion tensor tractography study. Frontiers in Human Neuroscience. 2014;**8**:366. DOI: 10.3389/fnhum.2014.00366

[119] Jang SH, Kwon HG. The ascending reticular activating system from pontine reticular formation to the hypothalamus in the human brain: A diffusion tensor imaging study. Neuroscience Letters. 2015;**590**:58-61. DOI: 10.1016/j.neulet.2015.01.071

4

Role of Fibrinogen in Vascular Cognitive Impairment in Traumatic Brain Injury

Nino Muradashvili, Suresh C. Tyagi and
David Lominadze

Abstract

Fibrinogen (Fg) is one of the biomarkers of inflammation and a high risk factor for many cardiovascular and cerebrovascular diseases. Elevated levels of Fg (hyperfibrinogenemia, HFg) are also associated with traumatic brain injury (TBI). HFg in blood alters vascular reactivity and compromises integrity of endothelial cell layer that ultimately can result in extravasation of Fg and other plasma proteins. Proteins deposited in extravascular space may form plaques which can lead to neurodegeneration. Among these plasma proteins are amyloid beta (Aβ) and/or cellular prion protein (PrP^C) that can form degradation resistant complexes with Fg and are known to be involved in memory impairment. The purpose of this chapter is to propose and discuss some possible mechanisms involved in HFg-mediated cerebrovascular dysfunction leading to neuronal degeneration during TBI.

Keywords: astrocytes, fibrinogen deposition, neuroinflammation, neurodegeneration, neurovascular unit

1. Introduction

Traumatic brain injury (TBI) is the devastating cause of death and disability worldwide, for which no effective treatment exists other than supportive care [1]. It is a heterogeneous disease that is classically classified as mild, moderate, and severe TBI according to clinical severity using the Glasgow coma scale (GCS) for evaluation [2]. According to epidemiological data falls are the leading cause of TBI, followed by vehicle accidents and physical assaults including sports-related head traumas along with blast injuries that mainly occur in war zones. Pathoanatomic classification of TBI includes penetrating (open) or closed (blunt) head injuries, hemorrhages (epidural, subdural, subarachnoid, intraparenchymal, intraventricular) as well as focal and diffuse patterns of lesions. Classification of TBI by outcome includes categories such as death, vegetative state, disability (severe or moderate) and good recovery. Etiologically TBI is subdivided into "primary" and "secondary" injury based on their triggering mechanisms. Thus, while "primary" injury occurs immediately after a direct physical impact of damaging force, the "secondary" injury is a result of adverse effects of responses in the parenchymal tissue developing due to the "primary" injury. Defining TBI classification is very important for further diagnostic, treatment, clinical management, and prevention and prediction of outcome in patients with TBI [3].

TBI is associated with systemic inflammation [4, 5] that includes elevation of plasma content of fibrinogen (Fg, called hyperfibrinogenemia, HFg). According to clinical data blood level of Fg is elevated after mild-to-moderate TBI (when vascular ruptures are minimal or nonexistent) [6]. It is known that formation of Fg-containing protein complexes is associated with memory reduction emphasizing role of this inflammatory protein. Therefore, in this chapter we propose and discuss possible mechanisms involved in alterations of neuronal function associated with systemic inflammation particularly with HFg during TBI. Since at elevated levels Fg affects vasculature and only then it is involved in vasculo-astrocyte uncoupling [7], the main emphases are given to neuronal degeneration or dysfunction that occurs due to changes in cerebrovascular properties.

2. Traumatic brain injury and blood-brain barrier

The harmful effects of TBI occur during primary injury and secondary complications. Primary damage is induced by a mechanical force that causes compression and physical damage of brain parenchyma that leads to changes in neurovascular unit (NVU) [8, 9]. The secondary complications can occur days or months or years after the initial insult due to further development of chronic inflammation, vascular impairment, chronic ischemia or progressive neurodegeneration [9, 10]. They may involve blood-brain barrier (BBB) impairment, cognitive decline, and memory deficiency [11]. Disruption of BBB has often been documented in patients with TBI [12], but the role of vascular pathology and its consequences in neurological dysfunction has only recently become a sphere of high interest.

BBB is the regulated interface between the peripheral circulation and the central nervous system (CNS). BBB is constituted by the cerebrovascular endothelial cells (ECs) and vascular smooth muscle cells, and together with astrocytes, pericytes, neurons, and associated extracellular matrix proteins represents a NVU [13]. Majority of CNS diseases are associated with mechanical and functional disruption in NVU. The changes and regulation of ion balance and homeostasis, oxygen and nutrition supply, transport of hormones and neurotransmitters depend on normal function of cerebral vessels and blood flow properties. Therefore, because of events initiated in the vasculature as a result of vascular dysfunction, alterations in blood flow and/or changes in blood component properties, which prompt or exacerbate neuronal dysfunction/degeneration, the term "vasculo-neuronal" dysfunction seems more appropriate to emphasize the source of destructive effect in CNS [10].

Studies have shown that increased BBB permeability is involved in initiation of pathological changes in the neuro-vascular network leading to neuronal dysfunction and degeneration.

BBB breakdown in patients with TBI usually confirmed with brain imaging results, and it is suggested to use it as a biomarker in the clinical studies and in drug trials.

The disruption of integrity of vascular walls caused by injury allows proteins such as thrombin, albumin, and/or Fg to enter CNS parenchyma. These proteins have the ability to activate astrocytes and microglia, which are the integral components of the NVU. These effects can be the cause of an increase in synthesis of pro-inflammatory cytokines, including tumor necrosis factor (TNF-α), interlukin-1 (IL-1), interlukin-6 (IL-6), and others [14].

3. Inflammatory markers during TBI

The inflammatory markers can be defined as pro- and anti-inflammatory. The most commonly observed pro-inflammatory cytokines such as TNF-a, IL-1, IL-6 are elevated during TBI [14]. Interestingly, levels of an anti-inflammatory interlukin-10 (IL-10) are also elevated during TBI [15].

TBI-induced inflammation activates acute-phase responses. One of the most known acute-phase proteins is C reactive protein (CRP), which perceptibly increases during inflammation and rapidly decreases after inflammation subsides [16]. On the other hand, blood level of another acute-phase protein—Fg increases slowly and returns to its normal level about 21 days post-inflammatory stimuli [16]. Since Fg itself results in inflammatory responses [17–26], besides being an inflammatory marker, it is considered as a pro-inflammatory protein.

In brain tissue, TNF-α, a well-known pro-inflammatory cytokine, is produced by microglia, astrocytes, endothelial cells, and neurons. The effects of TNF-α are associated with apoptotic/necrotic cell death induction [27]. TNF-α expression takes place shortly after neuronal injury and it is actively involved in process of neutrophil and monocyte recruitment to the site of the damage. The appearance of TNF-α varies from 1 to 24 h following the trauma (the peak is considered at 4–12 h following initial insult). Some scientists consider TNF-α as a marker of severe TBI [28]. There are data indicating a significant association of TNF-α with cognitive impairment during TBI [29]. However, it is known that in addition to induction of apoptotic/necrotic cell death, TNF-α is also involved in stimulation of cell growth and differentiation. Therefore, the role of TNF-α during TBI may still remain unclear since it has been shown to possess both neurotoxic and neuroprotective effects [27].

The main function of IL-1 is regulation and release of other cytokines. It is expressed in multiple cell types in the brain tissue. Expression of IL-1 is mostly associated with acute TBI [30]. There is a discrepancy in literature regarding the IL-1 detection in serum and cerebrospinal fluid (CSF) during TBI. One of the most reported isoforms of IL-1 family in TBI patients is IL-1β. It is highly involved in release of prostaglandins, apoptosis, leukocyte adhesion to ECs, BBB disruption, and edema formation. The use of IL-1 receptor antagonist, which improves cellular and behavioral outcomes emphasizes the basic pro-inflammatory and neurotoxic effect of IL-1 during TBI [30].

While some consider IL-6 a highly sensitive, but not specific biomarker for neurotrauma [28], others claim that it is not exclusively expressed in response of head trauma and predominantly indicates state of BBB integrity [31]. IL-6 is expressed by astrocytes, glial cells and neurons. Normally it is not detectable in serum and plasma but under pathological conditions level of IL-6 increases and points to mainly axonal injury [28]. Drastically increased levels of IL-6 are observed in CSF during severe TBI that reaches its maximum levels in about 3 to 6 days after the initial insult. The involvement of IL-6 in cognitive impairment during TBI in mice is shown [32]. However, although IL-6 can be a strong marker of TBI-induced inflammation, use of IL-6 as a possible therapeutic target is limited as it cannot readily cross the vascular wall [30].

Interlukin-8 (IL-8) belongs to chemokines, a special class of small cytokines. It is secreted by endothelial cells, glial cells, neurons, macrophages, lymphocytes and neutrophils [28]. IL-8 induces chemotaxis and neutrophil phagocytosis and causes its attraction to the site of damage and inflammation. Generally the persistence of the activated leukocytes in brain from 1 to 4 weeks after injury is neurotoxic, and exacerbates the ongoing neuronal damage [28]. The level of IL-8 in CSF is greater than in plasma or serum during head injuries.

The most well-known anti-inflammatory cytokine IL-10 serves as an inhibitor of pro-inflammatory mediators and regulates the cytokines. It is suggested that IL-10 reduces the neuroinflammation during TBI. It increases 24 hours after severe initial insult and coincides with decrease in TNF-α levels. In rat model of TBI, treatment with IL-10 results in reduction of IL-1β and TNF-α levels in brain tissue and improves neurological recovery [28].

Activation of transcription factor, nuclear factor kappa B (NF-kB) that is also considered as an inflammatory marker, has been shown to play a key role in inflammatory response, neuronal survival and signaling [33]. First appearance of NF-kB occurs in axons shortly after trauma (1–2 h), and then in neurons (24 h) and lasts up to 1 week. Later (24 hours after initial insult), activated NF-kB is detected in microglia, macrophages, and astrocytes in cortexes [33]. Activated NF-kB is also detected in ECs, as early as 1 h after initial insult, and persists there for up to 1 year [33]. Hence, it can be suggested that NF-kB activation plays a role in long-term inflammatory processes during TBI.

4. Fibrinogen (Fg)

One of the inflammatory mediators which is released after TBI-induced inflammation is Fg. It is a high molecular weight (~ 340 kD) plasma adhesion glycoprotein, that is primarily synthesized in hepatocytes. Inflammatory cytokines such as IL-1 and IL-6 are involved in Fg synthesis and stimulation of its synthesis, while increased plasma level of albumin suppresses it. Overexpression of these cytokines, that occurs during inflammation leads to HFg [34], which is a biomarker of inflammation and high risk factor for many cerebrovascular disorders [35–38]. Normally Fg concentration in blood is around 2 mg/ml. Higher content of Fg in blood is considered as a state of inflammation [39, 40] and it can be a cause of inflammatory responses [41]. It was shown that at high (≥4 mg/ml) levels Fg increases arteriolar constriction [18], regulates production of endothelin-1 (ET-1) [19], enhances vascular layer permeability [21] to proteins, and can itself leak through the EC layer [20]. Since Fg is synthesized in hepatocytes and circulates in blood, it may appear in extravascular space only after crossing the vascular wall. In brain, it may occur only if BBB is dysfunctional. Gradual deposition of Fg accelerates neurovascular damage and promotes neuroinflammation [42, 43].

Some clinical studies indicate that TBI is accompanied by hypo-fibrinogenemia, abnormally decreased blood level of Fg [44]. During severe brain injury that results in rapture of brain vessels and hemorrhage, blood cells and plasma components, including Fg come out of vessels. Particularly in the first 72 hours, the hemorrhage is an obvious cause of hypo-fibrinogenemia [44, 45]. In addition, activation of fibrinolytic system exacerbates hypo-fibrinogenemia [46]. However, 2 weeks after severe trauma and/or mild-to-moderate brain injury (when vascular ruptures are minimal or nonexistent), blood content of Fg increases [6, 47]. HFg can be noticeable in patients even 12 hours after initial insult [45]. Therefore, Fg crossing of vessel walls and its subsequent deposition in extravascular space, after the initial injury, can be a result of systemic or local inflammation.

5. Inflammation / vascular permeability / edema

Inflammation is a complex of different biological responses of vascular tissue to harmful stimuli. The actions of various inflammatory mediators cause significant vascular changes such as increased permeability (hyper-permeability), vasodilation, and worsening of hemorheology [48]. Majority of vascular diseases that are associated with inflammation include stroke [49], myocardial infarction [50], hypertension [51, 52], diabetes [53, 54], atherosclerosis [55], and TBI [4, 5, 12]. Inflammation is a key contributor to many vascular diseases and plays a major role in autoimmune diseases [56], allergic reactions [57], and cancer [58]. Neuroinflammation is one of the crucial stage of injury after brain trauma [28].

Inflammatory processes may induce endothelial dysfunction and vascular remodeling [51, 59]. The normal endothelium forms a stable anti-inflammatory interface between circulating blood components and cells within tissues. The endothelium builds a barrier, which along with its associated structures such as basement membrane and/or glycocalyx maintain the relatively constant plasma volume and venous return, and prevent tissue edema [60]. Maintaining tissue homeostasis and contributing the functions of the vessel wall by establishing communications between blood and adjacent tissue are the two pivotal functions of vascular endothelium, which functions as a barrier and a permeable filter at the same time [61].

Increase in vascular permeability is one of the indications of inflammation. In result of hyperpermeability, blood plasma substances and proteins move out of the blood stream and deposit in subendothelial matrix (SEM) and interstitium and may cause edema [41, 62]. This phenomena can occur during mainly an early stages of acute inflammation [63].

One of the most dangerous secondary consequences of TBI with significant morbidity and mortality is cerebral edema. It is an abnormal accumulation of fluid within the brain parenchyma and is classified as vasogenic and cytotoxic [31]. Vasogenic edema is defined as fluid originating from blood vessels that accumulates around cells. Cytotoxic edema is defined as fluid accumulating within cells as a result of injury. The most common cytotoxic edema occurs in cerebral ischemia. Heretofore, the edema specific to TBI has generally been considered to be of vasogenic origin, secondary to traumatic opening of the BBB. However, lately clinical studies showed the significant role of cytotoxic edema [31]. It is possible that both forms of edema can coexist. To define the type of edema (mostly by imaging technique) may be a decisive moment, as effective treatment will clearly depend on the major type of edema contributing to the brain swelling process.

6. Transvascular transport pathways

There are two major transport pathways for blood plasma components to pass through the endothelial barrier: transcellular and paracellular [62, 64, 65]. Paracellular pathway takes place when plasma components move between the ECs. It involves alterations in junction proteins and their interbinding forces [62]. It is implied that low molecular weight molecules take this pathway as oppose to transcellular transport of high molecular weight molecules such as proteins, which occurs mainly through the ECs and involves formation of functional caveolae (and/or fenestrae, and/or transendothelial channels [64]) and its motility [66]. Thus, movement of proteins across the vascular wall via transcellular transport pathway can be defined as caveolar transcytosis [67]. At elevated levels Fg can enhance caveolar transcytosis [68, 69]. The net transport of blood plasma substances in microcirculation is governed by the combination and the functional balance of transcellular and paracellular pathways.

Head injury-induced inflammation leads to an increased blood content of Fg [6, 47]. At elevated levels, Fg increases vascular permeability to other proteins and itself crosses the vascular wall [20, 47]. During majority of cardiovascular and cerebrovascular inflammatory diseases, increased levels and/or activity of the plasminogen system have not been observed. For example, activity of tissue plasminogen activator (tPA) is diminished in brains of patients with Alzheimer's disease (AD), mouse models of the disease [68], and during various inflammatory traumas [46]. Thus, an increased leakage of Fg, in the context of decreased or unaltered activity of the plasminogen system, leads to an enhanced deposition of Fg in extravascular space in pathologies such as TBI and AD. There, immobilized Fg can form different protein complexes [47, 70]. Furthermore, immobilized Fg is converted to fibrin by thrombin. Since protein fibrinolytic system can no longer counterbalance excess formation of fibrin, enhanced deposition of fibrin exacerbates neurovascular damage and neuroinflammation [42, 71].

7. Fg-containing complexes

After extravasation Fg deposits into parenchyma and makes complexes with other proteins. The most known is Fg amyloid beta (Aβ) protein complex, called amyloid plaque [72], which is a hallmark of AD and it is associated with loss of memory [73]. The defects in Aβ and its precursor protein (APP) are considered a cause of AD and dementia. The neurotoxic Aβ peptide (oligomers of Aβ) is derived from the APP and it is considered as a major constituent of the plaques. After deposition in SEM, Fg becomes readily available for binding to Aβ oligomers and even APP. The appearance of Fg-Aβ and/or Fg-APP complexes can be a result of vascular hyper-permeability leading to transcytosis of Fg to SEM [74]. It has been shown that binding of Aβ to Fg leads to its oligomerization [70], and Fg-Aβ complex is highly resistant to degradation [75]. Similarly, there is a strong evidence that Fg, which is found immobilized in extravascular space, besides being associated with Aβ, can also be associated with other proteins, such as collagen and cellular prion protein (PrP^C). Alteration of collagen content in SEM is one of the indications of vascular remodeling. Increased collagen level in cerebral microvessels during AD has been shown [76]. It was shown that collagen can serve as a substrate for Fg-Aβ complex deposition in SEM [74]. The present results indicate an increased formation of collagen along with increased expression of Aβ and enhanced deposition of Fg and Aβ. Data suggest that during inflammation, increased cerebrovascular permeability leads to an enhanced deposition of Fg on SEM collagen through formation of Fg-Aβ-collagen complex, which was found to be correlated with reduction of short-term memory [74].

Some studies indicate that Aβ has a limited effect on memory and point to a greater role of PrP^C [77, 78]. It was found that Fg interacts with non-digested scrapie prion protein [79]. Results of our studies also point to the role of PrP^C in memory impairment during HFg [80] and TBI [47]. Therefore, formation of Fg-Aβ and/or Fg-PrP^C complexes may indicate a mechanism for memory reduction seen in diseases such as TBI, associated with inflammatory cerebrovascular impairment. As a result, these findings highlight a new role of Fg during inflammation-induced impairment of vascular wall properties and thus, vasculo-neuronal unit dysfunction.

8. Oxidative damage and neurodegeneration

TBI-induced inflammation and increased cerebrovascular permeability lead to translocation of Fg from vessels to the extravascular space, and its deposition most likely in the vasculo-astrocyte endfeet interface, which may cause astrocyte activation and vascular and astrocyte physical and functional uncoupling [7]. This may result in neuronal degeneration and possible decline in short-term memory [7]. Possible mechanism for this vasculo-neuronal dysfunction can be an activation of astrocytes leading to tyrosine kinase receptor B (TrkB)-mediated enhanced production of reactive oxygen species (ROS) and nitric oxide (NO), which result in neuronal degeneration [81].

Oxidative damage and free radical formation remains one of the important contributors to the pathophysiology of TBI. Generation of ROS causes damage of neuronal membranes, which results in subsequent disruption in ion balance and homeostasis, mitochondrial function failure, and microvascular damage [82]. ROS such as hydrogen peroxide, hydroxyl radical, superoxide onion, peroxyl radical (hydroperoxyl), singlet oxygen, and NO are the highly reactive molecules produced during monocyte migration. They contribute to BBB impairment and inflammation in brain after trauma [83]. The cascade of ROS production begins immediately within the first hours after initial insult and lasts for several days [82]. The amplification of neurodegeneration can be caused by neuronal NO production. This process is highly dependent on TrkB receptor regulation on astrocytes. It was shown that depletion of TrkB protected experimental animals from neurodegeneration [81]. Fg prompts rapid microglial responses toward the cerebrovascular system and axonal damage during neuroinflammation [84]. Extravasation of Fg and deposited fibrin correlate with axonal damage and cause ROS formation in microglia [84]. In vitro, it was shown that astrocytes remove Fg coating from the growth surface that results in their activation and disappearance [85]. Reduction in astrocyte population may be due to their death. Fibrin activates astrocytes by transforming the growth factor beta receptor pathway and promotes astrocyte scar formation after vascular rupture during severe TBI [71]. These findings suggest that there is a strong interactive association between Fg/fibrin and astrocytes [7, 71].

9. Role of Fg in loss of memory during TBI

Cognitive impairment and particularly memory deficiency is a result of neurodegeneration and is one of the devastating problems of people with neurotrauma [86]. The role and contribution of Fg in development of AD is known [70, 72, 75]. Strong association of Fg-Aβ complex formation is linked to severity of AD [70, 72, 75]. Thus, deposition of Fg in extravascular space and formation of Fg-Aβ complexes can be a major indicator for memory reduction during TBI. Similarly, possible formation of Fg-PrP^C complexes may result in memory impairment.

The Prion diseases, one of the forms of encephalopathies, are the group of progressive neurodegenerative conditions with memory impairment. The role of PrP^C in cognitive dysfunction has been shown [77, 78]. Increased formation of Fg-PrP^C complex in mice during TBI was accompanied by reduction in short-term memory [47]. Combined, these results indicate that PrP^C alone as well as its possible association with Fg can have a role in memory reduction during inflammatory cerebrovascular diseases.

10. Conclusion

Thus, TBI-induced inflammation besides directly affecting neurons, leads to vasculo-neuronal dysfunction resulting in Fg deposition in extravascular space and formation of Fg-containing protein complexes between the vessels and astrocyte endfeet. Enhanced cerebrovascular permeability can be a first and the most important step in the process leading to alterations in cognitive function. Thus, at elevated levels, Fg can play a significant role in vascular cognitive impairment and dementia (VCID) (**Figure 1**). There is a great attention to the problems related to VCID in the past few years. Presented review indicates that Fg has a significant role in vascular permeability, neuroinflammation and cognitive impairment. Therefore, as a possible diagnostic or outcome predicting approach, it seems important to carefully monitor plasma levels of Fg during TBI. Simultaneously targeting multiple mechanistic components of an altered vasculo-neuronal interaction after head injury, such as blood level of Fg and PrP^C may be an effective therapeutic approach to ameliorate TBI-induced neurovascular inflammation.

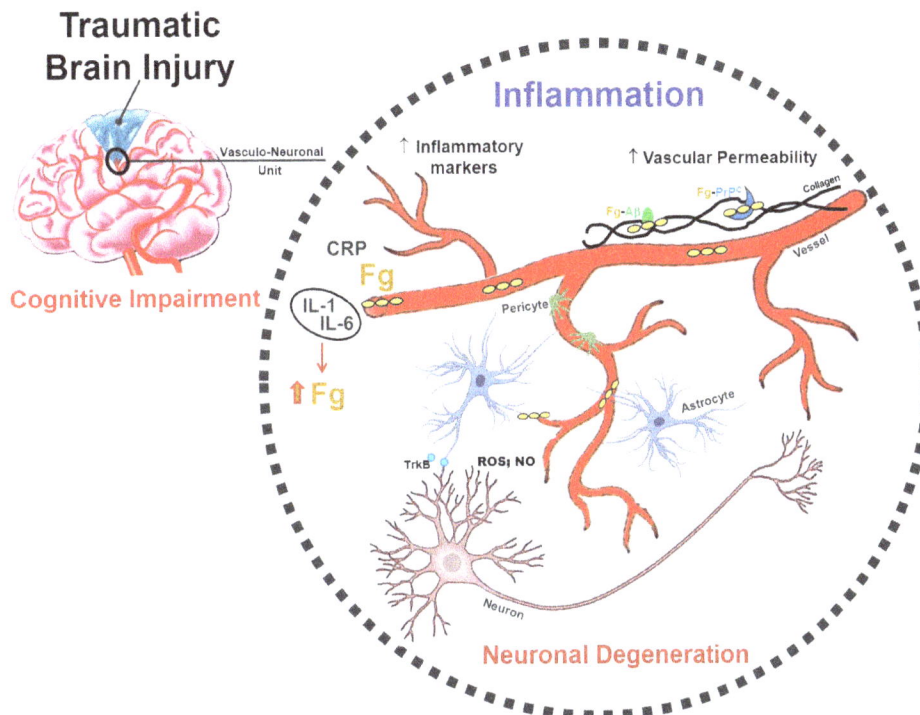

Figure 1. Possible mechanism of traumatic brain injury (TBI)-induced cognitive impairment. TBI causes inflammation leading to an increase in inflammatory markers including C reactive protein (CRP), interleukins 1 and 6 (IL-1 and IL-6, respectively) and fibrinogen (Fg). The latter exacerbates TBI-induced cerebrovascular permeability resulting in enhanced deposition of Fg in vasculo-astrocyte endfeet interface, and formation of Fg-containing complexes with proteins Aβ and PrP^C, which are known to be involved in cognitive decline. In addition, activation of astrocytes causing upregulation of tyrosine kinase receptor B (TrkB) results in formation of reactive oxygen species leading to neurodegeneration.

Author details

Nino Muradashvili, Suresh C. Tyagi and David Lominadze*

*Address all correspondence to: david.lominadze@louisville.edu

Department of Physiology, University of Louisville, School of Medicine, Louisville, KY, USA

References

[1] Brody D, Mac Donald C, Kessens C, Yuede C, Parsadanian M, Spinner M, Kim E, Schwetye K, Holtzman D, Bayly P. Electromagnetic controlled cortical impact device for precise, graded experimental traumatic brain injury. Journal of Neurotrauma. 2007;**24**:657-673

[2] Teasdale G, Jennett B. Assessment of coma and impaired consciousness: A practical scale. The Lancet. 1974;**304**:81-84

[3] Saatman KE, Duhaime A-C, Bullock R, Maas AIR, Valadka A, Manley GT. Classification of traumatic brain injury for targeted therapies. Journal of Neurotrauma. 2008;**25**:719-738

[4] Cederberg D, Siesjö P. What has inflammation to do with traumatic brain injury? Child's Nervous System. 2010;**26**:221-226

[5] Ziebell J, Morganti-Kossmann M. Involvement of pro- and anti-inflammatory cytokines and chemokines in the pathophysiology of traumatic brain injury. Neurotherapeutics. 2010;**7**:22-30

[6] Mansoor O, Cayol M, Gachon P, Boirie Y, Schoeffler P, Obled C, Beaufrère B. Albumin and fibrinogen syntheses increase while muscle protein synthesis decreases in head-injured patients. American Journal of Physiology. Endocrinology and Metabolism. 1997;**273**:E898-E902

[7] Muradashvili N, Tyagi SC, Lominadze D. Localization of fibrinogen in the vasculo-astrocyte interface after cortical contusion injury in mice. Brain Sciences. 2017;**7**:77

[8] Moppett I. Traumatic brain injury: Assessment, resuscitation and early management. British Journal of Anaesthesia. 2007;**99**:18-31

[9] Walker PA, Shah SK, Harting MT, Cox CS. Progenitor cell therapies for traumatic brain injury: Barriers and opportunities in translation. Disease Models & Mechanisms. 2009;**2**:23-38

[10] Muradashvili N, Lominadz D. Role of fibrinogen in cerebrovascular dysfunction after traumatic brain injury. Brain Injury. 2013;**27**:1508-1515

[11] Rostami R, Salamati P, Yarandi KK, Khoshnevisan A, Saadat S, Kamali ZS, Ghiasi S, Zaryabi A, Ghazi Mir Saeid SS, Arjipour M, Rezaee-Zavareh MS, Rahimi-Movaghar V. Effects of neurofeedback on the short-term memory and continuous attention of patients with moderate traumatic brain injury: A preliminary randomized controlled clinical trial. Chinese Journal of Traumatology. 2017;**20**:278-282

[12] Shlosberg D, Benifla M, Kaufer D, Friedman A. Blood-brain barrier breakdown as a therapeutic target in traumatic brain injury. Nature Reviews. Neurology. 2010;**6**:393-403

[13] Hawkins BT, Davis TP. The blood-brain barrier/neurovascular unit in health and disease. Pharmacological Reviews. 2005;**57**:173-185

[14] Chodobski A, Zink BJ, Szmydynger-Chodobska J. Blood-brain barrier pathophysiology in traumatic brain injury. Translational Stroke Research. 2011;**2**:492-516

[15] Garcia JM, Stillings SA, Leclerc JL, Phillips H, Edwards NJ, Robicsek SA, Hoh BL, Blackburn S, Doré S. Role of Interleukin-10 in acute brain injuries. Frontiers in Neurology. 2017;**8**:244

[16] Gabay C, Kushner I. Acute-phase proteins and other systemic responses to inflammation. The New England Journal of Medicine. 1999;**340**:448-454

[17] Muradashvili N, Qipshidze N, Munjal C, Givvimani S, Benton RL, Roberts AM, Tyagi SC, Lominadze D. Fibrinogen-induced increased pial venular permeability in mice. Journal of Cerebral Blood Flow and Metabolism. 2012;**32**:150-163

[18] Lominadze D, Tsakadze N, Sen U, Falcone JC, D'Souza SE. Fibrinogen- and fragment D-induced vascular constriction. American Journal of Physiology. 2005;**288**:H1257-H1264

[19] Sen U, Tyagi N, Patibandla PK, Dean WL, Tyagi SC, Roberts AM, Lominadze D. Fibrinogen-induced endothelin-1 production from endothelial cells. American Journal of Physiology. Cell Physiology. 2009;**296**:C840-C847

[20] Tyagi N, Roberts AM, Dean WL, Tyagi SC, Lominadze D. Fibrinogen induces endothelial cell permeability. Molecular and Cellular Biochemistry. 2008;**307**:13-22

[21] Patibandla PK, Tyagi N, Dean WL, Tyagi SC, Roberts AM, Lominadze D. Fibrinogen induces alterations of endothelial cell tight junction proteins. Journal of Cellular Physiology. 2009;**221**:195-203

[22] Muradashvili N, Tyagi N, Tyagi R, Munjal C, Lominadze D. Fibrinogen alters mouse brain endothelial cell layer integrity affecting vascular endothelial cadherin. Biochemical and Biophysical Research Communications. 2011;**413**:509-514

[23] Koenig W. Fibrin(ogen) in cardiovascular disease: An update. Thrombosis and Haemostasis. 2003;**89**:601-609

[24] Patibandla PK, Tyagi N, Tyagi SC, Dean WL, Roberts AM, Lominadze D. An elevated fibrinogen increases matrix metalloproteinases activity in cardiac microvascular endothelial cells. Experimental Biology. 2009;**23**:592, 10

[25] Davalos D, Akassoglou K. Fibrinogen as a key regulator of inflammation in disease. Seminars In Immunopathology. 2012;**34**:43-62

[26] Vitorino de Almeida V, Silva-Herdade A, Calado A, Rosário H, Saldanha C. Fibrinogen modulates leukocyte recruitment in vivo during the acute inflammatory response. Clinical Hemorheology and Microcirculation. 2015;**59**:97-106

[27] Longhi L, Perego C, Ortolano F, Aresi S, Fumagalli S, Zanier ER, Stocchetti N, Simoni M-GD. Tumor necrosis factor in traumatic brain injury: Effects of genetic deletion of p55 or p75 receptor. Journal of Cerebral Blood Flow and Metabolism. 2013;**33**:1182-1189

[28] Werhane ML, Evangelista ND, Clark AL, Sorg SF, Bangen KJ, Tran M, Schiehser DM, Delano-Wood L. Pathological vascular and inflammatory biomarkers of acute- and chronic-phase traumatic brain injury. Concussion. 2017;**2**:CNC30

[29] Baratz R, Tweedie D, Wang J-Y, Rubovitch V, Luo W, Hoffer BJ, Greig NH, Pick CG. Transiently lowering tumor necrosis factor-α synthesis ameliorates neuronal cell loss and cognitive impairments induced by minimal traumatic brain injury in mice. Journal of Neuroinflammation. 2015;**12**:45

[30] Woodcock T, Morganti-Kossmann C. The role of markers of inflammation in traumatic brain injury. Frontiers in Neurology. 2013;**4**:18

[31] Winkler EA, Minter D, Yue JK, Manley GT. Cerebral Edema in traumatic brain injury. Neurosurgery Clinics of North America. 2016;**27**:473-488

[32] Yang SH, Gustafson J, Gangidine M, Stepien D, Schuster R, Pritts TA, Goodman MD, Remick DG, Lentsch AB. A murine model of mild traumatic brain injury exhibiting cognitive and motor deficits. Journal of Surgical Research. 2013;**184**:981-988

[33] Nonaka M, Chen X-H, Pierce JES, Leoni MJ, McIntosh TK, Wolf JA, Smith DH. Prolonged activation of NF-κB following traumatic brain injury in rats. Journal of Neurotrauma. 1999;**16**:1023-1034

[34] Nakamura A, Kohsaka T, Johns EJ. Neuro-regulation of interleukin-6 gene expression in the spontaneously hypertensive rat kidney. Journal of Hypertension. 1996;**14**:839-845

[35] del Zoppo GJ, Levy DE, Wasiewski WW, Pancioli AM, Demchuk AM, Trammel J, Demaerschalk BM, Kaste M, Albers GW and Ringelstein EB. Hyperfibrinogenemia and functional outcome from acute ischemic stroke. Stroke 2009;**40**:1687-1691

[36] Lominadze D, Joshua IG, Schuschke DA. Increased erythrocyte aggregation in spontaneously hypertensive rats. American Journal of Hypertension. 1998;**11**:784-789

[37] Eidelman RS, Hennekens CH. Fibrinogen: A predictor of stroke and marker of atherosclerosis. European Heart Journal. 2003;**24**:499-500

[38] Ernst E, Resch KL. Fibrinogen as a cardiovascular risk factor: A meta-analysis and review of the literature. Annals of Internal Medicine. 1993;**118**:956-963

[39] Ross R. Mechanisms of disease - atherosclerosis - an inflammatory disease. The New England Journal of Medicine. 1999;**340**:115-126

[40] Danesh J, Lewington S, Thompson SG, Lowe GD, Collins R, Kostis JB, Wilson AC, Folsom AR, Wu K, Benderly M, Goldbourt U, Willeit J, Kiechl S, Yarnell JW, Sweetnam PM, Elwood PC, Cushman M, Psaty BM, Tracy RP, Tybjaerg-Hansen A, Haverkate F, de Maat MP, Fowkes FG, Lee AJ, Smith FB, Salomaa V, Harald K, Rasi R, Vahtera E, Jousilahti P, Pekkanen J, D'Agostino R, Kannel WB, Wilson PW, Tofler G, Arocha-Pinango CL, Rodriguez-Larralde A, Nagy E, Mijares M, Espinosa R, Rodriquez-Roa E, Ryder E, Diez-Ewald MP, Campos G, Fernandez V, Torres E, Coll E, Marchioli R, Valagussa F, Rosengren A, Wilhelmsen L, Lappas G, Eriksson H, Cremer P, Nagel D, Curb JD, Rodriguez B, Yano K, Salonen JT, Nyyssonen K, Tuomainen TP, Hedblad B, Lind P, Loewel H, Koenig W, Meade TW, Cooper JA, De Stavola B, Knottenbelt C, Miller GJ, Bauer KA, Rosenberg RD, Sato S, Kitamura A, Naito Y, Iso H, Rasi V, Palosuo T, Ducimetiere P, Amouyel P, Arveiler D, Evans AE, Ferrieres J, Juhan-Vague I, Bingham A, Schulte H, Assmann G, Cantin B, Lamarche B, Despres JP, Dagenais GR, Tunstall-Pedoe H, Woodward M, Ben Shlomo Y, Davey SG, Palmieri V, Yeh JL, Rudnicka A, Ridker P, Rodeghiero F, Tosetto A, Shepherd J, Ford I, Robertson M, Brunner E, Shipley M, Feskens EJ, Kromhout D, Fibrinogen SC. Plasma fibrinogen level and the risk of major cardiovascular diseases and nonvascular mortality: An individual participant meta-analysis. JAMA. 2005;**294**(14):1799-1809

[41] Lominadze D, Dean WL, Tyagi SC, Roberts AM. Mechanisms of fibrinogen-induced microvascular dysfunction during cardiovascular disease. Acta Physiologica Scandinavica. 2010;**198**:1-13

[42] Paul J, Strickland S, Melchor JP. Fibrin deposition accelerates neurovascular damage and neuroinflammation in mouse models of Alzheimer's disease. The Journal of Experimental Medicine. 2007;**204**:1999-2008

[43] Hay JR, Johnson VE, Young AM, Smith DH, Stewart W. Blood-brain barrier disruption is an early event that may persist for many years after traumatic brain injury in humans. Journal of Neuropathology and Experimental Neurology. 2015;**74**:1147-1157

[44] Bayir A, Kalkan E, Kocak S, Ak A, Cander B, Bodur S. Fibrinolytic markers and neurologic outcome in traumatic brain injury. Neurology India. 2006;**54**:363-365

[45] Nakae R, Takayama Y, Kuwamoto K, Naoe Y, Sato H, Yokota H. Time course of coagulation and Fibrinolytic parameters in patients with traumatic brain injury. Journal of Neurotrauma. 2016;**33**:688-695

[46] Hayakawa M. Dynamics of fibrinogen in acute phases of trauma. Journal of Intensive Care. 2017;**5**:3

[47] Muradashvili N, Benton RL, Saatman KE, Tyagi SC, Lominadze D. Ablation of matrix metalloproteinase-9 gene decreases cerebrovascular permeability and fibrinogen deposition post traumatic brain injury in mice. Metabolic Brain Disease. 2015;**30**:411-426

[48] Komarova Y, Malik AB. Regulation of endothelial permeability via paracellular and transcellular transport pathways. Annual Review of Physiology. 2010;**72**:463-493

[49] Nieswandt B, Kleinschnitz C, Stoll G. Ischaemic stroke: A thrombo-inflammatory disease? The Journal of Physiology. 2011;**589**:4115-4123

[50] Gonzales C, Pedrazzini T. Progenitor cell therapy for heart disease. Experimental Cell Research. 2009;**315**:3077-3085

[51] Savoia C, Schiffrin EL. Inflammation in hypertension. Current Opinion in Nephrology and Hypertension. 2006;**15**:152-158

[52] Wang TJ, Gona P, Larson MG, Levy D, Benjamin EJ, Tofler GH, Jacques PF, Meigs JB, Rifai N, Selhub J, Robins SJ, Newton-Cheh C, Vasan RS. Multiple biomarkers and the risk of incident hypertension. Hypertension. 2007;**49**:432-438

[53] Donath MY, Shoelson SE. Type 2 diabetes as an inflammatory disease. Nature Reviews. Immunology. 2011;**11**:98-107

[54] Pietropaolo M, Barinas-Mitchell E, Kuller LH. The heterogeneity of diabetes. Diabetes. 2007;**56**:1189-1197

[55] Ross R. Atherosclerosis - an inflammatory disease. The New England Journal of Medicine. 1999;**340**:115-126

[56] Abou-Raya A, Abou-Raya S. Inflammation: A pivotal link between autoimmune diseases and atherosclerosis. Autoimmunity Reviews. 2006;**5**:331-337

[57] Galli SJ, Tsai M, Piliponsky AM. The development of allergic inflammation. Nature. 2008;**454**:445-454

[58] Broderick L, Tourangeau LM, Kavanaugh A, Wasserman SI. Biologic modulators in allergic and autoinflammatory diseases. Current Opinion in Allergy and Clinical Immunology. 2011;**11**:355-360

[59] Savoia C, Sada L, Zezza L, Pucci L, Lauri FM, Befani A, Alonzo A, Volpe M. Vascular inflammation and endothelial dysfunction in experimental hypertension. International Journal of Hypertension. 2011;**2011**:281240-281247

[60] Curry F-RE, Noll T. Spotlight on microvascular permeability. Cardiovascular Research. 2010;**87**:195-197

[61] Bazzoni G. Endothelial tight junctions: Permeable barriers of the vessel wall. Thrombosis & Haemostasis. 2006;**95**:36-42

[62] Mehta D, Malik AB. Signaling mechanisms regulating endothelial permeability. Physiological Reviews. 2006;**86**:279-367

[63] Michel CC, Curry FE. Microvascular permeability. Physiological Reviews. 1999;**79**:703-761

[64] Simionescu M, Popov D, Sima A. Endothelial transcytosis in health and disease. Cell and Tissue Research. 2009;**335**:27-40

[65] Clark TM, Hayes TK, Beyenbach KW. Dose-dependent effects of CRF-like diuretic peptide on transcellular and paracellular transport pathways. American Journal of Physiology. Renal Physiology. 1998;**274**:F834-F840

[66] Stan R-V, Marion K, Palade GE. PV-1 is a component of the fenestral and stomatal diaphragms in fenestrated endothelia. Proceedings of the National Academy of Sciences of the United States of America. 1999;**96**:13203-13207

[67] Tuma PL, Hubbard AL. Transcytosis: Crossing cellular barriers. Physiological Reviews. 2003;**83**:871-932

[68] Ledesma MD, Da Silva JS, Crassaerts K, Delacourte A, De Strooper B, Dotti CG. Brain plasmin enhances APP alpha-cleavage and Abeta degradation and is reduced in Alzheimer's disease brains. EMBO Reports. 2000;**1**:530-535

[69] Muradashvili N, Khundmiri SJ, Tyagi R, Gartung A, Dean WL, Lee M-J, Lominadze D. Sphingolipids affect fibrinogen-induced caveolar transcytosis and cerebrovascular permeability. American Journal of Physiology. Cell Physiology. 2014;**307**:C169-C179

[70] Ahn HJ, Zamolodchikov D, Cortes-Canteli M, Norris EH, Glickman JF, Strickland S. Alzheimer's disease peptide β-amyloid interacts with fibrinogen and induces its oligomerization. Proceedings of the National Academy of Sciences of the United States of America. 2010;**107**:21812-21817

[71] Schachtrup C, Ryu JK, Helmrick MJ, Vagena E, Galanakis DK, Degen JL, Margolis RU, Akassoglou K. Fibrinogen triggers astrocyte scar formation by promoting the availability of active TGF-β after vascular damage. The Journal of Neuroscience. 2010;**30**:5843-5854

[72] Cortes-Canteli M, Strickland S. Fibrinogen, a possible key player in Alzheimer's disease. Journal of Thrombosis and Haemostasis. 2009;**7**:146-150

[73] Johnson VE, Stewart W, Smith DH. Traumatic brain injury and amyloid-[beta] pathology: A link to Alzheimer's disease? Nature Reviews. Neuroscience. 2010;**11**:361-370

[74] Muradashvili N, Tyagi R, Metreveli N, Tyagi SC, Lominadze D. Ablation of MMP9 gene ameliorates paracellular permeability and fibrinogen-amyloid beta complex formation during hyperhomocysteinemia. Journal of Cerebral Blood Flow and Metabolism. 2014;**34**:1472-1482

[75] Cortes-Canteli M, Paul J, Norris EH, Bronstein R, Ahn HJ, Zamolodchikov D, Bhuvanendran S, Fenz KM, Strickland S. Fibrinogen and β-amyloid association alters thrombosis and fibrinolysis: A possible contributing factor to Alzheimer's disease. Neuron. 2010;**66**:695-709

[76] Kalaria RN, Pax AB. Increased collagen content of cerebral microvessels in Alzheimer's disease. Brain Research. 1995;**705**:349-352

[77] Gimbel DA, Nygaard HB, Coffey EE, Gunther EC, Laurén J, Gimbel ZA, Strittmatter SM. Memory impairment in transgenic Alzheimer mice requires cellular prion protein. The Journal of Neuroscience. 2010;**30**:6367-6374

[78] Chung E, Ji Y, Sun Y, Kascsak R, Kascsak R, Mehta P, Strittmatter S, Wisniewski T. Anti-PrPC monoclonal antibody infusion as a novel treatment for cognitive deficits in an Alzheimer's disease model mouse. BMC Neuroscience. 2010;**11**:130

[79] Fischer MB, Roeckl C, Parizek P, Schwarz HP, Aguzzi A. Binding of disease-associated prion protein to plasminogen. Nature. 2000;**408**:479-483

[80] Muradashvili N, Tyagi R, Tyagi N, Tyagi SC, Lominadze D. Cerebrovascular disorders caused by hyperfibrinogenemia. The Journal of Physiology. 2016;**594**:5941-5957

[81] Colombo E, Cordiglieri C, Melli G, Newcombe J, Krumbholz M, Parada L, Medico E, Hohlfeld R, Meinl E, Farina C. Stimulation of the neurotrophin receptor TrkB on astrocytes drives nitric oxide production and neurodegeneration. The Journal of Experimental Medicine. 2012;**209**:521-535

[82] Bains M, Hall ED. Antioxidant therapies in traumatic brain and spinal cord injury. Biochimica et Biophysica Acta (BBA) - Molecular Basis of Disease. 2012;**1822**:675-684

[83] Schreibelt G, Kooij G, Reijerkerk A, van Doorn R, Gringhuis SI, van der Pol S, Weksler BB, Romero IA, Couraud P-O, Piontek J, Blasig IE, Dijkstra CD, Ronken E, de Vries HE. Reactive oxygen species alter brain endothelial tight junction dynamics via RhoA, PI3 kinase, and PKB signaling. The FASEB Journal 2007;**21**:3666-3676

[84] Davalos D, Kyu Ryu J, Merlini M, Baeten KM, Le Moan N, Petersen MA, Deerinck TJ, Smirnoff DS, Bedard C, Hakozaki H, Gonias Murray S, Ling JB, Lassmann H, Degen JL, Ellisman MH, Akassoglou K. Fibrinogen-induced perivascular microglial clustering is required for the development of axonal damage in neuroinflammation. Nature Communications. 2012;**3**:1227

[85] Hsiao TW, Swarup VP, Kuberan B, Tresco PA, Hlady V. Astrocytes specifically remove surface-adsorbed fibrinogen and locally express chondroitin sulfate proteoglycans. Acta Biomaterialia. 2013;**9**:7200-7208

[86] Cernich A, Kurtz S, Mordecai K, Ryan P. Cognitive rehabilitation in traumatic brain injury. Current Treatment Options in Neurology. 2010;**12**:412-423

5

Management of Intracranial Pressure in Traumatic Brain Injury

Christ Ordookhanian, Meena Nagappan,
Dina Elias and Paul E. Kaloostian

Abstract

Traumatic brain injury (TBI) is the result of an external force acting upon the head, causing damage to the brain. The severity of injury, mechanism by which the injury occurs, and the frequency of the high-force impact all play a role in the determination of a TBI. TBI describes a wide range of traumatic pathologies which is comprised of damage done to a multitude of cranial central nervous system components. TBI patients typically present with a series of symptoms are correlated with the presence of an intracranial injury, such as physical/cognitive difficulties. A major concern associated with intracranial injuries is the management of intracranial pressure (ICP), a resulting factor of a TBI which facilitates into intracranial hematoma and/or cerebral edema. These conditions have adverse effects on one's brain, and the immediate management and relief of intracranial pressure are crucial in avoiding hydrocephalus and brain herniation, conditions which lead to sensory loss and even death. In this chapter, we will begin by thoroughly understanding what a TBI is, its clinical presentation, and the first-tier examination to determine severity. Then, we will progress into the anatomy of the brain, followed by a thorough investigation into intracranial pressure management strategies and prognosis.

Keywords: intracranial, ICP, trauma, head injury, brain herniation, cerebral edema, hydrocephalus, shunt, skull, blood, cerebral fluid, pressure, relief

1. Introduction

The onset of increased intracranial pressure is often attributed to many pathologies such as large artery acute ischemic stroke, intracranial neoplasms, or disorders such as meningitis. The most common reason for which the onset of intracranial pressure is observed is due to traumatic brain injuries, such as colliding one's head into a hard object as a result of an accident. By definition, an intracranial pressure that exceeds 20 mm Hg is considered high and indicative for the need of immediate treatment [1]. Through the advancement of medicine and technology, the variety of treatment options available to relieve patients of increased intracranial pressure has grown tremendously. In practice today, there exists a multitude of treatment options ranging from nonsurgical interventions to surgical interventions [2, 3]. In this chapter, we will discuss the primary pathology of patients presenting with increased intracranial pressure (ICP) as a result of traumatic brain injuries (TBIs), and we will take a generalized perspective on this pathology by discussing a multitude of topics we find crucial to your understanding of the management of ICP in TBI patients.

2. Intracranial pressure management of traumatic brain injury

2.1. The occurrence of traumatic brain injury

Traumatic brain injury (TBI) is composed of an external mechanical force, whether it be a change in acceleration or impact by projectile that causes a temporary or at times a permanent brain function impairment as well as physical damage to the human brain anatomy. It is important that we establish a clear understanding of the term TBI and its partnering term non-TBI. A traumatic brain injury is brought on by the impact generated by an external force, while a nontraumatic brain injury is brought on by internal forces such as a stroke or infection. A traumatic brain injury, which we have now learned arises from external forces, can come in two pathological forms: penetrating and nonpenetrating. This classification presents as simply as it is defined. A penetrating TBI results in several lesions starting from one's head down to the cerebral level, and these often occur in severe accidents or injuries. A clear and prime example of a penetrating TBI is one that occurs all too often to members of our military, a foreign projectile being discharged from an external high-force machine, which then strikes a human head [4]. A nonpenetrating TBI is the form that we will cover more in depth within this chapter and results from an external force acting upon the head, but it does not penetrate any layer of human anatomy. Within the clinic, the formal classification of TBIs may be reduced to open-head injury for patients presenting with traumatic brain injuries of the penetrating type, and for patients presenting with a traumatic brain injury of the nonpenetrating type, the term closed head-injury may be assigned [5]. The simplification made to these terms adds an element of simplicity for when medical professionals present cases to patient's families and loved ones.

2.2. Anatomical description of the brain, relevant to penetrating traumatic brain injuries

To aid in our understanding of traumatic brain injuries and later on the rise of intracranial pressure, it is imperative we touch upon the anatomy of the human brain such that successive sections of this chapter can be understood with a greater degree of clarity. The human brain, the core of the central nervous system, controls a vast majority of bodily processes and functions. The center of knowledge and core processing is perhaps the most important regulator of human life, yet only weighs between three to five pounds. The first line of defense for the brain is called the cranium, often referred to as the skull, and this shields the brain with a tough bone structure [6]. The brain covering itself contains three layers: the dura, arachnoid and pia. Interestingly enough, there also exists a space between the pia and arachnoid referred to as the subarachnoid complex. This area houses a vast network of veins, arteries, and nerves, which channels both blood and electrochemical potential to the heart and back to the brain. This subarachnoid complex is prone to trauma as well as constriction or full blockage. Any trauma that may cause constriction or blockage will also pose a greater threat to the tissue of the brain. Thus far, we have discussed the cranium and the brain that it encloses; however, the brain does not fill the entire volume of the cranium, and the volume remaining is filled by cerebrospinal fluid (CSF), serving as a nutrient-rich cushion around the brain, and blood-vessels. It is important to note that the volume of the cranium is fixed, and the brain fills a fixed volume of the cranium and the cerebrospinal fluid (CSF); therefore, any trauma that may alter the volume of the cranial region can be devastating, a concept referred to as increased intracranial pressure (ICP), which we will discuss in immense detail throughout this chapter [7].

A common misconception we wish to clear up is the designation of the upper and lower brain, and it is often misunderstood that the brain is a term used only for the upper brain, the ovular shaped region; however, the lower brain that houses vital components such as the brainstem is also indeed part of the human brain. At the lowest point of the brain (brainstem), there exists a small circular opening for which the skull and the spinal cord merge to form the complete central nervous system. As we mentioned above, the brainstem in fact is one of the most important parts of the lower brain as it houses a plethora of intricate nerve fibers, which pass information from the brain to the spinal cord and to the body as a whole. Another crucial component of the lower brain is the cerebellum, a small mass of neuronal tissue that is responsible for the regulation and coordination of motor skills and balance. Without this region of the brain, the miracle of the human touch, whether it be the detailed touch of an artist or the intricate lifesaving work done at the microscopic level by a neurosurgeon, will not be possible. The ovular region of the human brain, known as the upper brain, is a large mass of neuronal tissue divided into white and gray matter. Gray matter houses neuronal cell bodies, axons, and dendrites, while white matter is entirely made up of axons, which connect other gray matter components together [8]. The upper brain is composed of the cerebral cortex, which is the largest component of the human brain, and this region is divided into two hemispheres: left and right. Uniquely enough, the right side of the brain will control left side of the body and vice versa. Despite the left and right hemisphere designations of the cerebral cortex, there are also various other designations called regional designations, and these include the frontal lobes, temporal lobe, parietal lobe, and occipital lobe. The frontal lobes are comprised of the left and right lobes, which are located directly behind the forehead, and these control one's intellectual abilities, decision making, behavior, and emotions. The temporal lobe is behind the ear and extends to the center of the head; from a bird's eye view of the brain, it is directly behind the frontal lobe and extends outward from both ears. This lobe controls speech, understanding, memory, and information retention [9]. Our ability to read, write, and understand spatial relationships is due to the efforts made by the parietal lobe, which is located at the rear of the head, specifically the upper section of the convex ovular protrusion site. Also at the rear of the head, but significantly lower, is the occipital lobe, which controls sight. While we have covered the brain as a whole, it is important to note that throughout the cerebral cortex there are also several sites that are denoted by specific names, which we will discuss when the pathology becomes relevant to those particular areas, and these sites are rich in nerves and also house nerve centers. These are called diencephalons; a more notable diencephalon is the hypothalamus, which regulates homeostasis of the body. These include control over body temperature, hunger, thirst, and arousal. Why discuss the anatomy of the brain to this extent? We hope that since we have discussed anatomy to this extent, the discussion of traumatic brain injury to regions of the brain can be better understood. Damage to any area of the brain can result in both impairment to the functions they regulate and permanent damage to the physical anatomy leading to cognitive deficiencies as well [10, 11].

2.3. Classifying traumatic brain injuries using GSC

The immediate identification of traumatic brain injuries is crucial for the positive-outlook prognosis of a patient, and injuries of this nature present in a spectrum of severities each consisting of unique clinical presentations. To simplify the spectra of severity, a classification system has been established that rates injuries in three categories: mild, moderate, and severe. This classification system is called the Glasgow Coma Scale (GSC), a system readily utilized for the classification of thousands of traumatic brain injury cases per year [12]. The Glasgow Coma Scale is used in evaluating a patient's level of consciousness based on a sum of several categories ranging between 3 and 15. Evaluation of patient consciousness is based upon his or her responsiveness to general verbal, visual, and motor stimuli [13]. The numerical score of this assessment will classify the severity of a patient's brain injury; a score closer to 15 demonstrates near-full neurological ability and consciousness, while a score closer to 3 demonstrates a case in which severe brain injury has occurred and the patient is in a deep coma. A Glasgow Coma Scale score of 13–15 indicates a mild brain injury, while a score of 9–12 indicates a moderate brain injury, and any patient scoring 8 or below is said to have incurred a severe brain injury [12, 14]. **Table 1** demonstrates the rating categories medical staff use to generate a Glasgow Coma Scale score.

To generate the Glasgow Coma Scale (GSC) score, a score will be determined for each category, followed by the summation of all three categories to generate a score between 3 and 15.

2.4. Introduction to intracranial pressure

An accumulation of pressure above the normal standard within the skull is denoted as elevated intracranial pressure (ICP), a severe condition that requires immediate remediation. While the

	1	2	3	4	5	6
Visual	Eyes closed	Eyes open to sharp stimuli	Eyes open to sounds	Eyes open without induced stimuli		
Motor	No movement	Movement to sharp stimuli	Muscle flexion to sharp stimuli	Muscle flexion and bodily movement	Able to localize touch	Appears to have normal movement
Verbal	No sounds	Slow intensity sounds	Incoherent words	Understandable words spoken	Normal conversation	

Table 1. The Glasgow Coma Scale (GSC) rating score sheet.

initial cause for the onset of ICP may vary greatly from patient to patient, the anatomical factors that play a role in intracranial pressure are simply the cranium, the brain, and the cerebrospinal fluid that fills the volume in between the cranium and the brain. Within medicine, the standard unit to measure pressure is "mm Hg," which stands for millimeters of mercury, the distance mercury travels in a closed system to indicate pressure. For a normal adult, at rest, and in good health, the intracranial pressure should remain between 6 and 16 mm Hg [15]. A unique high-order organismal advantage humans possess is the ability to maintain homeostasis, much like many functions of the body, and homeostasis is crucial to the long-term survival of the human. Within the brain, there are also many hemostatic mechanisms in place to maintain a healthy and acceptable pressure within the cranium. The management of intracranial pressure is in fact done through the regulation of the metabolism and production of cerebrospinal fluid (CSF). Since CSF is the only liquid occupying the volume between the cranium and brain, there is no other regulation factor that the body can maintain. The size of the brain and skull only grows slightly after birth and cannot be altered freely to reduce pressure; thus, the regulation of CSF metabolism and production are crucial in maintaining a healthy and acceptable intra-cranial pressure [16]. In the event that intracranial pressure rises to the limits of the normal and healthy range, immediate remediation is necessary. When the ICP reaches 17–18 mmHg, concern should be raised, and when ICP ranges between 19 and 25 mmHg, immediate relief of pressure is required to prevent damage to regions of the brain [17].

2.5. Monro-Kellie hypothesis

The Monro-Kellie hypothesis was proposed by Doctors Alexander Monro and George Kellie in correspondence to the impact cerebrospinal fluid (CSF) has on the pressure-volume relationship within the cranium. This particular hypothesis describes the intracranial volume-pressure rela-tionship, which we briefly mentioned above. According to the Monro-Kellie hypothesis, the fixed volume of the cranium is comprised of the brain, cerebrospinal fluid, blood, and the pressure of blood flowing to the brain called cerebral perfusion pressure (CPP). Within the fixed volume, the cranium and all components within come to form a state of equilibrium, which we discussed as homeostasis. This hypothesis states that an increase in volume of any one of the cranial con-stituents results in an increase of pressure within the cranium unless there is an equal or greater reduction of volume in another cranial constituent [18]. Buffers within the cranium respond to increases in cranial constituent volume in hopes to reduce pressure to avoid brain damage. In the event that cranial pressure rises, typically due to an increase in lesion volume, a decrease in blood and cerebrospinal fluid is observed in hopes to reduce intracranial pressure [19].

2.6. Rise of intracranial pressure resulting from brain injury

The most common cause of increased intracranial pressure, also known as intracranial hyper-tension, is traumatic brain injuries. The neurological complication that is accompanied by a traumatic brain injury is the loss of pathophysiologic regulators of the brain that results in deregulation of intracranial pressure management [20]. The volume of an average adult's skull is approximately 1500 mL, in which over 85% is occupied by the brain, 10% by arterial blood, and 5% by cerebrospinal fluid [21]. Cerebral profusion pressure (CPP), which we briefly mentioned above as the pressure created by cerebral blood flow, is dependent on two factors: both mean sys-temic arterial pressure (MAP) and ICP. Mean systemic arterial pressure (MAP) and intracranial pressure (ICP) are related to cerebral perfusion pressure (CPP) based on the relationship that: CPP = MAP − ICP. Mean systematic arterial pressure (MAP) is calculated by the summation of one-third systolic blood pressure (SBP) and two-thirds diastolic blood pressure (DBP), in abbreviated form as: MAP = 1/3 SBP + 2/3DBP [22]. In line with the Monro-Kellie hypothesis, an increase in intracranial pressure (ICP) is remediated physiologically by a decrease in cerebral perfusion pressure (CPP) [23]. Through the relationship we described above, a decrease in CPP dictates that there is a decrease in blood pressure and therefore autoregulation of intracranial pressure. While a decrease in CPP regulates ICP, it is also vital that a minimum CPP be maintained such that the brain can receive adequate amounts of blood. Normal CPP ranges between 50 and 165 mmHg, and in the event that CPP drops below 50 mmHg, the brain will not receive adequate amounts of blood, thus creating further complications with maintaining normal cerebral blood flow [24]. When the brain is subjected to injury, the physiological homeostatic functions of the brain may be deregulated or not functional at all. A normal pathology will maintain the normal CPP of 50–165 mmHg while regulating an appropriate ICP level as well. In the event that the intracranial pressure (ICP) rises past 16 mmHg, blood vessels within the brain will constrict to reduce the blood to flow to cranium thus lowering the intracranial pressure. Thus, when a traumatic brain injury occurs, to the extend where the brain's homeostatic functions are lost, intracranial pressure (ICP) increases and physiological regulatory functions are nonoperable [25].

2.7. Negative outlook of untreated increased intracranial pressure

The management of an increased intracranial pressure is vital for the successful outcome of the patient. In the event that an elevated intracranial pressure goes untreated, two major complications arise. The first is the temporary or permanent loss of vision (depending on severity) and the second is development of a severe headache that lasts for more than 48 hours [26]. Additionally, patients will also begin to exhibit irritability, lethargy, slow cognitive processes, as well as abnormal behavior. Untreated elevated intracranial pressure may subject the patient to enter a state of near-unconsciousness, coma, or even death [27]. Another concern for patients presenting with elevated intracranial pressure is the possibility for damage incurred through brain herniation. Brain herniation is a deadly condition that arises when the ICP is extremely high, and this condition presses the brain tissue against the hard cranium causing compression damage to the brain. This extreme pressure may also cause the brain to shift across vital structures that connect the brain to the spinal cord, such as the falx cerebri [28]. While brain herniation may also occur in the absence of an elevated ICP, it is more frequently seen in patients that do in fact present with a severely elevated ICP. High pressure within the cranium induces brain herniation and that can constrict or block arterial blood flow to various parts of the brain, proving to be fatal. In **Figure 1**, the CT scan of a patient presenting with left-side brain herniation of the parahippocampal gyrus, a structure of the brain that is paramount in memory encoding and memory retrieval, is shown, and damage to this area may result in memory disturbances and schizophrenia [29].

2.8. Clinical presentation of patients with ICP resulting from TBI

Patients presenting with elevated intracranial pressure (ICP) resulting from traumatic brain injury (TBI) exhibit symptoms very much similar to patients presenting solely with elevated ICP due to other factors. Traumatic brain injury patients, depending on severity, will present

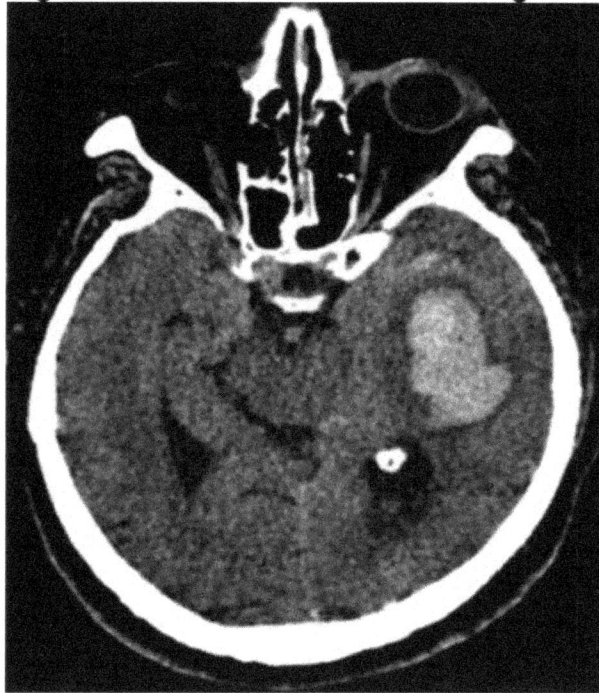

Figure 1. CT scan demonstrating brain herniation on left side due to temporal lobe hemorrhage [29].

with a series of symptoms that are generally along the lines of unconsciousness/coma, headache, vomiting, nausea, compromised motor function, blurred vision, headache, perception of noise that is not present (ringing sounds), as well as difficulty keeping balance. The one symptom we did not mentioned above that we will discuss in depth now is elevated intracranial pressure resulting from traumatic brain injury. Alongside all the symptoms a TBI patient will exhibit, ICP will also cause several symptoms to be present much similar to those already seen in TBI patients [30]. Typical elevated ICP patients present clinically with headache, vomiting, nausea, reduced state of consciousness, and vision blurriness. **Figure 3** demonstrates the overlap of the symptoms a TBI patient will exhibit versus symptoms an elevated ICP patient will exhibit. But do note that a common symptom of a TBI patient is in fact also elevated ICP, but elevated ICP in not only brought on my a TBI, and other factors may contribute to elevated ICP such as hydrocephalus and intracranial hemorrhage [33].

Now that we understand the clinical features of traumatic brain injury (TBI) patients as well as elevated intracranial pressure (ICP) patients, let us combine the two as one pathology, elevated intracranial pressure due to a traumatic brain injury. Referring back to **Table 2**, we know how similar the presenting symptoms may be; thus, let us briefly discuss how a diagnosis may be made. First and foremost, if the history of the patient prior to clinical presentation involves any form of trauma to the head, a TBI can be easily diagnosed. The next step will be to conduct a neurological evaluation, often using the Glasgow Coma Scale (GCS). A symptom of a TBI may be elevated intracranial pressure (ICP), which can be diagnosed primarily through a neurological exam conducted by a neurologist or neurological surgeon. Additionally, radiological imaging via computed topography (CT) scan and magnetic resonance imaging (MRI) can be utilized to determine the presence of the cause as well as the severity of the elevated intracranial pressure [34].

Clinical presentation	TBI patient	ICP patient
Coma—unconsciousness	Present	Present
Headache	Present	Present
Vomiting—nausea	Present	Present
Reduced motor function—balance	Present	Present
Vision deficits—blurriness	Present	Present
Ringing of ear	Present	Not Present
Elevated intracranial pressure (ICP)	Present	←Symptom of TBI

Table 2. Comparison of TBI and ICP symptoms.

Regions of common trends in radiological findings
Optic nerves
Bilateral venous sinus stenosis
Lesioned ventricles
Enlarged arachnoid
Cerebellar tonsil
Subdermal adipose tissue accumulation

Table 3. CT and MRI radiological findings for ICP resultant of TBI.

2.9. Radiology of intracranial pressure caused by TBI

Radiographic imaging to determine the presence of a traumatic brain injury that results in the onset of elevated intracranial pressure is crucial for the high-certainty diagnosis medical professionals seek to provide. Radiographic methods utilized in the diagnostic process are CT scans and MRI, and over the years, a series of common trends have been documented in regard to radiological findings, which we will discuss in this section. In **Table 3**, we highlight the core radiological findings that we will discuss in this section.

The second cranial nerve, also known as the optic nerve, transmits visual information from the retina through a complex nervous network to the brain. This cranial nerve develops from optic stalks during early embryonic development and is supported by nonneuronal glial cells [35]. In patients presenting with elevated intracranial pressure, the optic nerve region of the CT and MRI scan shows a clear area of prominence. Within this region, approximately 40% of elevated ICP patients present with optic nerve tortuosity, a condition in which optic nerve is twisted or alerted slightly from physiologically normal conditions [36, 37]. In approximately 45% of patients, the subarachnoid space surrounding the optic nerve is highly prominent and pro- trudes the space of the optic nerve [38]. This region is comprised of delicate connective tissue as well as channels that contain cerebrospinal fluid (CSF), and this region plays a role is creating channels for intercommunication between the arachnoid, the pia mater, and the CSF. The optic disk, also referred to as the optic nerve head, is the terminal point for ganglion cells leaving the eye. The region is a physiologically normal blind spot each eye possesses due to the lack of photoreceptors, rods, and cones in that region [39]. A condition involving the swelling of optic disk is called papilledema, and in patients that present with elevated ICP, this is a common occurrence [40]. Due to the fact that the optic disk is continuous with the subarachnoid space, swelling of this region contributes greatly to elevated intracranial pressure. This swelling can manifest itself into two forms: either as an intraocular protrusion of the optic nerve or as seen in a vast majority of papilledema patients, a flattening of the posterior white of the eye, sclera [41]. In **Figure 2**, the nodular enhancement of the optic nerves is seen, from a case study on irregular papilloedema [42]. The last pathology we will discuss in relevance to the optic nerve is the MRI enhancement of the intraocular optic nerve, which is anterior to the sclera's lamina cribrosa. This pathology is seen in approximately 50% of elevated ICP due to TBI and adds to the intracranial pressure via degeneration of optic nerves, causing damage to axonal components leading to increased ICP and irreversible blindness in a vast majority of glaucoma patients [43].

Another pathology consistent with the increase in intracranial pressure is bilateral venous sinus stenosis, which may be prevalent in segments of the transverse sinus. Stenosis involves the constriction of a venous tract, in this case of the sinus [44].

Pseudotumor cerebri (PTC) is a clinically relevant pathology that presents with increased intracranial pressure, but the etiology is not entirely understood. This syndrome tends to target women over men, and specifically obese women. PTC, as mentioned above, results from increased ICP and presents clinically with headaches, nausea, as well as changes in vision. Through radiographic efforts, this pathology is linked with elevated CSF, a connection that was dismissed in the earlier years of medicine. Interestingly enough, patients with elevated ICP who also present with PTC have the following pathologies: an empty sella, an enhancement of the optic nerve head, and a tortuosity of the optic nerve [45]. An empty sella, otherwise known as empty sella syndrome (ESS), is where the pituitary gland is physically altered, and thus the sella turcica becomes filled with CSF [46]; see **Figure 3**. ESS is usually highly indicative of an increased intracranial pressure.

Thus far, we have discussed three of the most common radiological findings, in a nonspecific order. The next pathology we will discuss is the enlargement of the arachnoid resulting from an increase of ICP due to TBI. ESS, or empty sella syndrome, we just discussed also plays

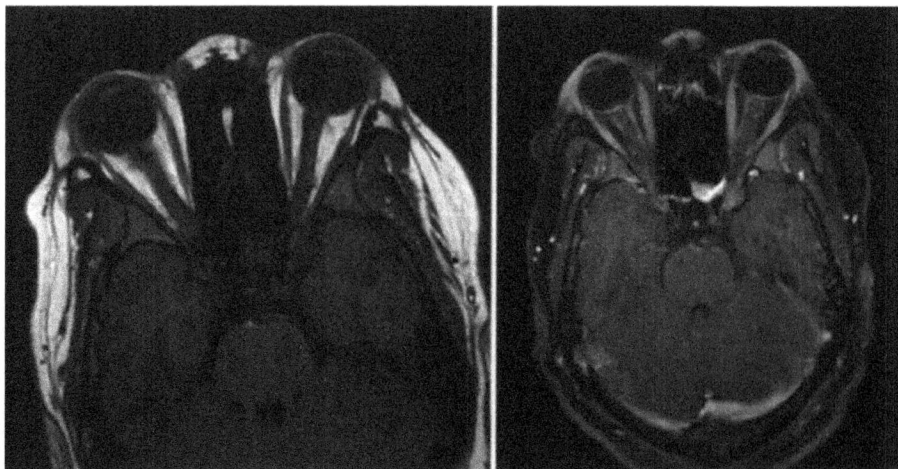

Figure 2. Papilledema, enhancement of optic nerve leading to increased ICP [42].

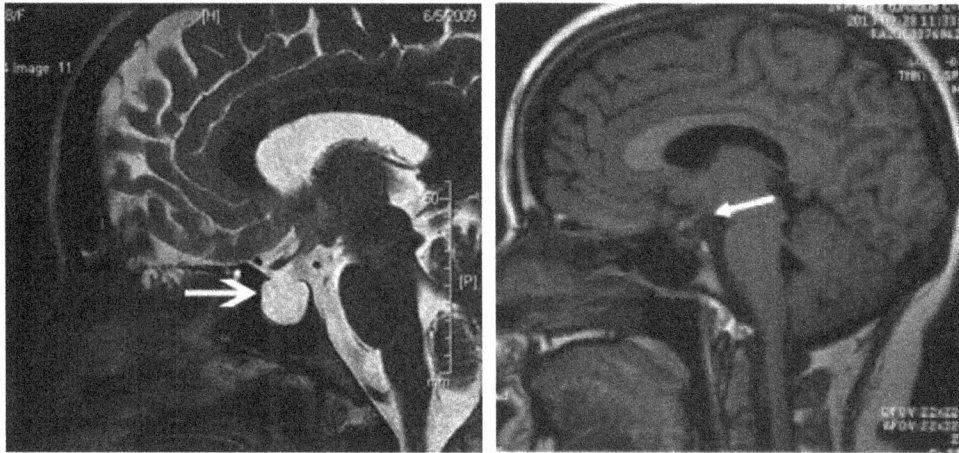

Figure 3. Sagittal T2-weighted image of ESS in an elevated ICP patient [31, 32]. (Left) Pathological findings of "empty sella syndrome" where the arrow points at a completely empty sella. (Right) Anatomically and pathologically healthy individual, for comparison.

a major role in the enlargement of the arachnoid. Actually, approximately 70% of enlarged arachnoid cases due to increased ICP are because of empty sella syndrome, replacing the void volume of the pituitary gland with CSF [47, 48]. Some cases of arachnoid enlargement are attributable to an enlarged Meckel cave [49]. The Meckel cave, previously known as the trigeminal cave, is a CSF-filled arachnoid pouch, which protrudes from the posterior cranial fossa, the most posterior segment of the cranium base where the cerebellum and brainstem reside. In the event of a TBI, cerebrospinal fluid (CSF) fills into this cavity, expanding the volume of this cavity, resulting in an increase of intracranial pressure due to the narrow and space-limited anatomy of this brain region [50, 51].

The next pathology that we will discuss that is commonly observed in radiological investigations of increased ICP in TBI patients is tonsillar ectopia, synonymous to cerebellar tonsils, a disorder of the papa-axial mesoderm. In this pathology, the cerebellar tonsils elongate due to pressure, leading the cerebellum to be pushed through the foramen magnum of the cranium resulting in additional increased intracranial pressure as well as tonsillar herniation [52]. This condition is life threatening, as cranial pressure is heavily diverted onto the medulla oblongata, a vital sector of the brain that controls cardiac and respiratory functions [53, 55].

As we have now discussed the most common radiological presentation for patients presenting with increased intracranial pressure due to a traumatic brain injury, we will begin our discussion on the treatment pathways to remediate these issues. Management and treatment for increased intracranial pressure can utilize both a nonsurgical and surgical intervention, and in the sections to follow, we will discuss both management options.

2.10. Nonsurgical care of increased intracranial pressure

Nonsurgical management of increased intracranial pressure can take on a multitude of forms. In this section, we will discuss the many medicinal options available to patients presenting with increased intracranial pressure resulting from a traumatic brain injury. The quickest and least invasive method to reduce a patient's ICP to a normal range is by elevating the patients head to 30° with respect to the horizontal plane [56]. The elevation of a patient's head does not directly act toward lowering the ICP; in fact, an elevated head aims to reduce CPP, which in turn reduces ICP by increasing venous drainage (based on the relationship we discussed in an earlier section of this chapter) [57]. A common practice typically conducted by first responders to patients that show clear signs of a traumatic brain injury and increased intracranial pressure in the field is to medically induce a state of minimal hyperventilation. In 1970, hyperventilation of a patient with an increased ICP was a common practice and used readily, and it was not until a study came out stating the adverse outcomes of a prolonged state of hyperventilation; in fact, it was shown to have caused cerebral ischemia, a condition where an insufficient amount of blood is delivered to the brain. Today, hyperventilation is still used in the treatment of an increased ICP but only to a pCO_2 level of 25 mmHg. Immediate initial treatment may call for the hyperventilation of a patient to pCO_2 levels of 30–40 mmHg but for no greater than 2–5 min, before returning back to 25 mmHg. More often than not, hyperventilation is not necessary for the treatment of an increased ICP, and there are better methods that were developed compared to the hyperventilation that was introduced in the 1970s [58, 59]. An organic biological medication, mannitol, which is a sugar alcohol typically administered intravenously is used to decrease high blood pressure in the eyes as well as to decrease intracranial pressure [60]. With effects seen 10–20 min after administration and lasting up to 8–10 h, mannitol is metabolized by the liver and excreted mostly by the kidney. Mannitol has a biological half-life of 100 min and is mostly a synthetic drug, with only a 7% bioavailability [61]. The biochemical mechanism by which mannitol acts on human physiology is bimodal, meaning the drug can mechanistically act in two ways. The first pathway is to lower osmotic diuresis through the reduction of swelling within the cerebral parenchyma. The second pathway is to lower the viscosity of the blood, therefore allowing for more laminar blood flow through veins and arteries eventually causing a state of vasoconstriction, which decreases the intracranial volume of blood and thus a lowered intracranial pressure [62, 63]. The mechanistic bimodal action by mannitol makes the drug a popular choice among patients presenting with an increased ICP due to TBI [64]. A class of drugs known as barbiturates has been widely debated in its effects on lowering intracranial pressure, while this class of drugs can successfully complete the task at hand, the use of barbiturates often causes a state of decreased myocardial function and decreased CPP, which can cause higher rates of morbidity and mortality if left unmonitored. Thus, we do not advocate the use of barbiturates as a drug for the treatment of elevated ICP, unless as a last resort option. For your understanding, a barbiturate is a synthetic chemical drug that acts as a depressant of the central nervous system capable of producing a wide spectrum of effects [65]. While barbiturates are not a recommended class of drugs to utilize in the treatment of elevated ICP due to TBI, it in fact can and has been utilized as a last resort option for a procedure called "barbiturate-induced coma," which aims to immediately reduce intracranial pressure in patients that are unresponsive to any other form of nonsurgical medical treatment. The barbiturate of choice for this procedure is pentobarbital, which requires electroencephalogram (EEG) monitor during intravenous use. While using this drug, it is of key importance to monitor the blood pressure of the patient such that the patient does not slip into a hypotensive state. Hypotension resulting from the use of a barbiturate dramatically increases the rate of mortality two-fold, from 25 to 50% mortality [66]. In addition to the intravenous medication administered to patients presenting with increased ICP due to TBI, the administration of a hypertonic solution to maintain a state of euvolemia, a condition in which bodily liquid volume, viscosity, and circulation are all normal, is also imperative. These hypertonic solutions depend on the results of a complete blood diagnostic panel and differ from patient to patient, and the most common intravenous hypertonic solution administered is a 0.8–8% NaCl solution [67]. In patients where intravenous euvolemia cannot be established and maintained, remediation of coagulopathy must be placed as a medical team's highest priority [68]. Coagulopathy is a state in which the blood's ability to coagulate is diminished or impaired, resulting in a variable viscosity of the blood and therefore further complications in the treatment of elevated intracranial pressure. Normal human physiology tightly regulates the viscosity of blood and its coagulating ability, and in patients that have suffered a traumatic brain injury, the release of biochemical pathway intermediate, thromboplastin, causes abnormal blood clotting. These abnormal clotting factors can be fatal if not remediated quickly; therefore, blood transfusions for these patients is the quickest and most preferred method in correcting blood coagulating abilities and eliminating coagulopathy. Patients on anticoagulating mediations due to high cholesterol, such as heparin or warfarin, who sustain a traumatic brain injury that results in elevated intracranial pressure are typically at risk and thus require immediate blood transfusion [69]. Approximately 1 in 10 TBI patients that present with elevated ICP also demonstrates a fever 24–48 hours after the initial injury, and this elevation in temperature is in fact part of the body's inflammatory response [70]. Often in patients where the hypothalamus has been damaged, elevated body temperature is noticed due to an underlying infection of the region. While the biochemical mechanism of this observation is not understood, what is understood is that immediate elimination of the infection is required for a successful recovery. This unexplained fever is often called "neurological fever," and unlike a fever caused by a cold or viral infection, neurological fever tremendously increases metabolic demand [71]. In patients with GCS scores less than or equal to 8 with imaging that demonstrates signs of cerebral edema, placement of external ventricular drain in a sterile fashion is recommended to allow CSF drainage. This procedure can be completed at bedside or in the operating room with the overall goal of decreasing cerebral edema by CSF drainage. In cases where intracranial pressure remains at or above 22 mmHg, despite all strategies discussed above, surgical intervention will need to be considered. In this section, we have discussed the nonsurgical and medicinal approach in resolving an elevated intracranial pressure; however, in any remedy for the management of ICP, it is important to remember that the overall goal is to reduce and prevent any agitation of the intracranial region. In the section to follow, we will discuss the surgical option for the management of intracranial pressure in the event that nonsurgical interventions do not remediate the issue.

2.11. Surgical care of increased intracranial pressure

Immediate and rapid surgical care of patients presenting with elevated intracranial pressure due to a traumatic brain injury is vital for the positive prognosis of the patient, especially if nonsurgical routes did not suffice in the remediation of intracranial pressure. Intracranial lesions resulting in an increased ICP typically present in patients as a state of reduced consciousness, and this pathology requires a surgical procedure called "rapid decompression." This surgery is self-explanatory at the elementary level, as the surgical efforts aim to reduce intracranial pressure ("decompress") and do so as soon as possible. Prior to operation, a complete patient profile must be reobtained, meaning that radiological evidence alone is not enough to proceed with decompression surgery; a neurological examination coupled with radiological evidence that is convincing without any doubt is what surgical staff must aim to achieve. Similar to many forms of surgery, patient age plays a major role. For decompression surgeries, patients that are young (12 years old or younger) or elder (70 years old or older) pose a greater risk to surgical harm, and this harm is referred to as intracranial hemorrhage, excessive bleeding from tissue and venous tract within the intracranial region [72]. The first form of decompression surgery that we will discuss is decompressive craniotomy, a procedure in which a segment of the cranium is removed to relieve intracranial pressure and to create additional room for the brain swelling. This decompressive surgery evolved from a primitive form of surgery called trephining. Today, this surgical practice is a last resort option and has been more successful in younger patients rather than in older patients, another surgical option is craniotomy for evacuation of focal hemorrhage which can be subdural, epidural or intraparenchymal in nature [73]. The next surgical practice we will discuss that is used in the treatment of elevated intracranial pressure due to a TBI, which causes an over production of CSF, is a ventriculoperitoneal (VP) shunt. A VP shunt is a medical device that relieves pressure from the brain due to fluid accumulation, and this shunt drains the excess fluid and allows it to be metabolized and reabsorbed. Normally, CSF will coat the brain and spinal cord and be reabsorbed into the blood, and in a disrupted flow, the CSF can build up and create pressure on the brain causing damage. A common source for deregulation for CSF production and reabsorption is traumatic brain injury, and in these cases, it is common for CSF to cause damage to the brain [74]. Prior to surgery, a patient will be instructed to halt any consumption of food and water by mouth (PO) at least 8–12 h before surgery. Then a surgical nurse will prepare the area behind the ear for surgical incision. The shunt is a catheter, a thin flexible but heavy-duty tube that is used to drain excess liquid. A neurological surgeon will then make a small incision behind the ear and using a burr-drill will create a small hole within the patient's scalp [75]. With the hole in the cranium, surgical staff will insert one catheter into the brain and another subdermal catheter will be placed behind the ear. A thin tube will travel down the patient's torso and into the abdominal cavity. The excess CSF will drain into the abdominal cavity relieving intracranial pressure [76]. In patients that present with intracranial pressure regularly, a pump may be placed to activate this channel when ICP rises. For the context in which we have been discussing, this shunt will be used to relieve patients of increased ICP following a TBI.

2.12. Medication utilization

Management of elevated intracranial pressure due to a traumatic brain injury requires the utilization of many forms of medication. Thus far, we have discussed a few drugs that directly target elevated intracranial pressure, but often these pathologies require surgical intervention. For that to occur, a wide variety of drugs must be utilized to stabilize the patient from common complications that arise. In this section, we will touch upon the class of drugs utilized prior to neurological surgery. The most prevalent presurgical complication presenting in medical centers today is intracranial hemorrhages; see **Figure 4**. Intracranial hemorrhages denote bleeding of the brain; medical personnel often utilize prophylactic anticonvulsants, and the term prophylactic refers to the act of committing an action before hand and the term anticonvulsants refers to a set of

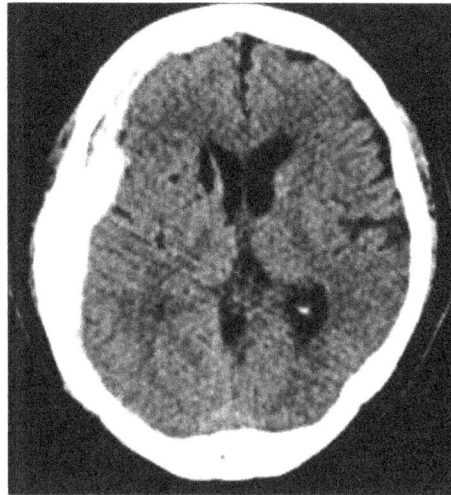

Figure 4. CT scan of subdural in a TBI patient presenting for surgical intervention [77]. Presentation of severe intracranial pressure buildup resulting from TBI. Images depict transverse CT images from ventral (left) to dorsal views (right), respectively, 5 h after injury with a Glasgow Coma Scale (GSC) score of 3 (an extremely severe form). This imaging depicts right focal subdural hematoma.

pharmacological drugs that block sodium channels or enhance GABA (gamma-aminobutyric acid) function [78, 79]. Physiologically, these drugs can save a life in the event of a seizure as well as reduce bleeding in the brain prior to surgery [80]. There are many drugs that can be used that are considered in this pharmacological class, and the first of its kind was discovered in 1882 (paraldehyde); today, the drug of choice is phenytoin or fosphenytoin [81]. In adults, a loading dose of phenytoin or fosphenytoin is administered, typically in adults 18 mg anticonvulsant per kilogram (kg) of patient body weight. Then, therapeutic levels of 20 milligram (mg) per deciliter (dL) are maintained until intracranial hemorrhage subsides [82]. Prolonged use of anticonvulsant drugs may result in gingival hyperplasia, an enlargement of one's gingiva (commonly known as gums) as well as randomized hair growth in men and unwanted male-hair growth in women, known as hirsutism [83–85]. In the unfortunate case where a pediatric patient is subjected to elevated intracranial pressure due to a traumatic brain injury that is accompanied by intracranial hemorrhage, the drug of choice changes to phenobarbital, where a 20 mg/1 kg body weight loading dose is given, followed by a therapeutic dose of 10–50 mg/dL.

2.13. Patient follow-up and future care

Many patients that present to medical centers for treatment of mild to severe traumatic brain injury and are subjected to an elevated intracranial pressure will tremendously benefit from numerous outpatient care options. As traumatic brain injury patients typically have difficulty with daily tasks, physical and occupation therapy is highly recommended as patients try to regain a normal lifestyle. Additionally, times following a traumatic incident can be hard emotionally and spiritually, and thus it is also beneficial for patients to receive counseling care from professional as well as from family and loved ones. The initial efforts to reestablish the life the patient once had is difficult and both mentally and physically taxing, and support and counseling are of key essence.

3. Conclusion

Throughout this chapter, we have discussed the many applications and forms of medical care pertaining to the presence of elevated intracranial pressure resulting from traumatic brain injury. Throughout this chapter, we hope that you have learned the key diagnostic characteristics, medical treatment, and future outcomes for patients experiencing this traumatic pathology. While we hope no patient has to suffer from TBI, we wish all medical staff best of luck in their efforts to remediate these conditions and for continual excellence in patient care.

Disclosure

All figures displayed within this manuscript were obtained through the Open Access Biomedical Image Search Engine, with the image owners receiving appropriate citation for the contributions. In accordance to the terms of the Creative Commons Attribution License, the reproduction and distribution of each figure used in this manuscript are accompanied by the citation of the original author(s) or licensors. Original publication within their respected journals is also cited. Our intended uses of these figures are in good and accepted academic practice.

Author details

Christ Ordookhanian[1], Meena Nagappan[2], Dina Elias[1] and Paul E. Kaloostian[1]*

*Address all correspondence to: paulkaloostian@hotmail.com

1 University of California, Riverside School of Medicine, Riverside, CA, United States

2 St. Georges School of Medicine, True Blue, Grenada

References

[1] Freeman WD. Management of intracranial pressure. Continuum (Minneap Minn). 2015;**21**(5 Neurocritical Care):1299-1323

[2] Stocchetti N, Zoerle T, Carbonara M. Intracranial pressure management in patients with traumatic brain injury: An update. Current Opinion in Critical Care. 2017;**23**(2):110-114

[3] Smith M. Monitoring intracranial pressure in traumatic brain injury. Anesthesia and Analgesia. 2008;**106**(1):240-248

[4] Jennett B. Epidemiology of head injury. Archives of Disease in Childhood. 1998;**78**(5): 403-406

[5] Blissitt PA. Care of the critically ill patient with penetrating head injury. Critical Care Nursing Clinics of North America. 2006;**18**(3):321-332

[6] Kalia M. Brain development: Anatomy, connectivity, adaptive plasticity, and toxicity. Metabolism. 2008;**57**(Suppl 2):S2-S5

[7] Andreasen NC et al. Intelligence and brain structure in normal individuals. The American Journal of Psychiatry. 1993;**150**(1):130-134

[8] O'Muircheartaigh J, Jbabdi S. Concurrent white matter bundles and grey matter networks using independent component analysis. NeuroImage. 2017

[9] Burruss JW et al. Functional neuroanatomy of the frontal lobe circuits. Radiology. 2000;**214**(1):227-230

[10] Grand W. The anatomy of the brain, by Thomas Willis. Neurosurgery. 1999;**45**(5):1234-1236 (discussion 1236-1237)

[11] Buckner RL, Andrews-Hanna JR, Schacter DL. The brain's default network: Anatomy, function, and relevance to disease. Annals of the New York Academy of Sciences. 2008; **1124**:1-38

[12] Saatman KE et al. Classification of traumatic brain injury for targeted therapies. Journal of Neurotrauma. 2008;**25**(7):719-738

[13] Sternbach GL. The Glasgow coma scale. The Journal of Emergency Medicine. 2000;**19**(1): 67-71

[14] McNarry AF, Goldhill DR. Simple bedside assessment of level of consciousness: Comparison of two simple assessment scales with the Glasgow coma scale. Anaesthesia. 2004;**59**(1):34-37

[15] Steiner LA, Andrews PJ. Monitoring the injured brain: ICP and CBF. British Journal of Anaesthesia. 2006;**97**(1):26-38

[16] Berdahl JP, Allingham RR. Intracranial pressure and glaucoma. Current Opinion in Ophthalmology. 2010;**21**(2):106-111

[17] Ghajar J. Traumatic brain injury. Lancet. 2000;**356**(9233):923-929

[18] Mokri B. The Monro-Kellie hypothesis: Applications in CSF volume depletion. Neurology. 2001;**56**(12):1746-1748

[19] Neff S, Subramaniam RP. Monro-Kellie doctrine. Journal of Neurosurgery. 1996;**85**(6):1195

[20] Dawes AJ et al. Intracranial pressure monitoring and inpatient mortality in severe traumatic brain injury: A propensity score-matched analysis. Journal of Trauma and Acute Care Surgery. 2015;**78**(3):492-501 discussion 501-2

[21] Rangel-Castillo L, Robertson CS. Management of intracranial hypertension. Critical Care Clinics. 2006;**22**(4):713-732 (abstract ix)

[22] Rosner MJ, Coley IB. Cerebral perfusion pressure, intracranial pressure, and head eleva-
      tion. Journal of Neurosurgery. 1986;**65**(5):636-641

[23] Lang EW, Chesnut RM. Intracranial pressure and cerebral perfusion pressure in severe
      head injury. New Horizons. 1995;**3**(3):400-409

[24] Peterson EC, Wang Z, Britz G. Regulation of cerebral blood flow. International Journal of
      Vascular Medicine. 2011;**2011**:823525

[25] Nakagawa K, Smith WS. Evaluation and management of increased intracranial pres-
      sure. Continuum (Minneap Minn). 2011;**17**(5 Neurologic Consultation in the Hospital):
      1077-1093

[26] Friedman DI, Rausch EA. Headache diagnoses in patients with treated idiopathic intra-
      cranial hypertension. Neurology. 2002;**58**(10):1551-1553

[27] Dunn LT. Raised intracranial pressure. Journal of Neurology, Neurosurgery, and
      Psychiatry. 2002;**73**(Suppl 1):i23-i27

[28] Rehman T et al. Rapid progression of traumatic bifrontal contusions to transtentorial
      herniation: A case report. Cases Journal. 2008;**1**(1):203

[29] Dahlqvist MB et al. Brain herniation in a patient with apparently normal intracranial
      pressure: A case report. Journal of Medical Case Reports. 2010;**4**:297

[30] McAllister TW. Neurobiological consequences of traumatic brain injury. Dialogues in
      Clinical Neuroscience. 2011;**13**(3):287-300

[31] Saifudheen K et al. Idiopathic intracranial hypertension presenting as CSF rhinorrhea.
      Annals of Indian Academy of Neurology. 2010;**13**(1):72-73

[32] Manousaki D et al. A 15-year-old adolescent with a rare pituitary lesion. Endocrinology,
      Diabetes & Metabolism Case Reports. 2014;**2014**:140010

[33] Round R, Keane JR. The minor symptoms of increased intracranial pressure: 101 patients
      with benign intracranial hypertension. Neurology. 1988;**38**(9):1461-1464

[34] Stocchetti N, Maas AI. Traumatic intracranial hypertension. The New England Journal
      of Medicine. 2014;**370**(22):2121-2130

[35] Selhorst JB, Chen Y. The optic nerve. Seminars in Neurology. 2009;**29**(1):29-35

[36] Armstrong GT et al. Defining optic nerve tortuosity. American Journal of Neuroradiology.
      2007;**28**(4):666-671

[37] Han HC. Twisted blood vessels: Symptoms, etiology and biomechanical mechanisms.
      Journal of Vascular Research. 2012;**49**(3):185-197

[38] Killer HE, Mironov A, Flammer J. Optic neuritis with marked distension of the optic
      nerve sheath due to local fluid congestion. The British Journal of Ophthalmology.
      2003;**87**(2):249

[39] Sadun AA, Wang MY. Abnormalities of the optic disc. Handbook of Clinical Neurology. 2011;**102**:117-157

[40] Passi N, Degnan AJ, Levy LM. MR imaging of papilledema and visual pathways: Effects of increased intracranial pressure and pathophysiologic mechanisms. American Journal of Neuroradiology. 2013;**34**(5):919-924

[41] Jinkins JR. "Papilledema": Neuroradiologic evaluation of optic disk protrusion with dynamic orbital CT. American Journal of Roentgenology. 1987;**149**(4):793-802

[42] Nguyen HS, Haider KM, Ackerman LL. Unusual causes of papilledema: Two illustrative cases. Surgical Neurology International. 2013;**4**:60

[43] Roy Chowdhury U, Fautsch MP. Intracranial pressure and its relationship to glaucoma: Current understanding and future directions. Medical Hypothesis, Discovery & Innovation Ophthalmology Journal. 2015;**4**(3):71-80

[44] Kelly LP et al. Does bilateral transverse cerebral venous sinus stenosis exist in patients without increased intracranial pressure? Clinical Neurology and Neurosurgery. 2013;**115**(8):1215-1219

[45] Degnan AJ, Levy LM. Pseudotumor cerebri: Brief review of clinical syndrome and imaging findings. American Journal of Neuroradiology. 2011;**32**(11):1986-1993

[46] Gonzalez-Tortosa J. Primary empty sella: symptoms, physiopathology, diagnosis and treatment. Neurocirugia (Astur). 2009;**20**(2):132-151

[47] Haughton VM et al. Recognizing the empty sella by CT: The infundibulum sign. American Journal of Roentgenology. 1981;**136**(2):293-295

[48] Zagardo MT et al. Reversible empty sella in idiopathic intracranial hypertension: An indicator of successful therapy? American Journal of Neuroradiology. 1996;**17**(10):1953-1956

[49] Bialer OY et al. Meningoceles in idiopathic intracranial hypertension. American Journal of Roentgenology. 2014;**202**(3):608-613

[50] Kamel HA, Toland J. Trigeminal nerve anatomy: Illustrated using examples of abnormalities. American Journal of Roentgenology. 2001;**176**(1):247-251

[51] San Millan D, Kohler R. Enlarged CSF spaces in pseudotumor cerebri. American Journal of Roentgenology. 2014;**203**(4):W457-W458

[52] Freeman MD et al. A case-control study of cerebellar tonsillar ectopia (Chiari) and head/neck trauma (whiplash). Brain Injury. 2010;**24**(7-8):988-994

[53] Aiken AH et al. Incidence of cerebellar tonsillar ectopia in idiopathic intracranial hypertension: A mimic of the Chiari I malformation. American Journal of Neuroradiology. 2012;**33**(10):1901-1906

[54] Lunge SB et al. Rhinocerebrocutaneous mucormycosis caused by Mucor species: A rare causation. Indian Dermatology Online Journal. 2015;**6**(3):189-192

[55] Sivasankar R et al. Imaging and interventions in idiopathic intracranial hypertension: A pictorial essay. Indian Journal of Radiology and Imaging. 2015;**25**(4):439-444

[56] Miller JD et al. Early insults to the injured brain. JAMA. 1978;**240**(5):439-442

[57] Rosner MJ, Daughton S. Cerebral perfusion pressure management in head injury. The Journal of Trauma. 1990;**30**(8):933-940 discussion 940-1

[58] Stein SC, Ross SE. Moderate head injury: A guide to initial management. Journal of Neurosurgery. 1992;**77**(4):562-564

[59] Muizelaar JP et al. Adverse effects of prolonged hyperventilation in patients with severe head injury: A randomized clinical trial. Journal of Neurosurgery. 1991;**75**(5):731-739

[60] Wakai A et al. Mannitol for acute traumatic brain injury. Cochrane Database of Systematic Reviews. 2013;**8**:CD001049

[61] Song SH, Vieille C. Recent advances in the biological production of mannitol. Applied Microbiology and Biotechnology. 2009;**84**(1):55-62

[62] Muizelaar JP et al. Mannitol causes compensatory cerebral vasoconstriction and vasodilation in response to blood viscosity changes. Journal of Neurosurgery. 1983;**59**(5):822-828

[63] Sakowitz OW et al. Effects of mannitol bolus administration on intracranial pressure, cerebral extracellular metabolites, and tissue oxygenation in severely head-injured patients. The Journal of Trauma. 2007;**62**(2):292-298

[64] Muizelaar JP, Lutz HA 3rd, Becker DP. Effect of mannitol on ICP and CBF and correlation with pressure autoregulation in severely head-injured patients. Journal of Neurosurgery. 1984;**61**(4):700-706

[65] Roberts I, Sydenham E. Barbiturates for acute traumatic brain injury. Cochrane Database of Systematic Reviews. 2012;**12**:CD000033

[66] Gopinath SP et al. Jugular venous desaturation and outcome after head injury. Journal of Neurology, Neurosurgery, and Psychiatry. 1994;**57**(6):717-723

[67] Wang H et al. The effect of hypertonic saline and mannitol on coagulation in moderate traumatic brain injury patients. The American Journal of Emergency Medicine. 2017

[68] Vassar MJ et al. 7.5% sodium chloride/dextran for resuscitation of trauma patients undergoing helicopter transport. Archives of Surgery. 1991;**126**(9):1065-1072

[69] Winter JP et al. Early fresh frozen plasma prophylaxis of abnormal coagulation parameters in the severely head-injured patient is not effective. Annals of Emergency Medicine. 1989;**18**(5):553-555

[70] Clinchot DM, Otis S, Colachis SC 3rd. Incidence of fever in the rehabilitation phase following brain injury. American Journal of Physical Medicine & Rehabilitation. 1997; **76**(4):323-327

[71] Cariou A et al. Targeted temperature management in the ICU: Guidelines from a French expert panel. Anaesthesia, Critical Care & Pain Medicine. 2017

[72] Alali AS et al. Intracranial pressure monitoring in severe traumatic brain injury: Results from the American College of Surgeons trauma quality improvement program. Journal of Neurotrauma. 2013;**30**(20):1737-1746

[73] Taylor A et al. A randomized trial of very early decompressive craniectomy in children with traumatic brain injury and sustained intracranial hypertension. Child's Nervous System. 2001;**17**(3):154-162

[74] Tribl G, Oder W. Outcome after shunt implantation in severe head injury with post-traumatic hydrocephalus. Brain Injury. 2000;**14**(4):345-354

[75] Reddy GK, Bollam P, Caldito G. Ventriculoperitoneal shunt surgery and the risk of shunt infection in patients with hydrocephalus: Long-term single institution experience. World Neurosurgery. 2012;**78**(1-2):155-163

[76] Nigim F et al. Ventriculoperitoneal shunting: Laparoscopically assisted versus conventional open surgical approaches. Asian Journal of Neurosurgery. 2014;**9**(2):72-81

[77] Chung P, Khan F. Mild traumatic brain injury presenting with delayed intracranial hemorrhage in warfarin therapy: A case report. Journal of Medical Case Reports. 2015;**9**:173

[78] Rogawski MA, Loscher W. The neurobiology of antiepileptic drugs. Nature Reviews. Neuroscience. 2004;**5**(7):553-564

[79] Meldrum BS, Rogawski MA. Molecular targets for antiepileptic drug development. Neurotherapeutics. 2007;**4**(1):18-61

[80] Kaminski RM, Rogawski MA, Klitgaard H. The potential of antiseizure drugs and agents that act on novel molecular targets as antiepileptogenic treatments. Neurotherapeutics. 2014;**11**(2):385-400

[81] French JA et al. Efficacy and tolerability of the new antiepileptic drugs, I: Treatment of new-onset epilepsy: Report of the TTA and QSS subcommittees of the American Academy of Neurology and the American Epilepsy Society. Epilepsia. 2004;**45**(5):401-409

[82] Troupin AS. Dose-related adverse effects of anticonvulsants. Drug Safety. 1996;**14**(5):299-328

[83] Nakazawa Y, Ohkawa T. Study of the side effects of long-term anticonvulsant treatment. Folia Psychiatrica et Neurologica Japonica. 1980;**34**(3):271-275

[84] Gaitatzis A, Sander JW. The long-term safety of antiepileptic drugs. CNS Drugs. 2013;**27**(6):435-455

[85] Conomy JP. Long-term use of the major anticonvulsant drugs. American Family Physician. 1978;**18**(4):107-116

6

Explosive Blast Mild Traumatic Brain Injury

John Magnuson and Geoffrey Ling

Abstract

In the recent wars in Iraq and Afghanistan, US military personnel have suffered over 333,000 traumatic brain injuries (TBIs), with over 85% being mild TBI. A variety of improvised munitions, such as improvised explosive devices (IEDs) and improvised rocket assisted mortars (IRAMs), have resulted in the explosive blast-induced TBI (bTBI). Due to its prevalence, TBI has been referred to as the signature wound of US warfighters in Afghanistan and Iraq. Explosive blast produces damage to the brain by creating a dynamic environment in forms of overpressure shock wave, heat impulse, blast-propelled projectiles, and debris, whose impact can cause complex injuries in the brain and other visceral organ systems, such as lung and bowel. Mechanisms of bTBI incorporate all forms of TBI such as falls, motor vehicle accidents, and coup-contrecoup injury. Some of the unique aspects of bTBI include the rate at which the injury occurs, the differential pressure load on and within the tissue, and the pressure-loaded tissue response. Mild bTBI is the most problematic injury within the US military in terms of number of warfighters affected and recognition of the injury. The pathobiology of mild bTBI is not fully understood. Here, we review mild bTBI injury, symptomology, and diagnosis. Finally, multi-modality testing is discussed, including functional, structural, and evidence-based evaluation with an intention to describe and diagnose mild bTBI affecting the US warfighter.

Keywords: brain injury, blast, concussion, TBI, military, IED, improvised explosive device

1. Introduction

Traumatic brain injury (TBI) in the most recent wars accounts for a significant percentage of combat-related injury. On average, about 1600 TBIs per month are suffered by US service members. The majority are due to explosive blast exposure. This is in spite of overall decreases in both combat-related injuries in general and increased wound survival rates. Active duty casualty reports compiled by the Defense Casualty Analysis System (DCAS) indicate that since the start of the Overseas Contingency Operations (OCO) in 2001, beginning with Operation Enduring Freedom (OEF) in Afghanistan, Operation Iraqi Freedom (OIF), to the current Operation Inherent Resolve (OIR) and Operation Freedom's Sentinel (OFS), US combat casualties have a 90.7% casualty survival rate [1, 2]. In comparison, DCAS data from the Vietnam and Korean conflicts indicate 76.8 and 78.9% casualty survival rate, respectively [3, 4]. Increased survival in OCO is due to advancements in vehicle and body armor, ballistic helmets, and lenses, combined with forward-deployed surgical teams, faster evacuation times, and improved/enhanced training of medics, corpsman, and combat lifesavers based on the concepts of Tactical Combat Casualty Care (TCCC) [5–7]. Explosive blast continues to injure US warfighters leaving many with a mild blast-induced TBI (bTBI) that is difficult to diagnose and to treat.

2. Explosive blast-induced traumatic brain injury

During OCO from 2001 to mid-2016, US military service members have suffered over 333,000 traumatic brain injuries (TBIs), with over 85% being mild TBI [8]. These TBI statistics are often confusing when compared to casualty data reported by the DCAS. It must be kept in mind that DCAS casualty reporting is for active duty casualties and does not list the specific type of injury. In contrast, the TBI data collected by the Defense and Veterans Brain Injury Center (DVBIC) pools from the Armed Forces Health Surveillance Branch and does provide TBI data. In order to support US military personnel, it is essential to uncover the pathobiology of mild bTBI and develop improved treatment options. Modern combat will continue to cause bTBI, decreasing fighting strength to the point a combat team cannot accomplish mission objectives.

Explosions from various improvised munitions, such as improvised explosive devices (IEDs) and improvised rocket-assisted mortars (IRAMs), have resulted in explosive blast induced TBI (bTBI) becoming the signature wound of US warfighters in Afghanistan and Iraq [7, 8]. Explosive blast overpressure creates a dynamic environment, which can cause complex injuries in multiple organ systems [5, 9–11]. Brain injury due to explosive blast exposure is often overlooked. Realizing this, the Department of Defense (DoD) mandates that any service member exposed to a mandatory event such as a blast, vehicle collision, head injury, and so on, to be screened for concussion, followed by a neurologic evaluation.

Furthermore, categorizing and describing the different types of blast-induced head injury must continually evolve in order to better diagnose and treat the injuries.

3. Categorization of bTBI

Categorization of bTBI can initially be described as open or closed based upon the integrity of the skull and overlying tissue. Open head injury (OHI) indicates that the skull has been fractured. This can be by a foreign body, such as a bomb fragment or bullet, or from depressed skull fragments pushed into the skull interior by impact. Penetrating TBI (pTBI) is often used synonymously with OHI, but here it is presented as a subcategory of OHI, as the brain is not necessarily involved. Bomb case fragments, shrapnel, and debris are all types of explosive ejecta, which can penetrate the brain, resulting in a pTBI. When severe, brain tissue is violated, extrusion of brain matter and cerebrospinal fluid (CSF) are often noted at the site of penetration [11]. When ejecta enters the brain, it may leave wound tracts and cavitation disproportionate to objects' size [12]. The resulting hemorrhage, edema, and macerated tissue are hallmarks of pTBI [11]. Further evaluation by CT imaging often indicates blood along the wound tract [11]. Presentation of the OHI may be as apparent as brain herniation or more subtle such as a linear skull fracture with intact skin and mild swelling. Closed head injury (CHI) is much more common. Most typically, it is due to blunt force. This causes the head to move. The brain moves slower than the head because it is surrounded by fluid, that is, CSF. This lag causes the faster moving skull to strike the brain, leading to a contusion. If the head rebounds, such as in an acceleration/deceleration injury, the brain will be struck on the opposite side as well, causing a coup-contrecoup injury pattern. During an explosive blast, the detonation generates an overpressure shock wave that moves rapidly through the air, striking the head. The pressure is transmitted through the skull to the brain. Consequently, the patient has an intact skull but underlying damage to the brain parenchyma. Both categories of bTBI can be caused by multiple injury mechanisms.

4. Explosive blast injury mechanisms

There are five injury mechanisms which contribute to bTBI individually or in combination: primary, secondary, tertiary, quaternary, and quinary injuries [13, 14]. Primary barotrauma (overpressure) injury results from the detonation/shock front impingement on and transmission through the tissue [15, 16]. Differential density of juxtaposed body structures can result in reflective waves and turbulent spalling effects within the tissue [16]. Secondary (ejecta/fragment) injury is caused by shrapnel, ejecta, and/or foreign body impact. Tertiary (acceleration) injury is due to the body being thrown by the explosive, which may result in the traditional coup-contrecoup injury and/or rotation stress causing tissue shearing or membrane disruption. Quaternary (burn) injury is caused by heat, chemicals, and/or toxidromes [17]. Finally, quinary (contaminant) injury is due to environment (infection from soil bacteria in the ejecta) or detonation (radiation) contamination [14]. Clinical identification of bTBI and severity stratification are based on post-event signs and clinical symptoms.

5. Mild bTBI severity criteria

According to VA/DoD Clinical Practice Guidelines, bTBI clinical diagnosis is primarily based on history of event (blast exposure) and any one of the following: any period of loss of consciousness (LOC), post-traumatic amnesia (PTA), alteration of consciousness/mental state (AOC), transient or persistent neurological deficits, and/or intracranial lesion [18]. Blast-induced TBI can further be categorized by severity based on degree or duration of LOC, PTA,

AOC, and imaging findings. Open head injury is considered a severe injury, while CHI severity can be classified as mild, moderate, or severe.

Mild bTBI is the most common explosive blast injury affecting US warfighters and is largely a diagnosis of exclusion. The patient may present with decreased LOC <30 min, AOC at event to <24 h, PTA <1d, best Glasgow coma scale (GCS) score within first 24 h [1, 3, 4], and no gross abnormalities on imaging such as CT [18]. For a more thorough discussion of TBI evaluation, the VA/DoD Clinical Guidelines for Management of Concussion/mTBI is suggested.

6. Mild bTBI symptoms and sequela

As with concussion, majority of mild bTBI patients recover within hours to days [18]. Often, warfighters are not aware they have suffered a bTBI or endure the symptoms to continue the mission and support fellow warfighters. It is important for all combat medical staff from the squad level to the company level and above to educate the team on the importance of prompt reporting and evaluation of those exposed to blast. Initial evaluation is the most important in order to determine severity of the injury and avoid obfuscating the classification with worsening PCS symptoms. Prompt medical evaluation of initial bTBI allows determination of timing for recovery, ensuring avoidance of a second head injury [9]. A head injury occurring within the recovery window can cause life threatening second impact syndrome (SIS) [11]. Military first providers are given the military acute concussion evaluation (MACE) as a screening tool. With the MACE is the standardized assessment of concussion (SAC). This is a paper-and-pencil clinical device that tests for alterations in attention, consciousness, memory, and orientation. If abnormal, the patient is referred to an advanced health care provider, typically the unit's physician, for diagnosis.

If concussed, patients are then placed into a Concussion Care Center for recovery. *Guidelines for Concussion Management* from the American Academy of Neurology lists recommended recovery periods [19]. A step-wise approach to rest, rehabilitation, and recovery is conducted in the Military Concussion Care Centers. Basically, patients are educated on their condition and reassured that they will likely recover quickly. Adequate sleep and rehydration are important. Behavior health issues such as post-traumatic stress disorder (PTSD) are also addressed. Once symptoms abate, the patient is allowed to resume mild physical activity and cognitive tasks. This progresses until the patient is able to conduct full physical and cognitive activities without symptom manifestation without the need for any medications. Fortunately, the vast majority of patients, over 95%, will fully recover without sequelae within a few days.

Unfortunately, some bTBI patients develop postconcussion syndrome (PCS) days after initial injury [20]. PCS is a set of symptoms (headaches, nausea, balance or coordination deficits, slurred speech, confusion, sensitivity to noise, sensitivity to light, tinnitus) that usually resolve within days to weeks after blast exposure. In general, the syndrome responds with patient reassurance and symptomatic treatment such as non-narcotic analgesics/antimigraine for headache and antidepressants for depression [11]. A subset of PCS suffers may continue to have persistent or chronic symptoms.

Persistent postconcussion syndrome (PPCS) has been identified in non-blast TBI as a condition of at least three nonresolving neurologic and behavioral PCS symptoms lasting longer than 3 months following the injury [21]. Clinical data from 181 blast-exposed veterans indicate that these criteria are inadequate to properly diagnose blast-related PPCS and that more focused testing is required [22]. The relative contribution of mild bTBI versus PTSD for PPCS is under investigation. Davenport et al. interviewed 122 veterans with a diagnosis of mild TBI, 88% having been exposed to explosive blast, and found that both mild bTBI and PTSD contribute to PPCS; however, the relative contribution of PTSD is substantially diminished after accounting for personality traits [23]. These data indicate timely description of the initial injury, correlation of ≥4 symptoms, and accounting for experience and personality traits aid in isolating diagnosis of PPCS.

Post-traumatic stress disorder and mild bTBI share many common symptoms such as difficulty in concentration, sleep disturbances, and mood alteration. However, there are differences. For example, bTBI patients typically complain of headaches and vertigo, whereas PTSD patients much less commonly complain of headaches and vertigo. Conversely, PTSD patients experience flashback, whereas bTBI patients typically do not. The American Psychiatric Association DMS V describes post-traumatic stress disorder as a mental health condition triggered by witnessing, experiencing, or learning a traumatic event. Symptoms of PTSD may include severe anxiety, flashbacks, nightmares, and uncontrolled thoughts about the event. Avoidance of stimuli about the event is common. Alteration in arousal may include outbursts, difficulty in concentration, hypervigilance, exaggerated startle response, and sleep disturbances [24]. All of these symptoms interfere with the person's ability to live a normal enjoyable life. Due to the extreme situations in which blast injuries occur, it is not surprising to find that mild bTBI and PTSD afflict the blast-injured patient.

7. Noninvasive evaluation of mild bTBI

Diagnosis of mild bTBI has been difficult due to limited understanding of its pathobiology. Inability to identify brain structural and functional changes in mild bTBI is a further complication. Traditional methods of imaging (CT, MRI) generally do not show gross changes for mild bTBI even though physiologic symptoms are present. Negative imaging with persistent symptoms likely indicates an injury below the limit of resolution of the image scanner. High-resolution imaging studies and electrophysiology recordings are two noninvasive tools that may aid in diagnosis of mild bTBI.

Cortical thinning on MRI scans has been noted in 11 active-duty military persons with a diagnosis of mild bTBI at an average of 1-month post-injury. Cortical thinning was identified in the superior temporal and superior frontal gyri and two areas in lateral orbitofrontal gyrus [25]. Another study of 38 veterans diagnosed with bTBI measured cortical thickness utilizing a T1 weighted 3-T MRI with 1-mm isotropic resolution and 8-channel birdcage head coil. The cortical thinning was noted in the inferior frontal, temporal, and insula regions [26]. The data is an important initial step toward a structurally relevant diagnosis and quantification of mild bTBI. Cooperation among radiologist, clinicians, and researchers could immediately establish a database for correlating mild bTBI events, presenting symptoms, PCS, PPCS, and PTSD with MRI cortical thinning.

Diffusion tensor imaging (DTI) can be used to image white mater (WM-) integrity, which may be a predictor of mild bTBI [27]. White matter in the brain constrains water and causes it to diffuse along the myelinated axons in an anisotropic pattern of diffusion. Large linear fractional anisotropy (FA) combined with a low mean diffusivity (MD) of water is characteristic of healthy WM. On the contrary, disruption in WM-integrity allows diffusion of water away from the WM, indicated by a decrease in FA and increases MD. There are several DTI studies of veterans where loss of WM-integrity predicts mTBI [28–30]. A study of 125 veterans, 2–5 years post-deployment, indicated that mild TBI was correlated with number of deployments and increased PCS, however, indicated normal WM-integrity on DTI [23]. In addition, veterans with PTSD initially showed a larger loss of WM-integrity, but the effect was negated when accounting for behavioral sequela. As indicated by other investigators, the relative contribution of mild bTBI, PCS, PTSD, and WM-integrity, during the chronic phase of injury, still needs to be determined [23].

Evidenced-based standardized approach to evaluation of head injury has been proposed by emergency medicine physicians so as to better describe and diagnose mild bTBI. Physical exam should look for neurological abnormalities, ocular dysfunction, vestibular dysfunction, cervical injury/tenderness, ocular motor performance, signs of vestibular dysfunction, and orthostatic blood pressure. All parameters can be evaluated at the initial clinical presentation and throughout treatment, which should enhance the traditional symptomology based MACE and SAC [31].

Electrocortical potentials generated by the pyramidal neurons of the cortex can be used to monitor brain function with transdermal electrodes. Passive recording of electroencephalograms (EEGs) is often used in sleep studies and aids in the diagnosis of epilepsy. The spatial resolution is inversely proportional to width of recording electrode and distance from cortex. Temporal resolution is good and an advantage of EEG recording. Evoke response recording provides a method to evaluate cortical activity in response sensory stimulus. Visual evoked responses (VERs) are well characterized and aid in diagnosis of multiple sclerosis. Pattern reversal and flash stimuli are two of many protocols, which can be used to evaluate retinal to visual cortex integrity. Auditory evoked responses (AERs) can be used to evaluate inner ear to auditory cortex [32]. Somatosensory evoked response (SER), olfactory evoke response (OER), and gustatory evoked response (GER) all can be used to evaluate the integrity of the sensory apparatus to the sensory cortex through repeated stimuli-responses [33]. The multiple and variable symptoms of mild bTBI presentation and later transient PCS and chronic PPCS suggest diffuse low-level injury. Multisensory evaluation, combined with repeated follow-up, will aid in bridging the gap for understanding the pathobiology of this insidious condition.

8. Conclusion

Mild bTBI still lacks sufficient understanding of the mechanisms that lead to structural and functional alterations of the brain. Multidisciplinary scientific and clinical investigation can provide the coordinated efforts required to sufficiently elucidate the pathobiology of mild bTBI. Identification of what is injured will allow development of effective treatments and protective strategies. Improvements in electroencephalography deconvolution, removable discrete electrode arrays, combined with multisensory-evoked response protocols, will make the electrophysiology techniques more clinically useful as diagnostic and, potentially, prognostic tools. Functional and structural imaging, evoked responses, and symptomology assessment are all useful in describing parts of TBI. The best approach is likely a multitest protocol to identify and diagnose the diffuse patterns of mild bTBI.

Acknowledgements

The authors acknowledge with gratitude the expert assistance rendered by Ms. Nicole Draghic.

Disclaimer

The opinions expressed herein belong solely to the authors. They do not and should not be interpreted as being those of, representative of, or endorsed by the Uniformed Services University of the Health Sciences, the Department of Defense, or any other agency of the US government.

Disclosures

The authors report no financial disclosures relevant to this work.

Author details

John Magnuson[1] and Geoffrey Ling[1,2,3]*

*Address all correspondence to: geoffrey.ling@usuhs.edu

1 Department of Neurology, Uniformed Services University of the Health Sciences, Bethesda, MD, United States

2 Inova Neuroscience and Spine Institute, Inova Fairfax Hospital, Fairfax, VA, United States

3 Department of Neurology, Johns Hopkins Medical Institutions, Baltimore, MD, United States

References

[1] Defense Casualty Analysis System. U.S. Military Casualties - OCO Casualty Summary by Casualty Type. 2016. https://www.dmdc.osd.mil/dcas/pages/report_sum_reason.xhtml

[2] Goldberg MS. Death and injury rates of U.S. military personnel in Iraq. Military Medicine. 2010;**175**:220-226

[3] Defense Casualty Analysis System. U.S. Military Casualties - Korean War Casualty Summary. 2016. https://www.dmdc.osd.mil/dcas/pages/report_korea_sum.xhtml

[4] Defense Casualty Analysis System. U.S. Military Casualties - Vietnam Conflict Casualty Summary. 2016. https://www.dmdc.osd.mil/dcas/pages/report_vietnam_sum.xhtml

[5] Banti M, Walter J, Hudak S, Soderdahl D. Improvised explosive device-related lower genitourinary trauma in current overseas combat operations. The Journal of Trauma and Acute Care Surgery. 2016;**80**:131-134

[6] Eastridge BJ, Mabry RL, Seguin P, Cantrell J, Tops T, et al. Death on the battlefield (2001-2011): implications for the future of combat casualty care. The Journal of Trauma and Acute Care Surgery. 2012;**73**:S431-S437

[7] Ling G, Bandak F, Armonda R, Grant G, Ecklund J. Explosive blast neurotrauma. Journal of Neurotrauma. 2009;**26**:815-825

[8] Defense and Veterans Brain Injury Center (DVBIC). DoD WorldwideTBI Numbers 2000-2016. Q1-Q2. http://dvbic.dcoe.mil/dod-worldwide-numbers-tbi

[9] Barzilai L, Harats M, Wiser I, Weissman O, Domniz N, et al. Characteristics of Improvised Explosive Device Trauma Casualties in the Gaza Strip and Other Combat Regions: The Israeli Experience. Wounds: A Compendium of Clinical Research and Practice. 2015;**27**:209-214

[10] de Lanerolle NC, Kim JH, Bandak FA. Neuropathology of traumatic brain injury: comparison of penetrating, nonpenetrating direct impact and explosive blast etiologies. Seminars in Neurology. 2015;**35**:12-19

[11] Ling G, Ecklund JM, Bandak FA. Brain injury from explosive blast: description and clinical management. Handbook of Clinical Neurology. 2015;**127**:173-180

[12] Magnuson J, Leonessa F, Ling GS. Neuropathology of explosive blast traumatic brain injury. Current Neurology and Neuroscience Reports. 2012;**12**:570-579

[13] de Candole CA. Blast injury. Canadian Medical Association Journal. 1967;**96**:207-214

[14] Department of Defense. Medical Research for Prevention, Mitigation, and Treatment of Blast Injuries. ed. Do Defense. US Department of Defense Blast Injury Research Program 2006. p. 10

[15] Feng K, Zhang L, Jin X, Chen C, Kallakuri S, et al. Biomechanical responses of the brain in swine subject to free-field blasts. Frontiers in Neurology. 2016;**7**:179

[16] Nakagawa A, Manley GT, Gean AD, Ohtani K, Armonda R, et al. Mechanisms of primary blast-induced traumatic brain injury: Insights from shock-wave research. Journal of Neurotrauma. 2011;**28**:1101-1119

[17] CDC. Explosions and Blast Injuries: A Primer for Clinicians. Atlanta, GA: Centers for Disease Control and Prevention; 2006

[18] The Management of Concussion/mTBI Working Group. VA/DoD Clinical Practice Guidelines For Management of Concussion/mild Traumatic Brain Injury. 2009. http://www.healthquality.va.gov/guidelines/Rehab/mtbi/concussion_mtbi_full_1_0.pdf

[19] Giza CC, Kutcher JS, Ashwal S, Barth J, Getchius TS, et al. Summary of evidence-based guideline update: evaluation and management of concussion in sports: Report of the Guideline Development Subcommittee of the American Academy of Neurology. Neurology. 2013;80:2250-2257

[20] Ling G, Maher C. U.S. neurologists in Iraq: Personal perspective. Neurology. 2006;67:14-17

[21] Bigler ED. Neuropsychology and clinical neuroscience of persistent post-concussive syndrome. Journal of the International Neuropsychological Society : JINS. 2008;14:1-22

[22] Franke LM, Czarnota JN, Ketchum JM, Walker WC. Factor analysis of persistent post-concussive symptoms within a military sample with blast exposure. The Journal of Head Trauma Rehabilitation. 2015;30:E34-E46

[23] Davenport ND, Lim KO, Sponheim SR. Personality and neuroimaging measures differentiate PTSD from mTBI in veterans. Brain Imaging and Behavior. 2015;9:472-483

[24] American Psychiatric Publishing. American Psychiatric Association: Diagnostic and Statistical Manual of Mental Disorders. Arlington, VA: American Psychiatric Association; 2013. pp. 271-272 2 pp

[25] Tate DF, York GE, Reid MW, Cooper DB, Jones L, et al. Preliminary findings of cortical thickness abnormalities in blast injured service members and their relationship to clinical findings. Brain Imaging and Behavior. 2014;8:102-109

[26] Michael AP, Stout J, Roskos PT, Bolzenius J, Gfeller J, et al. Evaluation of cortical thickness after traumatic brain injury in military veterans. Journal of Neurotrauma. 2015;32:1751-1758

[27] Adam O, Mac Donald CL, Rivet D, Ritter J, May T, et al. Clinical and imaging assessment of acute combat mild traumatic brain injury in Afghanistan. Neurology. 2015;85:219-227

[28] Davenport ND, Lim KO, Armstrong MT, Sponheim SR. Diffuse and spatially variable white matter disruptions are associated with blast-related mild traumatic brain injury. NeuroImage. 2012;59:2017-2024

[29] Mac Donald CL, Johnson AM, Cooper D, Nelson EC, Werner NJ, et al. Detection of blast-related traumatic brain injury in U.S. military personnel. The New England Journal of Medicine. 2011;364:2091-2100

[30] Yeh PH, Wang B, Oakes TR, French LM, Pan H, et al. Postconcussional disorder and PTSD symptoms of military-related traumatic brain injury associated with compromised neurocircuitry. Human Brain Mapping. 2014;35:2652-2673

[31] Willer BS, Leddy JJ. Time to change from a symptom-based concussion assessment to a structured physical examination. Academic Emergency Medicine: Official Journal of the Society for Academic Emergency Medicine. 2016;**23**:495-496

[32] Bressler S, Goldberg H, Shinn-Cunningham B. Sensory coding and cognitive processing of sound in Veterans with blast exposure. Hearing Research. 2017;**349**:98-110

[33] Rombaux P, Mouraux A, Bertrand B, Guerit JM, Hummel T. Assessment of olfactory and trigeminal function using chemosensory event-related potentials. Neurophysiologie Clinique. 2006;**36**:53-62

7

Perfusion Computed Tomography in Traumatic Brain Injury

Cino Bendinelli, Shannon Cooper, Christian Abel,
Andrew Bivard and Zsolt J. Balogh

Abstract

Introduction: Almost 50 years ago, computed tomography (CT) revolutionized the management of traumatic brain injury (TBI) by imagining intracranial hematomas. This allowed prompt and accurate selection of patients who would benefit from surgical evacuation. Since then, unenhanced CT has been the gold standard imaging modality for patients with acute TBI. Today, multidetector CT can track intravenous contrasts flowing through brain creating maps that depict the speed and the amount of blood at capillary level. This imaging modality takes the name of perfusion CT. Perfusion CT is routinely used during the hyperacute phase of patients suffering from stroke to diagnose areas of penumbra (poorly perfused but still viable brain tissue) that may benefit from revascularization. Here, we summarize the current status of the research on the role of perfusion CT in patients suffering from TBI.

Methods: Inclusive literature research conducted on PubMed using the keywords "perfusion," "computed tomography" and "traumatic brain injury." Only articles published in English were considered for this review.

Conclusion: With a minimal logistic effort, perfusion CT provides clinicians with a multitude of additional information. Most patients with TBI show altered perfusion patterns. The maps generated with perfusion CT can predict the final size of cerebral contusions better than unenhanced CT. These maps can be used to clarify the status of brain autoregulation and possibly guide targeted therapies for intracranial hypertension. The integrity of the blood–brain barrier can also be evaluated with this technology and this might be crucial to predict and treat brain edema. Furthermore, perfusion maps can help physician to promptly and accurately predict the long-term functional outcomes of patients suffering from both mild and severe TBI.

Keywords: perfusion CT, severe traumatic brain injury, neuroimaging
Subject area: neuroimaging in traumatic brain injury

1. Introduction

Traumatic brain injury (TBI) remains a major cause of death and disability [1]. The heterogeneity of TBI is considered to be a one of the most significant obstacles to the development of effective therapeutic interventions [2, 3]. Physicians in order to understand, treat and prognosticate patients suffering from TBI do rely mainly on three parameters: [1] the Glasgow Coma Scale (GCS) is a rapid and reproducible test, which assesses overall neurologic function; [2] the unenhanced CT findings, which can detect skull fractures, hematomas, cerebral contusions and some indirect sign of brain swelling (i.e., ventricles size, midline shift, uncal herniation); [3] the intracerebral pressure (ICP) monitoring, which requires a quite invasive intracerebral or intraventricular probe, to calculate and help maintaining adequate cerebral perfusion pressure (CPP) [2–10]. This information routinely utilized in clinical management algorithms tend to compromise accuracy for simplicity and suffer from several weaknesses. For example, all patients with GCS below nine will be diagnosed as having a severe degree of TBI and, as such, will be admitted to intensive care intubated and pharmacologically sedated. Instead, patients with GCS higher than nine are most often discharged home or admitted to low intensity wards (especially if screening unenhanced CT appears normal). But GCS can also be affected by drug/alcohol assumption, and by systemic hypoperfusion making decision based on GCS alone often inaccurate [5]. Similarly unenhanced CT, despite its status of "gold standard imaging" for acute TBI, deprives clinicians from crucial information on brain tissue vascularity, perfusion and viability. Unenhanced CT underestimates the ultimate size of parenchymal lesions and does not afford insight into secondary ischemic injuries related to systemic hypotension, traumatic cerebral edema and intracranial hypertension [8]. Lastly, the clinical use of ICP monitors in patients at risk of brain swelling, which is often burdened by complications from its invasiveness, can often only provide an inaccurate reading. Calculating CPP using ICP and mean systemic arterial pressure (MAP) does not take into account cerebral vasculature autoregulation or cerebral regional differences often observed with more advanced technology [9, 10]. The efficacy of ICP monitoring-based treatment has been recently challenged in a large-scale randomized trial on more than 300 severe TBI patients. It appeared that ICP-based treatment (focused on maintaining ICP < 20 mmHg) was not superior to that based on imaging and clinical examinations alone in terms of survival and functional outcome [9].

It is of no wonder that these three pillars of TBI management have come under scrutiny recently, making sensible and grounded clinical decisions based on these limited and biased information alone resemble a dangerous gamble. As a possible result, most interventional studies investigating otherwise sensible therapeutic options have failed to identify successful treatments [4].

In terms of imaging, several relatively new technologies are available to better understand the complexity of TBI. Many are still research tools; some require long acquisition times and some others are poorly available and/or logistically difficult to organize in critically ill ventilated patients. Perfusion CT instead is a not logistically demanding imaging technique that provides detailed maps of intracerebral vascular flow and brain tissue perfusion and affords direct insight into cerebral infarct and penumbra. Today, perfusion CT is routinely used in the early care of patients with acute stroke and other cerebrovascular disorders [11].

The aim of this chapter is to evaluate potential benefits and limitation of perfusion CT as advanced diagnostic modality for patients suffering from TBI. Specifically, we overview the technical aspects, present published research and try to predict the future role of this diagnostic approach in patients suffering from TBI.

2. Description of perfusion CT technology

Several advanced imaging techniques exist, which can provide information about cerebral perfusion, such as stable xenon-enhanced CT (Xe-CT), single photon emission CT (SPECT) and perfusion-weighted magnetic resonance imaging (MRI) [12]. These techniques have logistic barriers to routine universal clinical use as they require specialized equipment and staffing and are burdened by long acquisition times [12]. Some, such as the 33% xenon mix used in Xe-CT that causes transitory ICP raise, can also be deleterious for patients [13]. These constrains are particularly relevant during the acute phase of severe TBI; when patients, often seriously injured polytrauma patients are intubated and ventilated, with ongoing needs for blood transfusions, vasoconstrictors. These patients need prompt and straightforward imaging to guide subsequent therapeutic options. Perfusion CT provides information about brain circulation and cerebral perfusion which can be obtained rapidly using wildly diffuse multidetector CT scanners [11, 14]. A perfusion CT can be obtained in few minutes utilizing a standard of care (more so in trauma centers) multidetector CT scanners (and dedicated post processing software) and does not require specialized technologists. The effective dose of ionizing radiation required for a head perfusion CT is about 5 mSv. The radiation-associated risks are believed to be low and approximately equivalent to about 2 years of background radiation [equates to an excess lifetime cancer risk = 0.025% (about 1:4000)] [15].

Acquisition of perfusion CT involves the administration of intravenous iodine contrast with concurrent acquisition of images using a helical CT multidetector scanner in cine mode. This allows for measurement of the movement of contrast material through the vessels and tissues over time. Perfusion data are obtained by monitoring the first pass of a contrast material bolus through the cerebral vessels. The relationship between the contrast agent concentration and attenuation can be used to calculate the amount of contrast agent in a region. Time versus contrast concentration curves are generated for a reference arterial region and venous region as well as each pixel of the scan [11, 15]. Post processing of the data allows the generation of color coded maps and quantification of the perfusion parameters of cerebral blood flow (CBF), cerebral blood volume (CBV) and mean transit time (MTT) [16]. The CBF for each area is calculated as CBV/MTT. CBF is measured in milliliters per 100 g of tissue per minute (ml/100 g/min), and normal tissue has values around 40 ml/100 g/min while values of 20 ml/100 g/min or less are diagnostic for ischemia. The CBV is calculated as the area under the curve in a parenchymal pixel divided by the area under the curve in the reference venous pixel. CBV is measured in

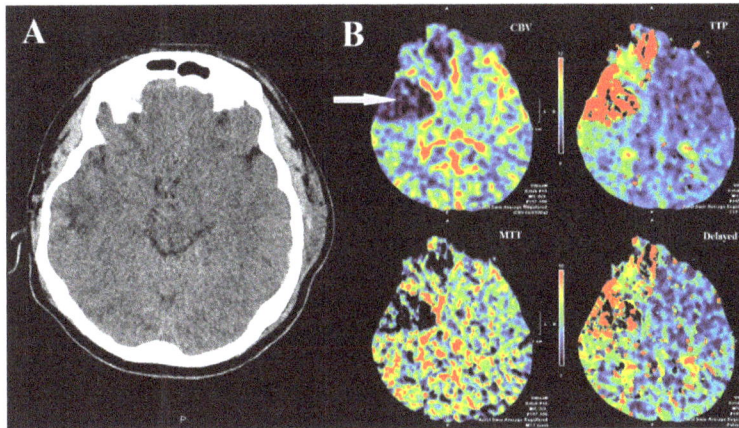

Figure 1. Axial computed tomography (CT) obtained 18 h from admission following a motor vehicle accident in a young male. (A) Noncontrast CT shows a left subgaleal hematoma, but no intracranial pathology. (B) Perfusion CT identifies an area of reduced perfusion on the right temporo-frontal lobe (white arrow): Cerebral blood volume (CBV) is reduced as per darker color, time-to-peak (TTP) is increased as per lighter color, and mean transient time (MTT) is decreased as per darker color. The axial image on the bottom right represents the delayed phase (which can be utilized by specific software to extrapolate permeability of brain–blood barrier).

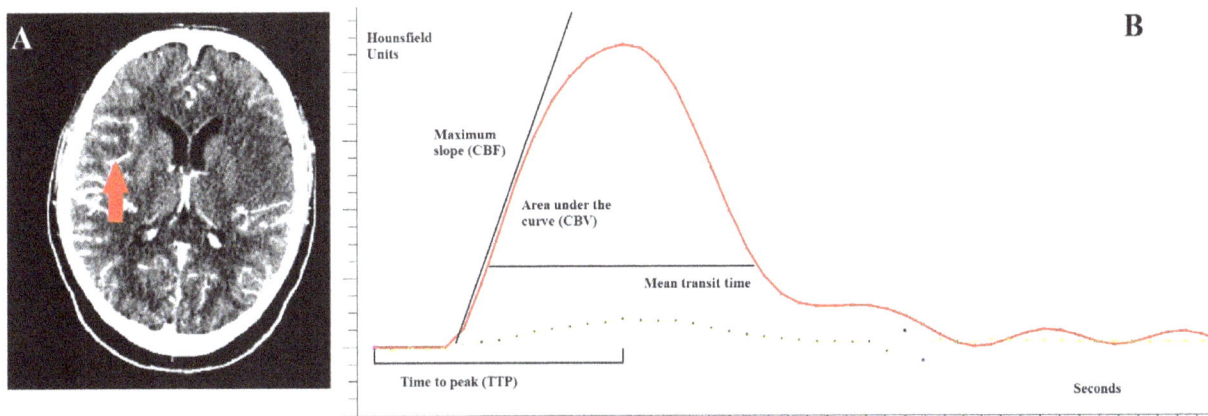

Figure 2. (A) An arterial input function (AIF, arrow on the axial CT scan) is used to calibrate the whole brain contrast change when post processing a CT perfusion. (B) the drawing depicts the rise and fall of the contrast over time (in seconds). The time from the start of the scan to the peak signal intensity is the time-to-peak (TTP); the maximum slope of the contrast enhancement being measured is the cerebral blood flow (CBF); and the area under the curve of the whole AIF is the cerebral blood volume (CBV). The time it takes for contrast to enter and leave the voxel is the mean transit time (MTT).

milliliters per 100 g of tissue (ml/100 g) and normal tissue has values around 4 ml/100 g, while values of 2 ml/100 g are indicative for a degree of ischemia. MTT is the average time taken by blood to cross the capillary network and is calculated from a deconvolution operation from the time concentration curve of each particular voxel and the arterial reference region. MTT is measured in seconds, and normal tissue has values around 5 s while values above 8 s are the rule in ischemic areas [11]. Perfusion CT thus provides a readily available means of examining brain perfusion and, by calculating MTT, CBV and CBF for different areas, can identify areas of abnormal perfusion and ischemia (**Figures 1** and **2**).

3. Perfusion CT and traumatic brain injury

Perfusion CT has revolutionized the diagnostic and therapeutic approach to acute ischemic stroke [17]. The prompt availability of perfusion maps and CT angiogram has transformed an irreversible condition requiring only supportive care and rehabilitation to a treatable neurological emergency. Neurologists use perfusion CT maps to define areas of ischemic penumbra and guide decisions on thrombolytic therapy [17]. As such, perfusion CT has now a well-established role in the acute management of stroke.

The potential role for perfusion CT in the management of TBI is still under investigation. A literature research including the terms "traumatic brain injury" and "perfusion CT" or "perfusion computed tomography" returned 185 results. Critical screening of the abstracts selected 18 papers that were considered as pertinent and relevant to this review and therefore they were analyzed and discussed in detail [16, 18–33]. **Table 1** illustrates the studies' characteristics and main findings. It appears that the published experience with perfusion CT in patients suffering from TBI is quite limited with a total of 540 patients investigated. Only three papers, including a total of 50 patients, were prospectively designed [24, 31, 33]. Almost all papers

First author, journal, year	Patients	Severity of TBI	Timing of CTP	Covered cerebral tissue	Studies' main findings
Wintermark [18] Radiology, 2004	130	Severe TBI	Admission	2 × 10 mm thick sections	Outcome prognostication Predicts raised ICP
Wintermark [19] Crit Care Med, 2004	42 subgroup [18]	Severe TBI and ICP monitor	Admission follow-up	2 × 10 mm thick sections	Correlation between CPP and CTP diagnose preserved or impaired autoregulation
Soustiel [20] Neuroradiology, 2008	30	Severe TBI and cerebral contusion	Within 48 h	4 × 6 mm thick sections	CBV maps depict pericontusion penumbra that later results in necrosis
Metting [21] Ann Neurol 2009	76	Mild TBI with normal CT	Admission	2 × 14 mm thick sections	Decreased CBF and CBV in frontal regions is associated with worse functional outcome
Escudero [16] Neurocrit Care, 2009	26	TBI or cardiac arrest	Unknown	4 × 8 mm thick sections	CTP can confirm brain death
Huang [22] J Trauma, 2011	22	Contusion on unenhanced CT	Admission	Not specified	Contrast extravasation predicts hemorrhage progression
Bendinelli [23] Injury, 2013	30 subgroup [31]	Severe TBI	Within 48 h	Whole brain 5-mm thick sections	CTP provided additional diagnostic information in 60% of patients

First author, journal, year	Patients	Severity of TBI	Timing of CTP	Covered cerebral tissue	Studies' main findings
Metting [24] PLoS One, 2013	18	Mild TBI with normal CT	Admission	2 × 14 mm thick section	CTP maps can predict brain dysfunction
Sarubbo [25] Neurorad, 2014	6	Cranioplasty after craniectomy	Before and after	Not specified	Cortical perfusion progressively declines after craniectomy
Wen [26] Brain In, (2015)	9	Cranioplasty after craniectomy	Before and after	Not specified	Cranioplasty increases CBF
Honda [27] Neurol Med, 2015	90	Severe TBI	Not specified	50-mm thick section	Higher CBF and lower MTT predictive for improved functional outcome
Jungner [28] Minerva Anest, 2016	17	Severe TBI or cerebral contusion	24 h	Whole brain 5-mm thick sections	Tracer extravasation shows altered blood–brain barrier around contusion
Trofimov [29] Adv Exp Med, 2016	25	Dishomogenous TBI patients	Not specified	Single 32 mm section	Positive correlation between cerebral oxygen saturation and CBV in frontal lobe
Songara [30] W Neurosurg, 2016	8	Cranioplasty after craniectomy	Before and after	Unclear	Brain perfusion improvement after cranioplasty
Bendinelli [31] W J Surg, 2017	50	Severe TBI	Within 48 h	Whole brain 5-mm thick sections	Perfusion abnormalities predict poor functional outcome at 6 months
Honda [32] Neurocrit Care, 2017	25	Severe TBI with ICP monitor	Within 7 days	Single slice	Cerebral perfusion disturbance when ICP >20 mmHg
Cooper [33] Injury, (submitted)	28 subgroup [31]	Severe TBI with ICP monitor	Within 48 h	Whole brain 5-mm thick sections	Perfusion disturbance predicts therapeutic requirement for intracerebral hypertension

Table 1. Studies published in English on the use of perfusion CT in patients with traumatic brain injury (in chronologic order of publication).

obtained a perfusion CT on admission following the standard of care unenhanced brain CT [18, 19, 21, 22, 24], while some timed the perfusion CT at the time of the first follow-up unenhanced CT [24, 31, 33], and two just before and after cranioplasty [25, 26]. Patients with severe TBI were most often investigated, with only one group investigating a total of 94 patients suffering from mild to moderate TBI [21, 24]. Most studies report perfusion CT maps produced using 64-slice multidetector CT scanner, which are limited to a small portion of the brain (usually two or four adjacent slabs taken just above the orbit), while a few and more recent papers benefited from technology improvements (320-slice CT scanner) and investigated the whole brain [23, 28, 31, 33].

4. Outcome prediction

Several authors have investigated the role of perfusion CT to help functional outcome prediction in the heterogeneous population of patients suffering TBI. Wintermark et al. investigated with perfusion CT performed at admission a consecutive series of 130 patients with severe TBI (following standard unenhanced CT). The perfusion maps, specifically the number of arterial territories with oligemia (reduced regional CBV and CBF but not to the severity of ischemia), predicted poor functional outcome at 3 months, while hyperemia (increased regional CBV and CBF) was associated with a favorable functional outcome [18]. The subcohort of these patients who received an ICP monitor were presented in a subsequent study: perfusion parameters were correlated with CPP allowing to discriminate between patients with preserved or disrupted vascular autoregulation, and this was associated with functional outcome at 3-month follow-up [19].

A prospectively designed study aimed at investigating the relationship between whole brain perfusion CT and functional outcome [31]. Fifty patients with severe TBI and who required follow-up unenhanced CT within 48 h from admission (the design selected the sickest TBI patients, excluding those whose neurology improved quickly, and did not require follow-up imaging) were examined with whole brain perfusion CT. This was a selected severe TBI population burdened by high (14%) mortality, and the perfusion maps were found to be often (67%) abnormal with areas of ischemia in 35% of patients. Poor functional outcome (defined as a Glasgow outcome scale-extended of four or less at 6-month follow-up) occurred to more than half of the population and was best predicted by perfusion CT findings. Logistic regression analysis showed that, among the most commonly used parameters used for outcome prognostication, preintubation GCS was a moderate predictor (AUC = 0.74), thus confirming several prior studies, but the inclusion of perfusion CT variables (specifically the presence of abnormal findings) in the model improved the performance of the prediction model to AUC = 0.92 [31]. Similarly, a study on 90 patients with severe TBI investigated with Xe-CT and perfusion CT confirmed that perfusion abnormalities (specifically low CBF and high MTT) were predictive for poor functional outcome [32].

Furthermore, overall absence of CBF has helped a prompt diagnosis of brain death as demonstrated in a study on 27 patients investigated with perfusion CT and CT angiogram [16].

The role of perfusion CT in outcome prediction of patients with mild-to-moderate TBI has been investigated by the van der Naalt group [21, 24]. In 76 patients with mild TBI and normal unenhanced CT, a perfusion CT was obtained on admission. Perfusion maps with decreased CBF and CBV in the frontal and occipital gray matter were associated on logistic regression analysis with a poorer functional outcome at 6-month follow-up [21]. Furthermore, when compared to the healthy controls, patients with post-traumatic amnesia were found to have reduced CBF in frontal gray matter and caudate nucleus [24]. Similarly, when neuropsychological tests were obtained in a subgroup of these patients, reduced perfusion of the frontal and parietotemporal regions was associated with impairment in executive functioning and emotion [24].

Taken together, these studies suggest a potential role for perfusion CT in early prediction of functional outcome in both the severe and less severe TBI population. These promising results are burdened by the limited experience but are consistent with similar previous studies, which utilized Xe-CT to prove the concept that an insight in cerebral circulation allows a more accurate functional outcome prediction [34, 35].

5. Perfusion CT and cerebral contusion

The role of perfusion CT in patients with cerebral contusions has been investigated by Soustiel et al. [20]. In this retrospective study on 30 patients, perfusion maps obtained 48 hours from injury predicted contusions progression better than unenhanced CT. Specifically, areas of hypoperfusion around the contusions resulted in areas of brain necrosis at follow-up unenhanced CT (CBV-derived maps showed congruence with the unenhanced CT at 7 days in 60% of lesions). This small study confirms the presence of a degree of ischemia around cerebral contusion (a regional secondary brain injury), which without perfusion CT would run completely undiagnosed till fully established and irreversible, and therefore, visible on unenhanced CT. Although not investigated in this study, it is foreseeable that overall intracerebral pressures (as measured by an ICP monitor) would be completely normal in these patients as the remaining brain adapts to the localized swelling. This kind of findings is exactly what physicians treating TBI patient need in order to craft appropriate and individualized therapeutic options. For example, in a recent study on 22 TBI patients with cerebral contusions, who were investigated acutely with contrast-enhanced CT and perfusion CT, the presence of contrast extravasation (identified in 40%) was predictive for hemorrhage progression [22]. Usually, hemorrhage progressions are otherwise diagnosed either by observing increased ICP (if monitored) or worsening GCS (if not three already) or by scheduling follow-up unenhanced CT (which may cause deleterious delays to diagnosis and treatment).

6. Cerebral perfusion pressure and perfusion CT

Wintermark et al. [19], in a subgroup of the previously mentioned severe TBI patients, studied the correlation between invasive ICP, CPP and perfusion CT findings. About 60% of patients were shown to have a weak dependence between CBF and corresponding CPP values (most likely due to preserved autoregulation), while the rest of the patients showed a strong dependence between CPP and CBF (disrupted autoregulation group). The relationship between perfusion CT findings and invasive ICP and calculated CPP has been more recently investigated by Honda et al. [27]. The perfusion maps of 25 patients with severe TBI and ICP monitor were obtained with combination of Xe-CT and perfusion CT. The CPP values were positively correlated with CBF, negatively correlated with MTT and did not correlate with CBV. If this well reflects the expected physiology and Monro-Kellie hypothesis, it is interesting to notice that the correlation between CPP and CBF was disturbed by intracerebral hypertension (defined as ICP above 20 mmHg). In patients without intracerebral hypertension, CBF values did not correlate with CPP (preserved autoregulation), while in patients with cerebral hypertension, the CBF negatively correlated with the CPP value (disrupted autoregulation). In our experience, with 28 patients with severe TBI and ICP monitor investigated with perfusion CT within 48 h from trauma, the presence of abnormalities on perfusion maps (specifically, the presence of ischemia) was associated with the requirement for increased level of intervention for cerebral hypertension [33]. Two small studies investigated the functional outcomes before and after cranioplasty in patients suffering from severe TBI treated with decompressive craniectomy. An improvement of neurocognitive functions was observed after cranioplasty (especially if done within 3 months from trauma). Interestingly, serial perfusion CTs (performed in a subgroup of nine patients) also confirmed an improvement in cerebral perfusion in both the operated and the contralateral side [26, 30].

It certainly appears that we have a very limited understanding of the degree and location of perfusion abnormalities and that we do not know how to act once these are identified and quantified; it also appears that physicians tend to treat severe TBI patients and their CPP very homogenously despite quite obvious differences in autoregulation mechanisms and degree of hypoperfusion and ischemia. These interesting studies, albeit preliminary, certainly suggest a potential crucial role for perfusion CT. Perfusion maps will clarify almost real time the extent and the degree of perfusion deficits and the association with MAP and CPP. This will help physicians to diagnose disrupted autoregulation and predicting patients who will benefit from ICP monitors and aggressive treatment of cerebral hypertension.

7. Cerebral oxygen saturation and perfusion CT

The relationship between cerebral oxygen saturation and brain perfusion maps has been investigated in a heterogeneous cohort of patients with a degree of TBI ranging from severe to moderate [29]. The authors obtained perfusion maps using single slice technology and compared with frontal cerebral oximetry in 25 patients (16 with cerebral ischemia on perfusion CT maps). A proportional dependence was observed between cerebral tissue oxygenation and CBV, but not with CBF and MTT. Possibly, vasospasm and cerebral autoregulation were responsible for the lack of maintained relationship between cerebral oxygenation and CBF (which should otherwise be observed considering that CBF=CBV/MTT) [29].

8. Cerebral permeability perfusion CT

When the blood–brain barrier is altered, contrast material extravasation can be observed during the delayed phase of perfusion CT. This has been observed in stroke patients and recently in a small study of TBI patients. Seventeen patients with severe TBI and three controls were investigated with perfusion CT within 48 h from admission. Increased permeability was observed in the pericontusional area in patients who later developed increased ICP [28]. This is extremely relevant as small molecular permeability will influence capillary hydrostatic and oncotic pressures and influence edema development. Possibly, osmotic treatment (such as hypertonic saline) might be efficient only when all or most of the brain has an intact blood–brain barrier. The implications of understanding and diagnosing blood–brain barrier dysfunction are huge. Potentially perfusion CT might help selecting patients for osmotic therapy rather than the use of sedation agents and/or craniectomy.

9. Future of perfusion CT

The routine imaging protocol for multiple injured trauma patients includes an unenhanced cerebral and cervical CT and an enhanced thoracic-abdominal-pelvic CT. Routinely, also patients with risk factors for cerebrovascular injuries (deceleration, seatbelt mark on the neck, massive facial bleeding) will have the neck and cerebral vasculature evaluated by enhanced CT. Early detection of cerebrovascular injuries is crucial as these arterial injuries can be repaired, stented or otherwise medically treated to minimize the risk or the extent of embolic strokes. We can foresee a near future in which brain perfusion CT becomes part of admission imaging for patients with TBI. The prompt availability of brain perfusion maps might have a huge impact on understanding and treating TBI. With or without the involvement of neurologist and interventional neurologist, these patients might be offered a better targeted treatment and their families are made aware of long-term outcomes by making decisions such as palliation or further treatment based on a more thorough understanding of cerebral perfusion and secondary brain injury.

10. Conclusion

In this chapter, we have identified, reviewed and discussed several aspects of implementation of perfusion CT in clinical diagnostics and research of TBI disease. These include assessment of TBI pathogenesis and prediction of functional outcomes, development of guidance for osmotic treatment, selection of patients for trial inclusion and development of regiments for surgical intervention. Perfusion CT imaging is a technology readily available and ripe for use in the vast majority of patients suffering from TBI. Perfusion CT should be considered in the context of audited research in patients with clinically proven severe TBI and possibly in patients with a less severe degree of TBI. Evidently, perfusion CT possesses eminent potentials and demonstrates a superior efficacy when compared to traditional noncontrast CT.

Author details

Cino Bendinelli[1], Shannon Cooper[1], Christian Abel[1], Andrew Bivard[2] and Zsolt J. Balogh[1]*

*Address all correspondence to: zsolt.balogh@hnehealth.nsw.gov.au

1 John Hunter Hospital, University of Newcastle, Newcastle, NSW, AU

2 Hunter Medical Research Institute, University of Newcastle, Newcastle, NSW, AU

References

[1] Evans JA, van Wessem KJ, McDougall D, Lee KA, Lyons T, Balogh ZJ. Epidemiology of traumatic deaths: Comprehensive population-based assessment. World Journal of Surgery. 2010;**34**:158-163

[2] Brain Trauma Foundation, American Association of Neurological Surgeons, Congress of Neurological Surgeons. Guidelines for the management of severe traumatic brain injury. Journal of Neurotrauma. 2007;**24**:S1-106

[3] Haddad SH, Arabi YM. Critical care management of severe traumatic brain injury in adults. Scandinavian Journal of Trauma, Resuscitation and Emergency. 2012;**20**:15

[4] Carney N, Totten AM, O'Reilly C, Ullman JS, Hawryluk GWJ, Bell MJ, et al. Guidelines for the management of severe traumatic brain injury, fourth edition. Neurosurgery. 2017;**80**:6-15

[5] Foreman BP, Caesar R, Parks J, Madden C, Gentilello LM, Shafi S, et al. Usefulness of the abbreviated injury score and the injury severity score in comparison to the Glasgow coma scale in predicting outcome after traumatic brain injury. Journal of Trauma. 2007;**62**:946-950

[6] Kubal WS. Updated imaging of traumatic brain injury. Radiology Clinics of North America. 2012;**50**:15-41

[7] Yuh EL, Cooper SR, Ferguson AR, Manley GT. Quantitative CT improves outcome prediction in acute traumatic brain injury. Journal of Neurotrauma. 2012;**29**:735-746

[8] Jacobs B, Beems T, van der Vliet TM, van Vugt AB, Hoedemaekers C, Horn J, et al. Outcome prediction in moderate and severe traumatic brain injury: A focus on computed tomography variables. Neurocritic Care. 2013;**19**:79-89

[9] Chesnut RM, Temkin N, Carney N, Dikmen S, Rondina C, Videtta W, et al. A trial of intracranial-pressure monitoring in traumatic brain injury. New England Journal of Medicine. 2012;**367**:2471-2481

[10] Shen L, Wang Z, Su Z, Qiu S, Xu J, Zhou Y, et al. Effects of intracranial pressure monitoring on mortality in patients with severe traumatic brain injury: A meta-analysis. PLoS One. 2016:111-115

[11] Huang AP, Tsai JC, Kuo LT, Lee CW, Lai HS, Tsai LK, Huang SJ, Chen CM, Chen YS, Chuang HY, Wintermark M. Clinical application of perfusion computed tomography in neurosurgery. Journal of Neurosurgery. 2014;**120**:473-488

[12] Wintermark M, Sanelli PC, Anzai Y, Tsiouris AJ, Whitlow CT. Imaging evidence and recommendations for traumatic brain injury: Advanced neuro- and neurovascular imaging techniques. AJNR American Journal of Neuroradiology. 2015;**36**:E1-E11

[13] Plougmann J, Astrup J, Pedersen J, Gyldensted C. Effect of stable xenon inhalation on intracranial pressure during measurement of cerebral blood flow in head injury. Journal of Neurosurgery. 1994;**81**:822-828

[14] Metting Z, Rodiger LA, Keyser JD, Jvd N. Structural and functional neuroimaging in mild-to-moderate head injury. Lancet Neurology. 2007;**6**:699-710

[15] Shankar JJS, Lum C, Sharma M. Whole-brain perfusion imaging with 320-MDCT scanner: Reducing radiation dose by increasing sampling interval. American Journal of Roentgenology. 2010;**195**:1183-1186

[16] Escudero D, Otero J, Marqués L, Parra D, Gonzalo JA, Albaiceta GM, Cofiño L, Blanco A, Vega P, Murias E, Meilan A, Roger RL, Taboada F. Diagnosing brain death by CT perfusion and multislice CT angiography. Neurocritical Care. 2009;**11**:261-271

[17] Bivard A, Levi C, Krishnamurthy V, McElduff P, Miteff F, Spratt NJ, Bateman G, Donnan G, Davis S, Parsons M. Perfusion computed tomography to assist decision making for stroke thrombolysis. Brain. 2015;**138**:1919-1931

[18] Wintermark M, Gv M, Schnyder P, Revelly J-P, Porchet F, Regali L, et al. Admission perfusion CT: Prognostic value in patients with severe head trauma. Radiology. 2004;**232**:211-220

[19] Wintermark M, Chiolero R, Melle Gv, Revelly JP, Porchet F, Regali L, et al. Relationship between brain perfusion computed tomography variables and cerebral perfusion pressure in severe head trauma patients. Critical Care Medicine. 2004;**32**:1579-1587

[20] Soustiel JF, Mahamid E, Goldsher D, Zaaroor M. Perfusion-CT for early assessment of traumatic cerebral contusions. Neuroradiology. 2008;**50**:189-196

[21] Metting Z, Rodiger LA, Stewart RE, Oudkerk M, Keyser JD, Naalt Jvd. Perfusion computed tomography in the acute phase of mild head injury: Regional dysfunction and prognostic value. Annals of Neurology. 2009;**66**:809-816

[22] Huang AP, Lee CW, Hsieh HJ, Yang CC, Tsai YH, Tsuang FY, Kuo LT, Chen YS, YK T, Huang SJ, Liu HM, Tsai JC. Early parenchymal contrast extravasation predicts subsequent hemorrhage progression, clinical deterioration, and need for surgery in patients with traumatic cerebral contusion. The Journal of Trauma and Acute Care Surgery. 2011;**71**:1593-1599

[23] Bendinelli C, Bivard A, Nebauer S, Parsons MW, Balogh ZJ. Brain CT perfusion provides additional useful information in severe traumatic brain injury. Injury. 2013;**44**:1208-1212

[24] Metting Z1, Cerliani L, Rödiger LA, van der Naalt Jvd. Pathophysiological concepts in mild traumatic brain injury: Diffusion tensor imaging related to acute perfusion CT imaging. PLoS One. 2013;**21**:8. 64461

[25] Sarubbo S, Latini F, Ceruti S, Chieregato A, d'Esterre C, Lee TY, Cavallo M, Fainardi E. Temporal changes in CT perfusion values before and after cranioplasty in patients without symptoms related to external decompression: A pilot study. Neuroradiology. 2014;**56**: 237-234

[26] Wen L, Lou HY, Xu J, Wang H, Huang X, Gong JB, Xiong B, Yang XF. The impact of cranioplasty on cerebral blood perfusion in patients treated with decompressive craniectomy for severe traumatic brain injury. Brain Injury. 2015;**29**:1654-1660

[27] Honda M, Ichibayashi R, Yokomuro H, Yoshihara K, Masuda H, Haga D, Seiki Y, Kudoh C, Kishi T. Early cerebral circulation disturbance in patients suffering from severe traumatic brain injury (TBI): A xenon CT and perfusion CT study. Neurologia Medico-Chirurgica (Tokyo). 2016;**56**:501-509

[28] Jungner M, Siemund R, Venturoli D, Reinstrup P, SCHALéN W, Bentzer P. Blood-brain barrier permeability following traumatic brain injury. Minerva Anestesiologica. 2016;**82**: 525-533

[29] Trofimov AO, Kalentiev G, Voennov O, Grigoryeva V. Comparison of cerebral oxygen saturation and cerebral perfusion computed tomography in cerebral blood flow in patients with brain injury. Advances in Experimental Medicine and Biology. 2016;**876**:145-149

[30] Songara A, Gupta R, Jain N, Rege S, Masand R. Early cranioplasty in patients with post-traumatic decompressive craniectomy and its correlation with changes in cerebral perfusion parameters and neurocognitive outcome. World Neurosurgery. 2016;**94**:303-308

[31] Bendinelli C, Cooper S, Evans T, Bivard A, Pacey D, Parsons M, Balough ZJ. Perfusion abnormalities are frequently detected by early CT perfusion and predict unfavourable outcome following severe traumatic brain injury. World Journal of Surgery. 2017

[32] Honda M, Ichibayashi R, Suzuki G, Yokomuro H, Seiki Y, Sase S, Kishi T. Consideration of the intracranial pressure threshold value for the initiation of traumatic brain injury treatment: A xenon CT and perfusion CT study. Neurocritical Care. 2017

[33] Shannon C, Bendinelli C, Bivard A, Parson M, Balogh Z. Brain perfusion disturbances predict therapeutic requirements for management of intracerebral hypertension. Injury (submitted for publication)

[34] Fridley J, Robertson C, Gopinath S. Quantitative lobar cerebral blood flow for outcome prediction after traumatic brain injury. Journal of Neurotrauma. 2015;**32**:75-82

[35] Kaloostian P, Robertson C, Gopinath SP, Stippler M, King CC, Qualls C, Yonas H, Nemoto EM. Outcome prediction within twelve hours after severe traumatic brain injury by quantitative cerebral blood flow. Journal of Neurotrauma. 2012;**29**:727-734

8

Metabolic Responses and Profiling of Bioorganic Phosphates and Phosphate Metabolites in Traumatic Brain Injury

Noam Naphatali Tal, Tesla Yudhistira,
Woo Hyun Lee, Youngsam Kim and
David G. Churchill

Abstract

This chapter constitutes a review of the recent literature on metabolic response and profiling of bioorganic phosphates and phosphate metabolites in disease related to traumatic brain injury (TBI). In this report we emphasize the emerging role of advanced imaging techniques in both the translational research of TBI biology and in the development of new modalities for the diagnosis and therapy of TBI-related diseases. To date, several neuroimaging techniques have been used for assessing phosphate metabolites related to TBI. These techniques include ^{31}P-MRI/MRS imaging, magnetic resonance imaging, and incorporation of phosphate derivative hydrogels, all of which are of particular interest in identifying TBI. These advanced neuroimaging techniques are currently under investigation in an attempt to optimize properties for therapeutics purposes. In addition, this chapter also discusses the role of endogenous and exogenous phosphates related to TBI. TBI imaging is a rapidly evolving field, and a number of the recommendations presented will be updated in the future to reflect the advances in medical knowledge.

Keywords: phosphate, TBI, molecular imaging, phosphorylation, brain edema, MRI contrast agents

1. Introduction

As progress of medical science/technology and imaging accelerates into the future, this work is intended as an important review regarding the related chemistry and biochemistry of traumatic brain injury (TBI). While some pertinent reviews have also appeared [1], we review what is known regarding phosphate chemistry. This is of critical importance for future researchers, and relates to brain-related injury, especially TBI. We sought to cover phosphates and phosphorylation in this context. From a database search, a list of keywords (phosphate, phosphonate, phosphorylation, traumatic brain injury, and probe, imaging, or sensor) and approximately 35 references have been acquired (ISI Web of Science, accessed in 2017). [1–35]. Instrumental techniques are also critically important and certain physical techniques are introduced and described as well (**Figures 1** and **2**). Reviews of biological phosphate imaging have emerged in the literature [36–39] and a combination of clinical and research aspects are presented. In addition, critically important phosphate species, probes, proteins, and related medicinal molecules are illustrated (**Figures 3–6**).

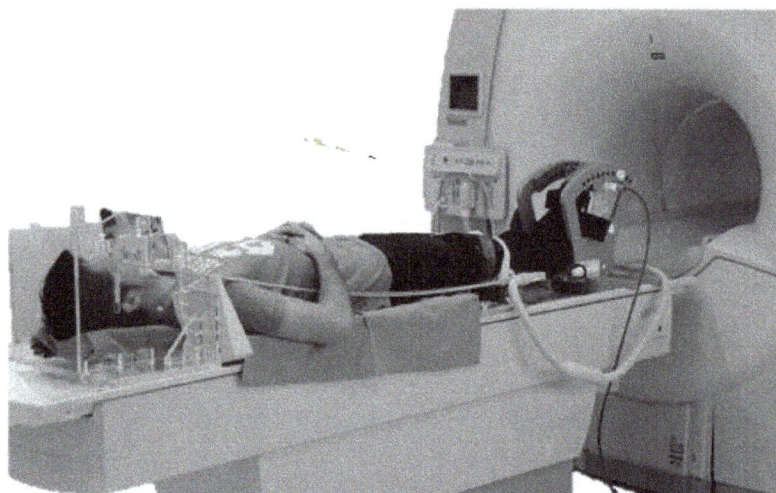

Figure 1. Dynamic 31P-magnetic resonance spectroscopy (http://www.mrtm.ethz.ch/research/mr-spectroscopy/physiological-projects/muscle-physiology.html).

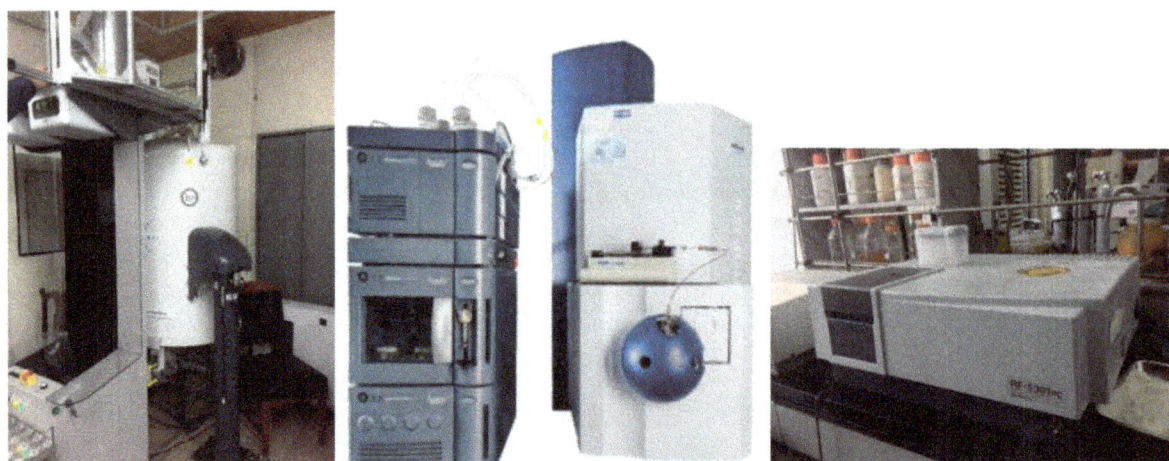

Figure 2. Instruments used in the scientific laboratory such as the multinuclear NMR spectrometer (left), high-resolution mass spectrometer (middle), and fluorimeter (right). (Photos acquired at KAIST (Daejeon, Korea); high-resolutionmass spectrometer photo taken from kara.kaist.ac.kr.).

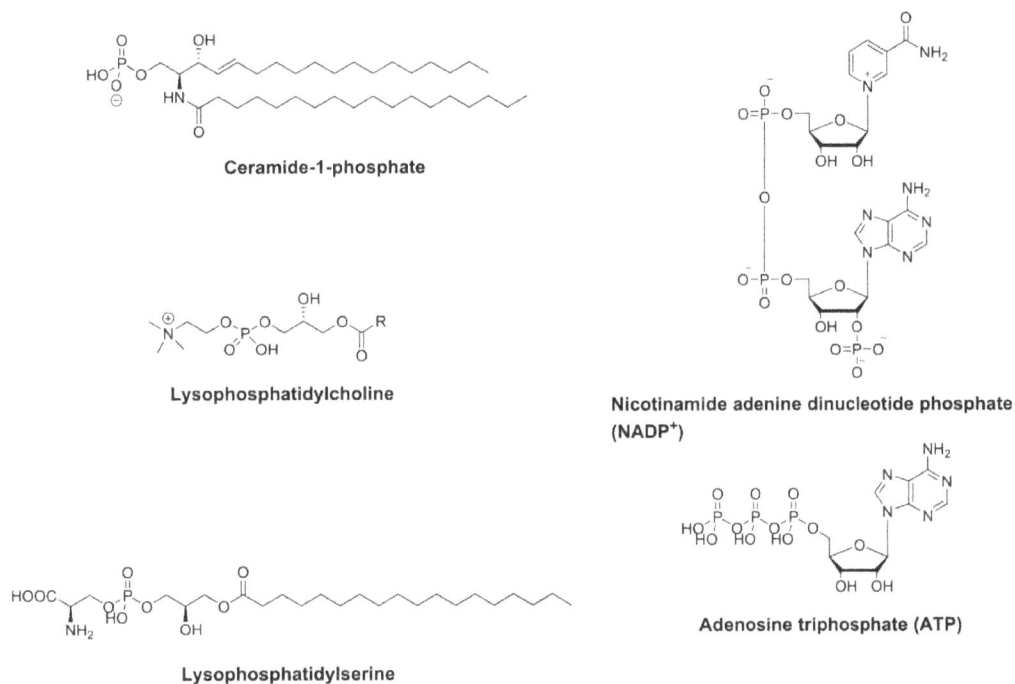

Figure 3. Phosphates under discussion in this review.

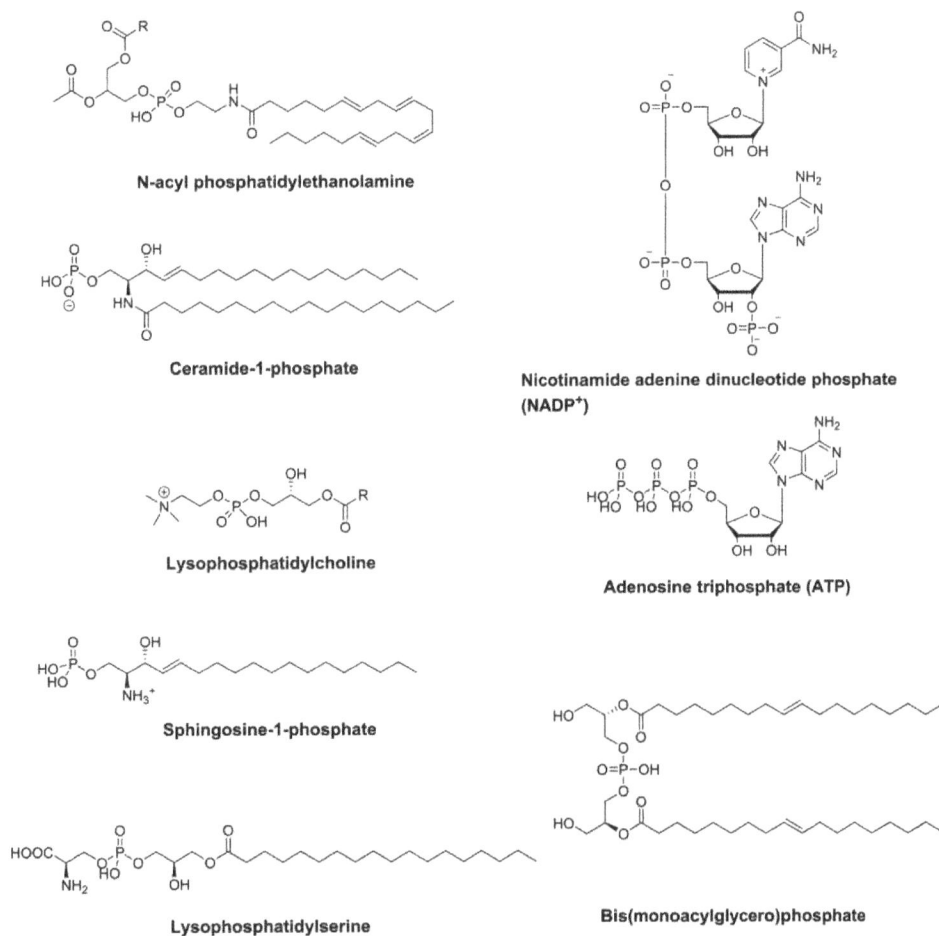

Figure 4. Phosphates under discussion in this review.

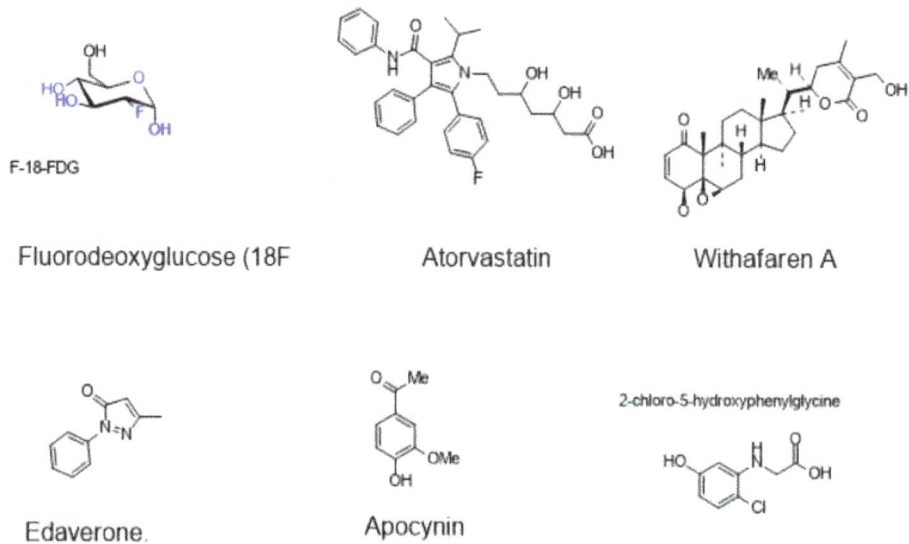

F-18-FDG

Fluorodeoxyglucose (18F   Atorvastatin   Withafaren A

Edaverone.   Apocynin   2-chloro-5-hydroxyphenylglycine

Figure 5. Therapeutic agents studied in the context of TBI and related studies. The nicotinamide adenine dinucleotide phosphate (NADP) oxidase inhibitor.

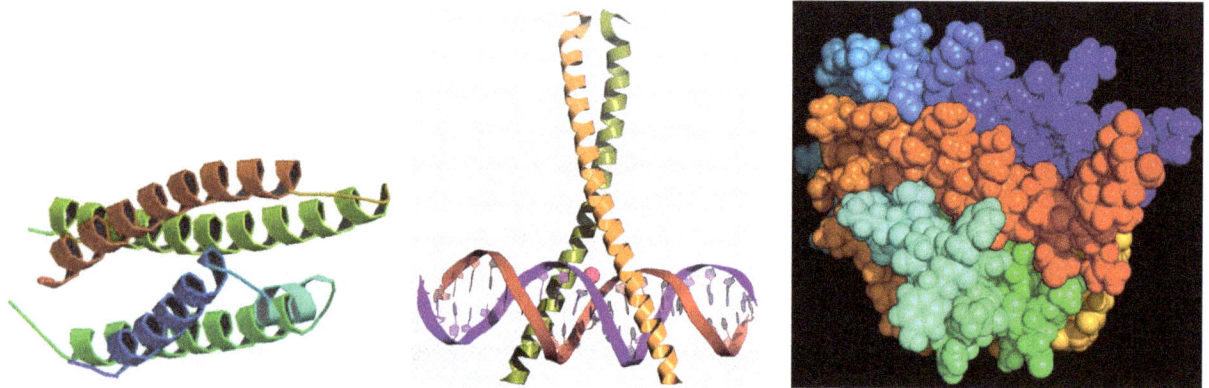

Figure 6. Some of the important proteins under discussion including apolipoprotein (APOE), the CREB protein, etc. (Copied without permission from the Internet, accessed in September 2017, Wikipedia.). CREB (top) is a transcription factor capable of binding DNA (bottom) and regulating gene expression.

2. TBI introduction

According to the US Centers for Disease Control and Prevention (CDC), every year in the United States approximately 1.7 million individuals receive an injury classified as a TBI), and 52,000 of these cases led to death [40]. TBI can be defined as alterations in brain functions and brain metabolism due to head collision with a stationary or moving object, or striking of a physical subject or coupling of an external mechanical force (e.g., g-force, blast shockwave) with the head [41–44]. Research has revealed that TBI can be associated with a variety of outcomes, from mild shock upon a single impact, to developing chronic traumatic encephalopathy (CTE) at a later time, a neurodegenerative disorder linked to repetitive brain injuries [45]. Each damaging event may lead to a specific clinical condition, which requires specific observation and care to prevent long-term neurological damage.

Related head injuries can involve different motions of the event that ultimately impose a stretching force on neurons, commonly resulting in the dangerous formation of edema in the tissue, which increases tissue volume. Brain edema is influenced by complex molecular and cellular changes in blood–brain barrier (BBB) function, as well as cell volume regulation. These changes may also develop into pathological pathways. Edema resulting from the original sustained injury has a devastating impact on morbidity and mortality. These downstream effects of TBI increase intracranial pressure, impair cerebral perfusion and oxygenation, and contribute to additional ischemic injuries [46]. Therefore, these changes may also develop into pathological pathways. Other issues related to cerebral hypoperfusion range from loss of consciousness to devastating neuronal damage. The reason for these symptoms is the lack of high-energy phosphate compounds and high-energy metabolic demand caused by disruption of the continuous oxygen supply in the blood to the brain.

In general, there are three major types of traumatic brain edema. The first is *vasogenic* due to disruption of the BBB, which results in extracellular water accumulation. The second is *cytotoxic/cellular* due to sustained intracellular water collection. The third is called *osmotic* brain edema, which happens because of osmotic imbalances between blood and tissue. Rarely after TBI do we encounter a "hydrocephalic edema/interstitial" brain edema related to an obstruction of cerebrospinal fluid outflow [47]. Various detailed case studies have emerged that continue to raise the alarm and grab the attention of researchers to understand the effects of TBI. For many repeated types of injuries to the head, in certain individuals CTE has similarities to age-related neurodegenerative diseases [1]. Model systems such as rats [4, 6, 12, 13, 15, 17, 28, 29, 32, 33] and mice [5, 9, 11, 12, 18, 20, 25] have been employed to better understand the mechanisms of TBI.

Phosphorus is a very important element in the body and is responsible for approximately 1.1% of total body mass. In the body, almost all of the phosphorus is combined with oxygen, forming phosphate. Phosphate acts as a body's electrolytes, carrying an electric charge in body fluids such as blood. The majority of phosphate in the body (85%) comes from bone [48]. The rest is stored as high-energy phosphate or in its free form, where it acts as a substrate for adenosine triphosphate (ATP) production. Even though phosphate metabolism in trauma has not been well studied, there are some interesting reports on phosphate in TBI that involve hypophosphatemia. In 2010 Lindsey et al studied 25 patients with TBI and found out that these individuals had a lower serum phosphorus concentration than those without TBI, suggesting ongoing phosphate loss in the TBI patients [49].

To date, conventional computed tomography (CT) is the main technique for the evaluation of TBI for patients' diagnoses. However, CT and magnetic resonance imaging (MRI) still cannot be used to predict neurocognitive functional deficits at any stage of TBI, because they do not image the functional pathology for the neurocognitive outcome [50]. Therefore, other techniques such as ^{31}P-magnetic resonance imaging/spectroscopy (^{31}P-MRI/MRS) and positron emission tomography (PET) are used as alternatives to provide insight into the metabolic changes that arise from TBI and to reveal the damage that contributes to short- and long-term impairment. In this chapter, a review of several relevant contributions of neuroimaging towards an improved understanding of TBI is presented, using both PET and ^{31}P-MRI/MRS.

3. MRI techniques for TBI that involve phosphates

In terms of MRI for TBI, various techniques have been employed (**Figures 1** and **2**). For example, T_2-weighted MRI has been used [5]. Interestingly, in 1990 Heiss et al. used PET of [18F]fluorodeoxyglucose (FDG)coupled with 31P-MRS to diagnose tumors in the brain. The study suggested that both methods can examine different aspects of tumors in the brain and can be used as a tool for further classification of brain tumors or diseases related to the brain such as TBI [51]. A further study in 2002 by Greenman et al. used a method called three-dimensional rapid acquisition with relaxation enhancement (RARE) pulse sequence for direct measurement of phosphocreatine (PCr) images of the human myocardium. The aim of this study was to assess the metabolic state of myocardial tissue in several disease states and determine the efficacy of therapeutic mediation [52]. Then, in 2005, Greenman et al. published a work related to 31P-MRS to evaluate the metatarsal head region of the foot in neuropathic diabetic patients. The study concluded that a very uniform net magnetization can be achieved and the use of double-tuned birdcage radiofrequency coils can improve the quality of MRI/MRS examinations [50]. A study in 2018 conducted by Chen et al. using in vivo 31P-MRS magnetization transfer (MT) suggested that MRS provides a direct measure of neuronal activity at the metabolic level by investigating the change in cerebral ATP metabolic rates in healthy adults upon repeated stimulation [45]. 31P-MRS has also proven effective in detecting a selective saturation sequence for ATP and phospholipids. Thus, the 31P-MRS-MT technique at 3 T is a good candidate for neurological and neuropsychiatric disorders because of the noninvasive nature of NMR studies. Additionally, 31P-MRS was reported and discussed in 2004 by Cernak et al. [6] The technique involving metals such as manganese is also applicable: manganese-enhanced MRI was used in a 2011 study by Tang et al. [29] Additionally, ex vivo diffusion tensor imaging was implemented in a study in 2012 by Jin and coworkers [5].

1H, 31P, and 13C in vivo MRS are complementary techniques that allow noninvasive measurement of different aspects of brain metabolism that may contribute to the clinical management of patients with acute TBI [53]. 13C-MRS measures the breakdown of intake of 13C-labeled sugar (e.g., glucose) via glycolysis and the tricarboxylic acid cycle. Even though not many 13C-MRS studies have been conducted, the development of in vivo hyperpolarized techniques shows a potential to detect TBI. On the other hand, 31P-MRS allows measurement of high-energy phosphates (ATP and PCr) produced by oxidative phosphorylation and creatine kinase in mitochondria [54]. Changes in these metabolites have been noted in several patients and animal studies (further study might reveal the role of the high-energy phosphates). 1H-MRS is the most commonly used MRS technique for studying brain metabolism following TBI. It has the potential to measure various metabolites: some are associated such as lactate, Glu and Gln, which can also be measured by 13C-MRS. Creatine and N-acetylaspartic acid are associated with the ATP and PCr, which can also be measured with 31P-MRS. Thus, the ratios of high-energy phosphates are thought to represent a balance in the brain. In addition, the chemical shift difference between inorganic phosphate and PCr enables calculation of intracellular pH. 13C-MRS detects the 13C isotope of carbon in brain metabolites [55].

4. Molecules of importance

There are various small molecules used either as diagnostic agents or potential therapies in the context of phosphate TBI studies. We can also consider small molecule probes and those coupled with the use of pharmaceuticals (**Figures 3–6**).

5. PET imaging

PET is an important clinically used instrumental technique that requires an administration of artificial diagnostic agents (**Figure 1**). The artificial agents used involve one disintegrating atom such as the ^{18}F or ^{11}C isotope. The isotope is generated and then covalently attached (by a simple chemical reaction and protocol) to a small molecule prior to nuclear medical examination [13, 21].

PET imaging is well known for its sensitivity for small molecular changes (nanogram scale) compared to milligram or microgram for MRI or CT. PET also is able to provide important information on brain metabolism. As a result, PET imaging is used to measure a change in the glucose metabolism after TBI. The magnitude and duration have been correlated with worse behavioral and cognitive outcomes [56]. These results regarding cerebral glucose utilization were obtained using deoxyglucose (DG) labeled with ^{14}C and autoradiography [57]. DG was chosen because DG is phosphorylated but not further metabolized, becoming trapped in the cell with a slow clearance rate. For noninvasive imaging, a positron-emitting isotope such as ^{18}F can be incorporated within DG, resulting in the production of [^{18}F]FDG; this then accumulates in brain tissue in proportion to glucose uptake and the level of phosphorylation and is quantifiable using the technique of PET imaging [58].

For more information on nuclear chemistry and the mechanism of positron/electron capture as well as the preparative chemistry, please see other sources.

6. Phosphate species

There is a range of phosphate species used in biology. In some ways, the phosphates are central to the discussion, but in other ways they are peripheral to the thrusts of literature reports. The phosphates under discussion are shown in **Figure 3** and listed below.

7. Phosphorylation

Phosphorylation of proteins (serine, threonine, and tyrosine), for example, is an essential theme in biology. It is a constantly monitored and investigated process in biological systems, and continues as a vital aspect in the study of neurodegenerative disease research because it relates to kinase and phosphatase activity (**Figure 3**). For example, tau protein has been central in Alzheimer's disease (AD) hypotheses for many years. Hyperphosphorylation is considered to be an important step in disease pathology [59].

Among many kinases proteins, mitogen-activated protein kinases (MAPKs), protein kinase B (also known as Akt), and glycogen synthase kinase (GSK) are the major kinases involved in cellular signaling, and as confirmed by the study from Joseph T. Neary, MAPKs, Akt, and GSK respond to trauma of the central nervous system (CNS). Therefore, it is very important to conduct further studies of these proteins to provide a better understanding of their role in the pathogenesis of many disorders, including traumatic injuries of the brain [58]. A study by Naoki Otani et al. showed that the extracellular signal-regulated kinase (ERK) pathway is triggered in lesions in regions of selective vulnerability after TBI and has a devastating effect on the hippocampus. The results show that pretreatment with U0126 (an ERK inhibitor) decreases neuronal cell loss after TBI [60]. Meanwhile, a study conducted by Noshita et al. also suggested that phosphorylation of Akt at serine-473 and DNA fragmentation after TBI in mice showed that phospho-Akt was decreased in the injured cortex 1 h after TBI and temporarily increased at 4 h in the perifocal damaged cortex. They concluded that the degree of Akt phosphorylation is dependent on the intensity of cellular damage after TBI [61].

Another study revealed that MAPKs are involved in pathophysiological TBI. Thus, regulating the MAPK pathway-mediated cerebral damage after acute injury could be a direction for the development of the novel therapeutic target in TBI [62–64]. Study of a simple chemical compound, sodium selenite, was performed. Sodium selenite was found to upregulate proteins that help to remove the phosphorylation group from its position on the amino acids in particular proteins. The specific enzyme is called PP2A/PR55 (protein phosphatase 2A regulatory subunit PR55). In a study from 2014 by Zhu et al., phosphorylation of various molecules was considered as a result of cerebral contusion (mouse model). The following molecules were studied: Akt, mTOR (mammalian target of rapamycin), and S6RP [35]. For example, the Thr308 and Ser473 sites of Akt are important phosphorylation sites for activating Akt. Thr308 becomes phosphorylated by PKD1 and other enzymes, including PDK2 phosphorylate Ser473. Activated Akt mediates several responses, including phosphorylating a range of intracellular proteins. mToR and S6RP are downstream targets of the PI3K/Akt pathway. Phosphorylation of a precursor stimulates activation of mTOR and S6RP [65–67]. Some phospholipids are ubiquitous and have been the subject of imaging regarding cell membrane dynamics.

8. Other phosphates

Various free, small, and organically bound phosphates are encountered in the phosphate imaging TBI literature:

- Pentose phosphate (see **Figure 3**)

- ATP and its dynamics [8]

- Reduced nicotinamide adenine dinucleotide phosphate (NADPH)

- *N*-acyl-phosphatidylethanolamines [20]

- Lysophosphatidylcholine [20]

- Ceramide phosphate [20]

- Bis(monoacylglycero)phosphate [20]

- Sphingosine-1-phosphate [20]

- Lysophosphatidylserine [20]

- *N*-acylethanolamine phospholipids

The result from Emily V. Mesev et al. proposes that the endogenous production of ceramide-1-phosphate (C1P) via ceramide kinase in brain tissue increases the basal activity of P-glycoprotein and contributes to general neuroprotection in healthy brains within the BBB. In cases of cellular injury or stress, it is possible that increases in C1P would act as a neuroprotector [68].

A study from Alice E. Pasvogel et al. showed that following TBI, membrane integrity of neurons and neuroglia is compromised resulting in elevated phospholipid levels in the cerebrospinal fluid. The pattern of change and the concentration of each of the phospholipids were different for those who died and those who survived following TBI. In conclusion, the study found the increase concentration of lysophosphatidylcholine in those who died. These findings give a preliminary proof of greater disruption of central nervous system membrane phospholipids in patients who died after TBI [69, 70].

9. Extracellular phosphates

In addition to the endogenous phosphate species that are produced in the biological system, there are also exogenous or xenobiological compounds that can be discussed. Chitosan combined with β-glycerophosphate disodium (β-GP) for use as a thermosensitive hydrogel was first reported by Chenite in 2000. This gel-forming biopolymer can be used for the development of therapeutic implants. Further study by Dong et al. from 2015 involved a hydrogel that consisted of derivatives of phosphate groups [10]. The result suggests that an injectable thermosensitive chitosan/gelatin/β-glycerol phosphate (C/G/GP) hydrogel could release the phenolic antioxidant ferulic acid (FA), which can inhibit the neurological oxidative stress and effectively protect the brain from further impairments. Another study from Ibrahim Jalloh et al. in 2015 also suggested that there was a shift in glucose metabolism from glycolysis to pentose phosphate pathways (PPPs) with decreasing brain tissue oxygen concentrations after TBI. This finding gives another perspective on the roles of PPPs and glycolysis after TBI, and whether they can be manipulated to enhance the potentially antioxidant role of PPPs and give better outcome to TBI patients [71].

In 2014, Brend L. Fiebich et al. suggested that prostaglandin E2 (PGE2), produced by the enzymatic activity of cyclooxygenases (COX) 1 and 2, is the common mediator for the inflammatory brain that leads to TBI. The group proposed a two-hit model for neuronal injury. First, an initial localized inflammation mediated by PGE2 was then followed by the release of ATP by injured cells (second hit). In this study, it was concluded that by inhibiting the P2 receptor in the second hit using P2 receptor-based antiinflammatory drugs (PBAIDs) the activity of specific ectonucleotidases and release of excessive ATP could be increased and is another approach to counter neuroinflammation [72, 73].

10. MRI contrast agents

In TBI phosphate literature, MRI contrast agents have been previously described [31]. Structural information about the brain can be quantified using brain volume based on T_1-weighted MRI. Even though the most common contrast agents are based on gadolinium, new pharmaceuticals (for example, gadobenate benate dimeglumine (Gd-BOPTA)) have been developed with higher T_1 and T_2 relaxivity to improve signal intensity enhancement and thereby improve lesion visualization [74]. Garcia-Martin et al. used a phosphonated Gd^{3+}-based contrast agent to measure intravascular acidification in rat gliomas. To distinguish the differences in pH, [75, 76] the contrast agent used undergoes changes in T_1 relaxivity over a broad range from pH 6 to 8 [77]. This application is an example of an alternative for TBI symptom detection.

Another study using manganese-enhanced MRI (MEMRI), in which the manganese ion acts as an MRI contrast agent, was used to study rats subjected to a controlled cortical impact. The results suggest that MEMRI detected early indications of excitotoxic injury and BBB disruption that preceded vasogenic edema in the hyperacute phase and offer a novel contrast that complements conventional MRI in the study of TBI [78, 79]. In 2009 Chapon et al. revealed that MRI contrast agent can detect the inflammatory progression by radiolabeled peptide (IELLQAR) to target E-selectin, an important intercellular adhesion molecule involved in the leukocyte cycle [78].

11. Therapeutics tested

Small molecules are at the heart of medically treating people who have received TBI. (R,S)-2-Chloro-5-hydroxyphenylglycine (CHPG [5]) was studied. This compound has been studied by David J loane et al. in 2013 [80] and the result in mice model demonstrate that activation of mGluR5 using the selective agonist and CHPG, within 30 minutes after the moderate-level TBI significantly improved sensorimotor and cognitive function recovery and reduced TBI-induced lesion volumes in the mice model. Next, edaverone (**Figure 5**) was used [11]; it was found to be effective in the mouse model under study. The theme of concussion-induced depression is elucidated in this paper [11].

12. Proteins and enzymes

There are also related proteins in these studies. Perhaps the most central protein in a discussion of neurodegeneration is the beta amyloid protein (Aβ)—one of the hallmarks of AD. It can be used as a baseline measurement. Studies by the Smith [81] and Sharp groups [82] showed that Aβ plaques may be found within TBI patients. The study also suggests that rapid Aβ plaque formation may result from the accumulation of amyloid precursor protein in damaged axons and a disturbed balance between Aβ genesis and catabolism during the process of TBI. In this study, the authors took an image of Aβ plaque burden in long-term survivors of TBI and made determinations to generate a correlation between traumatic axonal injury and Aβ concentration. By comparing the distribution of Aβ to AD, they found that Aβ-comprised plaque in the TBI survivors decreased in neocortical regions but increased in another brain region, the cerebellum. This then suggested that TBI may dispose one to an AD-like fate [25]. There are also phosphate-related reports involving studying the reduction of certain proteins after the onset of TBI. Such proteins include CREB and PSD95 [26]. Then there is carbamylated erythropoietin (EPO) [4]; EPO is a pleiotropic cytokine that identified its role in erythropoiesis (the process by which red blood cells are produced) [83]. EPO was recognized for its hematopoietic properties; however, many researchers around the globe were attracted by its function as a tissue protector. In 2004, a study from Leist et al. showed that the carbamylation of EPO formed a kind of nonhematopoietic derivative, cEpo. This reaction surprisingly eliminated its erythropoietic effects; however, it keeps its function in tissue protection [84]. These results led to another study conducted by Fiordaliso et al. from 2004, which suggested that the erythropoietic and tissue-protective effects of EPO were based on different receptors [85]. These discoveries have brought many researchers to design and synthesize EPO derivatives with tissue-protective effects only. To date, there are two major, developed, modified EPO molecules that have tissue-protective effects: cEpo and asialoerythroprotein (asialoEpo). Interestingly, the first modification of EPO through carbamylation was reported by Leist et al.; however, the method of producing cEpo was described in a patent by Warren Pharmaceuticals [86]. This newly reported research may shed new light on the development and application of cEpo, a prospective drug candidate for neuroprotection. There are studies that involve delayed mGluR5 activation and targeting of intermediate proteins [3]. One study found that activation of metabotropic glutamate receptor 5 (mGluR5) by CHPG decreases microglial activation and release of associated proinflammatory factors in vitro, which is mediated, in part, through inhibition of reduced NADPH oxidase. These results suggested that treatment with CHPG may significantly limit lesion progression in TBI through mGluR5 receptors [87].

13. Conclusions and future outlook

There are various ways that the wide variety of phosphates that exist in biology are involved in health and disease; ions such as phosphates can be exploited in many prospective ways in the future and in particular they could be imaged in new ways. This review concerned phosphates and TBI reports in which the discussion or study involved molecular imaging. The reports were clinical and involved laboratory studies. Animal models were often used. A great deal of biochemistry was described; often, enzyme activities were monitored and these trends were published.

This fresh review was intended to help medicinal chemists make new connections. *The major goals are intended to help achieve future innovation of potential treatment of TBI with chemical or biological agents. Administration within the "golden hour" for the best efficacy is an essential point to make.* In terms of imaging there are new MRI techniques and experiments that are available as well. Some of the most important instrument manufacturers such as GE Healthcare (Milwaukee, WI), Bruker, Hitachi Medical Corporation, Phillips, and Toshiba Medical Corporation provide the current hardware for the task at hand [88–92]. However, biochemistry can allow for additional innovative imaging to be undertaken. Below are a few detailed aspects for future study with regard to TBI and phosphate research.

13.1. Future

More commonly, research in the future will prominently feature the effects on phosphate metabolism. With phosphate metabolism still in its infancy [93], a fuller treatment would involve a great deal of related research. Therefore, we have described some related papers that involve important points about phosphates.

- Much research effort involves the status of enzyme activity. The importance of accurately carrying out immunohistochemistry involving phosphorylated proteins can be underscored [16, 47]. How well Western blots and other related assays are prepared and conducted by laboratory personnel and how they can be best carried out and executed are extremely important for the field.

- The theme of subcellular redistribution of phosphates can be made more pronounced [16]. Novel chemical probes that can "chase" the constituents between different cellular compartments can be designed and studied.

- The importance of the maintenance of vasculature and smooth muscle cells that help constitute the microvessels within neurological tissue can be further studied. How these structures are effected by TBI in, e.g., mouse models can be further determined [16].

- Overabundant Reactive Oxygen Species (ROS) concentration driven by Fenton reaction has major role in the transformation of many highly radical species such as ROS/RNS. These highly reactive species, can lead to many disturbances such as TBI. See references herein and elsewhere for an introduction to ROS and their analysis. MRI is a very common theme in research [1, 15, 28, 29, 31], as well as the closely related instrumental technique of NMR spectroscopy.

- How phosphates are interrelated (via brain injury) with the range of ROS is an important quest in basic science.

- More research about phosphates in *gliosis* needs to be researched. How can gliosis best be imaged and can it relate to the homeostasis of phosphates?

- What is the range of factors that delays mGluR5 activation and how do phosphates or phosphonates become involved?

- How can researchers parse between *secondary* and *primary* pathology at the chemical level regarding both experimental and clinical research of TBI phosphate activity?

- What divergent effects might arise from prior organophosphate/organophosphonate pesticide exposure (a history of exposure) in which phosphonates are located where phosphorylation usually takes place? How does this effect hinder or perhaps help in etiology? How can medicine take advantage of this artificial preloading?

Abbreviations

AD	Alzheimer's disease
ADP	adenosine diphosphate.
ATP	adenosine triphosphate
Akt	protein kinase B
APOE	apolipoprotein
BBB	blood brain barrier
C1P	ceramide-1-phosphate
CBF	cerebral blood flow.
COX	cyclooxygenases
CREB	cAMP response element-binding protein
CTE	chronic traumatic encephalopathy
Gd-BOPTA	gadolinium benate dimeglumine
Gln	glutamine
Glu	glutamic acid
HR-MS	high resolution–mass spectroscopy.
KCl	potassium chloride.
KH_2PO_4	monopotassium phosphate.
MEMRI	manganese-enhanced MRI
mGluR5	metabotropic glutamate receptor 5
MRI	magnetic resonance imaging
MRS	magnetic resonance spectroscopy
mTOR	mammalian target of rapamycin
NAA	*N*-acetylaspartic acid
NADPH	nicotinamide adenine dinucleotide phosphate
NaCl	sodium chloride.
Na_2HPO_4	sodium hydrogen phosphate.

NMR	nuclear mass resonance
NOX2	nicotinamide adenine dinucleotide phosphate oxidase.
PGE2	prostaglandin E2
PBAID	P2 receptor-based antiinflammatory drugs
PBS	phosphate buffered saline.
PET	positron emission tomography
PP2A/PR55	protein phosphatase 2A regulatory subunit PR55
PSD95	postsynaptic density protein 95
TBI	traumatic brain injury
Tg mice	transgenic mice.
TP	triphosphate
S6RP	phosphorylation of S6 ribosomal protein

Author details

Noam Naphatali Tal[1], Tesla Yudhistira[2,4], Woo Hyun Lee[2], Youngsam Kim[2,3] and David G. Churchill[2,3,5*]

*Address all correspondence to: dchurchill@kaist.ac.kr

1 Independent Scientist and Former student, Department of Medical Device Technology, Maltash College, Tel Aviv, Israel

2 Molecular Logic Gate Laboratory, Department of Chemistry, Korea Advanced Institute of Science and Technology (KAIST), Daejeon, Republic of Korea

3 Center for Catalytic Hydrocarbon Functionalizations, Institute for Basic Science (IBS), Daejeon, Republic of Korea

4 Lembaga Pengelola Dana Pendidikan (LPDP), Indonesia Endowment Fund for Education, Kementrian Keuangan Republik Indonesia, Jakarta, Indonesia

5 Schulich Faculty of Chemistry at Technion, Israel Institute of Technology, Haifa, Israel

References

[1] Nisenbaum EJ, Novikov DS, Lui YW. The presence and role of iron in mild traumatic brain injury: an imaging perspective. Journal of Neurotrauma. 2014;**31**(4):301

[2] Antonenko YN, Denisov SS, Silachev DN, Khailova LS, Jankauskas SS, Rokitskaya TI, Danilina TI, Kotova EA, Korshunova GA, Plotnikov EY, et al. A long-linker conjugate of fluorescein and triphenylphosphonium as mitochondria-targeted uncoupler and fluorescent neuro- and nephroprotector. Biochimica et Biophysica Acta - General Subjects. 2016;**1860**(11):2463

[3] Bargagna-Mohan P, Paranthan RR, Hamza A, Dimova N, Trucchi B, Srinivasan C, Elliott GI, Zhan CG, Lau DL, Zhu HY, et al. Withaferin A targets intermediate filaments glial fibrillary acidic protein and vimentin in a model of retinal gliosis. Journal of Biological Chemistry. 2010;**285**(10):7657

[4] Bouzat P, Francony G, Thomas S, Valable S, Mauconduit F, Fevre MC, Barbier EL, Bernaudin M, Lahrech H, Payen JF. Reduced brain edema and functional deficits after treatment of diffuse traumatic brain injury by carbamylated erythropoietin derivative. Critical Care Medicine. 2011;**39**(9):2099

[5] Jin H, Wu G, Hu S, Hua Y, Keep RF, Wu J, Xi G. T2 and T2* magnetic resonance imaging sequences predict brain injury after intracerebral hemorrhage in rats. Acta Neurochirurgica Supplement. 2013;**118**:151

[6] Cernak I, Vink R, Zapple DN, Cruz MI, Ahmed F, Chang T, Fricke ST, Faden AI. The pathobiology of moderate diffuse traumatic brain injury as identified using a new experimental model of injury in rats. Neurobiology of Disease. 2004;**17**(1):29

[7] Chantong B, Kratschmar DV, Lister A, Odermatt A. Inhibition of metabotropic glutamate receptor 5 induces cellular stress through pertussis toxin-sensitive Gi-proteins in murine BV-2 microglia cells. Journal of Neuroinflammation. 2014;**11**:16

[8] Connolly NMC, Prehn JHM. The metabolic response to excitotoxicity—lessons from single-cell imaging. Journal of Bioenergetics and Biomembranes. 2015;**47**(1–2):75

[9] DellaValle B. GLP-1 receptor activation improves neurological outcome after murine brain trauma (vol 1, pg 1, 2014). Annals of Clinical and Translational Neurology. 2016;**3**(8):664

[10] Dong GC, Kuan CY, Subramaniam S, Zhao JY, Sivasubramaniam S, Chang HY, Lin FH. A potent inhibition of oxidative stress induced gene expression in neural cells by sustained ferulic acid release from chitosan based hydrogel. Materials Science and Engineering C: Materials for Biological Applications. 2015;**49**:691

[11] Higashi Y, Hoshijima M, Yawata T, Nobumoto A, Tsuda M, Shimizu T, Saito M, Ueba T. Suppression of oxidative stress and 5-lipoxygenase activation by edaravone improves depressive-like behavior after concussion. Journal of Neurotrauma. 2014;**31**(20):1689

[12] Hill JL, Kobori N, Zhao J, Rozas NS, Hylin MJ, Moore AN, Dash PK. Traumatic brain injury decreases AMP-activated protein kinase activity and pharmacological enhancement of its activity improves cognitive outcome. Journal of Neurochemistry. 2016;**139**(1):106

[13] Hwang H, Jeong HS, Oh PS, Na KS, Kwon J, Kim J, Lim S, Sohn MH, Jeong HJ. Improving cerebral blood flow through liposomal delivery of angiogenic peptides: potential of

F-18-FDG PET imaging in ischemic stroke treatment. The Journal of Nuclear Medicine. 2015;**56**(7):1106

[14] Jin Y, Sui HJ, Dong Y, Ding Q, Qu WH, Yu SX, Jin YX. Atorvastatin enhances neurite outgrowth in cortical neurons in vitro via up-regulating the Akt/mTOR and Akt/GSK-3 beta signaling pathways. Acta Pharmacologica Sinica. 2012;**33**(7):861

[15] Karki K, Knight RA, Han YX, Yang DM, Zhang JF, Ledbetter KA, Chopp M, Seyfried DM. Simvastatin and atorvastatin improve neurological outcome after experimental intracerebral hemorrhage. Stroke. 2009;**40**(10):3384

[16] Kreipke CW, Morgan RL, Petrov T, Rafols JA. Subcellular redistribution of calponin underlies sustained vascular contractility following traumatic brain injury. Neurological Research. 2007;**29**(6):604

[17] Krishnappa IK, Contant CF, Robertson CS. Regional changes in cerebral extracellular glucose and lactate concentrations following severe cortical impact injury and secondary ischemia in rats. Journal of Neurotrauma. 1999;**16**(3):213

[18] Kumar A, Alvarez-Croda DM, Stoica BA, Faden AI, Loane DJ. Microglial/macrophage polarization dynamics following traumatic brain injury. Journal of Neurotrauma. 2016;**33**(19):1732

[19] Mannix R, Meehan WP, Mandeville J, Grant PE, Gray T, Berglass J, Zhang J, Bryant J, Rezaie S, Chung JY, et al. Clinical correlates in an experimental model of repetitive mild brain injury. Annals of Neurology. 2013;**74**(1):65

[20] Nielsen MMB, Lambertsen KL, Clausen BH, Meyer M, Bhandari DR, Larsen ST, Poulsen SS, Spengler B, Janfelt C, Hansen HS. Mass spectrometry imaging of biomarker lipids for phagocytosis and signalling during focal cerebral ischaemia. Scientific Reports. 2016;**6**:14

[21] Nortje J, Coles JP, Timofeev I, Fryer TD, Aigbirhio FI, Smielewski P, Outtrim JG, Chatfield DA, Pickard JD, Hutchinson PJ, et al. Effect of hyperoxia on regional oxygenation and metabolism after severe traumatic brain injury: preliminary findings. Critical Care Medicine. 2008;**36**(1):273

[22] Papisov MI, Belov VV, Gannon KS. Physiology of the intrathecal bolus: the leptomeningeal route for macromolecule and particle delivery to CNS. Molecular Pharmaceutics. 2013;**10**(5):1522

[23] Park J, Zhang J, Qiu JH, Zhu XX, Degterev A, Lo EH, Whalen MJ. Combination therapy targeting Akt and mammalian target of rapamycin improves functional outcome after controlled cortical impact in mice. Journal of Cerebral Blood Flow & Metabolism. 2012;**32**(2):330

[24] Patrick MM, Grillot JM, Derden ZM, Paul DW. Long-term drifts in sensitivity caused by biofouling of an amperometric oxygen sensor. Electroanalysis. 2017;**29**(4):998

[25] Schwetye KE, Cirrito JR, Esparza TJ, MacDonald CL, Holtzman DM, Brody DL. Traumatic brain injury reduces soluble extracellular amyloid-beta in mice: a methodologically novel combined microdialysis-controlled cortical impact study. Neurobiology of Disease. 2010;**40**(3):555

[26] Sen T, Gupta R, Kaiser H, Sen N. Activation of PERK elicits memory impairment through inactivation of CREB and downregulation of PSD95 after traumatic brain injury. The Journal of Neuroscience. 2017;**37**(24):5900

[27] Starkov AA, Polster BM, Fiskum G. Regulation of hydrogen peroxide production by brain mitochondria by calcium and Bax. Journal of Neurochemistry. 2002;**83**(1):220

[28] Tan XL, Wright DK, Liu SJ, Hovens C, O'Brien TJ, Shultz SR. Sodium selenate, a protein phosphatase 2A activator, mitigates hyperphosphorylated tau and improves repeated mild traumatic brain injury outcomes. Neuropharmacology. 2016;**108**:382

[29] Tang HL, Sun HP, Wu X, Sha HY, Feng XY, Zhu JH. Detection of neural stem cells function in rats with traumatic brain injury by manganese-enhanced magnetic resonance imaging. Chinese Medical Journal. 2011;**124**(12):1848

[30] Valable S, Francony G, Bouzat P, Fevre MC, Mahious N, Bouet V, Farion R, Barbier E, Lahrech H, Remy C, et al. The impact of erythropoietin on short-term changes in phosphorylation of brain protein kinases in a rat model of traumatic brain injury. Journal of Cerebral Blood Flow & Metabolism. 2010;**30**(2):361

[31] Van Horn JD, Bhattrai A, Irimia A. Multimodal imaging of neurometabolic pathology due to traumatic brain injury. Trends in Neurosciences. 2017;**40**(1):39

[32] Wu JG, Li H, Wang DS, Xu DS, Wang W. Intravenous adipose-derived stem cells transplantation ameliorates memory impairment in moderate traumatic brain injury rats via the phosphorylation of extracellular signal-regulated kinase 1/2. International Journal of Clinical and Experimental Medicine. 2016;**9**(7):12649

[33] Yu TG, Feng Y, Feng XY, Dai JZ, Qian HJ, Huang Z. Prognostic factor from MR spectroscopy in rat with astrocytic tumour during radiation therapy. The British Journal of Radiology. 2015;**88**(1045):10

[34] Zemlan FP, Rosenberg WS, Luebbe PA, Campbell TA, Dean GE, Weiner NE, Cohen JA, Rudick RA, Woo D. Quantification of axonal damage in traumatic brain injury: affinity purification and characterization of cerebrospinal fluid tau proteins. Journal of Neurochemistry. 1999;**72**(2):741

[35] Zhu XX, Park J, Golinski J, Qiu JH, Khuman J, Lee CCH, Lo EH, Degterev A, Whalen MJ. Role of Akt and mammalian target of rapamycin in functional outcome after concussive brain injury in mice. Journal of Cerebral Blood Flow & Metabolism. 2014;**34**(9):1531

[36] Liu B, Wang H, Yang D, Tan R, Zhao RR, Rui X, Zhang JZ, Zhang JF, Ying Z. A cyanine-based colorimetric and fluorescent probe for highly selective sensing and bioimaging of phosphate ions. Dyes and Pigments. 2016;**133**:127

[37] Resa S, Orte A, Miguel D, Paredes JM, Muñoz VP, Salto R, Giron MD, Rama MJR, Cuerva JM, Pez JMA, Crovetto L. New dual fluorescent probe for simultaneous biothiol and phosphate bioimaging. Chemistry: A European Journal. 2015;**21**:14772

[38] Paredes JM, Giron MD, Rama MJR, Orte A, Crovetto L, Talavera EM, Salto R, Pez JMA. Real-time phosphate sensing in living cells using fluorescence lifetime imaging microscopy (FLIM). Journal of Physical Chemistry B. 2013;**117**(27):8143

[39] Banerjee S, Versaw WK, Garcia LR. Imaging cellular inorganic phosphate in Caenorhabditis elegans using a genetically encoded FRET-based biosensor. PLoS One. 2015;**10**(10):1

[40] Janich K, Nguyen HS, Patel M, Shabani S, Montoure A, Doan N. Management of adult traumatic brain injury: a review. Journal of Trauma and Treatment. 2016;**5**:1

[41] Weaver CS, Sloan BK, Brizendine EJ, Bock H. An analysis of maximum vehicle g forces and brain injury in motorsports crashes. Medicine & Science in Sports & Exercise. 2006;**38**:246

[42] Nakagawa A, Fujimura M, Kato K, Okuyama H, Hashimoto T, Takayama K, Tominaga T. Shock wave-induced brain injury in rat: novel traumatic brain injury animal model. Acta Neurochirurgica Supplement. 2008;**102**:421

[43] Nakagawa A, Manley GT, Gean AD, Ohtani K, Armonda R, Tsukamoto A, Yamamoto H, Takayama K, Tominaga T. Mechanisms of primary blast-induced traumatic brain injury: insights from shock-wave research. Journal of Neurotrauma. 2011;**28**:1101

[44] Wang H, Zhang YP, Cai J, Shields LB, Tuchek CA, Shi R, Li J, Shields CB, Xu XM. Compact blast-induced traumatic brain injury model in mice. Journal of Neuropathology & Experimental Neurology. 2016;**75**:183

[45] Chen C, Stephenson MC, Peters A, Morris PG, Francis ST, Gowland PA. 31P magnetization transfer magnetic resonance spectroscopy: assessing the activation induced change in cerebral ATP metabolic rates at 3 T. Magnetic Resonance in Medicine. 2018;**79**:22

[46] Unterberg AW, Stover J, Kress B, Kiening KL. Edema and brain trauma. Neuroscience. 2004;**129**:1021

[47] Arur S, Schedl T. Generation and purification of highly-specific antibodies for detecting post-translationally modified proteins in vivo. Nature Protocols. 2014;**9**(2):375

[48] Penido MGMG, Alon US. Phosphate homeostasis and its role in bone health. Pediatric Nephrology (Berlin, Germany). 2012;**27**:2039-2048

[49] Lindsey KA, Brown RO, Maish GO 3rd, et al. Influence of traumatic brain injury on potassium and phosphorus homeostasis in critically ill multiple trauma patients. Nutrition (Burbank, Los Angeles County, Calif). 2010;**26**:784-790

[50] Greenman RL, Rakow-Penner R. Evaluation of the RF field uniformity of a double-tuned 31P/1H birdcage RF coil for spin-echo MRI/MRS of the diabetic foot. Journal of Magnetic Resonance Imaging. 2005;**22**:427

[51] Heiss WD, Heindel W, Herholz K, Rudolf J, Bunke J, Jeske J, Friedmann G. Positron emission tomography of fluorine-18-deoxyglucose and image-guided phosphorus 31 magnetic resonance spectroscopy in brain tumors. Journal of Nuclear Medicine. 1990;**31**:302

[52] Greenman RL, Axel L, Ferrari VA, Lenkinski RE. Fast imaging of phosphocreatine in the normal human myocardium using a three-dimensional RARE pulse sequence at 4 Tesla. Journal of Magnetic Resonance Imaging. 2002;**15**:467

[53] Mountford CE, Stanwell P, Lin A, Ramadan S, Ross B. Neurospectroscopy: The past, present and future. Chemical Reviews. 2010;**110**(5):3060

[54] Cernak I, Vink R, Zapple DN, Cruz MI, Ahmed F, Chang T, Fricke ST, Faden AI. The pathobiology of moderate diffuse traumatic brain injury as identified using a new experimental model of injury in rats. Neurobiology of Disease. 2004;**17**:29

[55] Stovell MG, Yan JL, Sleigh A, Mada MO, Carpenter TA, Hutchinson PJA, Carpenter KLH. Assessing metabolism and injury in acute human traumatic brain injury with magnetic resonance spectroscopy: current and future applications. Frontiers in Neurology. 2017;**8**:426

[56] Giza CC, Hovda DA. The neurometabolic cascade of concussion. Journal of Athletic Training. 2001;**36**:228

[57] Sokoloff L, Reivich M, Kennedy C, Des Rosiers MH, Patlak CS, Pettigrew KD. The [14C] deoxyglucose method for the measurement of local cerebral glucose utilization: theory, procedure, and normal values in the conscious and anesthetized albino rat. Journal of Neurochemistry. 1977;**28**:897-916

[58] Neary JT. Protein kinase signaling cascades in CNS trauma. IUBMB Life. 2005;**57**:711

[59] Franke H, Verkhratsky A, Burnstock G, Illes P. Pathophysiology of astroglial purinergic signalling. Purinergic Signalling. 2012;**3**:629

[60] Otani N, Nawashiro H, Fukui S, Ooigawa H, Ohsumi A, Toyooka T, Shima K. Role of the activated extracellular signal-regulated kinase pathway on histological and behavioral outcome after traumatic brain injury in rats. Journal of Clinical Neuroscience. 2007;**14**:42

[61] Noshita N, Lewén A, Sugawara T, Chan PH. Akt phosphorylation and neuronal survival after traumatic brain injury in mice. Neurobiology of Disease. 2002;**9**:294

[62] Mori T, Wang X, Jung JC, Sumii T, Singhal AB, Fini ME, Dixon E, Alessandrini A, Lo EH. Mitogen-activated protein kinase inhibition in traumatic brain injury: in vitro and in vivo effects. Journal of Cerebral Blood Flow & Metabolism. 2002;**22**:444

[63] Walker CL, Liu NK, Xu XM. PTEN/PI3K and MAPK signaling in protection and pathology following CNS injuries. Frontiers in Biology (Beijing). 2013;**8**:1

[64] Otani N, Nawashiro H, Fukui S, Nomura N, Yano A, Miyazawa T, Shima K. Differential activation of mitogen-activated protein kinase pathways after traumatic brain injury in the rat hippocampus. Journal of Cerebral Blood Flow & Metabolism. 2002;**22**:327

[65] Manning BD, Cantley LC. AKT/PKB signaling: navigating downstream. Cell. 2007;**129**: 1261

[66] Nicholson KM, Anderson NG. The protein kinase B/Akt signaling pathway in human malignancy. Cellular Signalling. 2002;**14**:381

[67] Hay N, Sonenberg N. Upstream and downstream of mTOR. Genes & Development. 2004;**18**:1926

[68] Mesev EV, Miller DS, Cannon RE. Ceramide-1-phosphate increases P-glycoprotein transport activity at the blood-brain barrier via prostaglandin E2 signaling. Molecular Pharmacology. 2017;**91**:373

[69] Pasvogel AE, Miketova P, Moore IM. Differences in CSF phospholipid concentration by traumatic brain injury outcome. Biological Research for Nursing. 2010;**11**:325

[70] Pasvogel A, Miketova P, Moore IM. Cerebrospinal fluid phospholipid changes following traumatic brain injury. Biological Research for Nursing. 2008;**10**:113

[71] Jalloh I, Carpenter KLH, Grice P, Howe DJ, Mason A, Gallagher CN, Helmy A, Murphy MP, Menon DK, Carpenter TA, Pickard JD, Hutchinson PJ. Glycolysis and the pentose phosphate pathway after human traumatic brain injury: microdialysis studies using 1,2-13C2 glucose. Journal of Cerebral Blood Flow & Metabolism. 2015;**35**:111

[72] Fiebich BL, Akter S, Akundi RS. The two-hit hypothesis for neuroinflammation: role of exogenous ATP in modulating inflammation in the brain. Frontiers in Cellular Neuroscience. 2014;**8**:1

[73] Franke H, Illes P. Nucleotide signaling in astrogliosis. Neuroscience Letters. 2014;**565**:14

[74] Maravilla KR. Gadobenate dimeglumine-enhanced MR imaging of patients with CNS diseases. European Radiology. 2006;**16**:8

[75] Chapon C, Franconi F, Lacoeuille F, Hindré F, Saulnier P, Benoit JP, Le Jeune JJ, Lemaire L. Imaging E-selectin expression following traumatic brain injury in the rat using a targeted USPIO contrast agent. Magnetic Resonance Materials in Physics, Biology and Medicine. 2009;**22**:167

[76] Garcia-Martin ML, Martinez GV, Raghunand N, Sherry AD, Zhang S, Gillies RJ. High resolution pH(e) imaging of rat glioma using pH-dependent relaxivity. Magnetic Resonance in Medicine. 2006;**55**:309

[77] Raghunand N, Zhang S, Sherry AD, Gillies RJ. In vivo magnetic resonance imaging of tissue pH using a novel pH-sensitive contrast agent, GdDOTA-4AmP. Academic Radiology. 2002;**9**:481

[78] Watts LT, Shen Q, Deng S, Chemello J, Duong TQ. Manganese-enhanced magnetic resonance imaging of traumatic brain injury. Journal of Neurotrauma. 2015;**32**:1001

[79] Jasanoff A. MRI contrast agents for functional molecular imaging of brain activity. Current Opinion in Neurobiology. 2007;**17**:593

[80] Loane DJ, Stoica BA, Byrnes KR, Jeong W, Faden AI. Activation of mglur5 and inhibition of nadph oxidase improves functional recovery after traumatic brain injury. Journal of Neurotrauma. 2013;**30**(5):403-412. http://doi.org/10.1089/neu.2012.2589

[81] Johnson VE, Stewart W, Smith DH. Traumatic brain injury and amyloid-β pathology: a link to Alzheimer's disease? Nature Reviews Neuroscience. 2010;**11**(5):361

[82] Scott G, Ramlackhansingh AF, Edison P, Hellyer P, Cole J, Veronese M, Leech R, Greenwood RJ, Turkheimer FE, Gentleman SM, Heckemann RA, Matthews PM, Brooks DJ, Sharp DJ. Amyloid pathology and axonal injury after brain trauma. Neurology. 2016;**86**(9):821

[83] Chen J, Yang Z, Zhang X. Carbamylated erythropoietin: a prospective drug candidate for neuroprotection. Biochemistry Insights. 2015;**8**:25

[84] Torup L. Neuroprotection with or without erythropoiesis; sometimes less is more. British Journal of Pharmacology. 2007;**151**(8):1141

[85] Brines M, Grasso G, Fiordaliso F. Erythropoietin mediates tissue protection through an erythropoietin and common beta-subunit heteroreceptor. Proceedings of the National Academy of Sciences of the United States of America. 2004;**101**(41):14907

[86] Warren Pharmaceuticals. Novel carbamylated EPO and method for its production. WO2006/014466; 2006

[87] Byrnes KR, Loane DJ, Stoica BA, Zhang J, Faden AI. Delayed mGluR5 activation limits neuroinflammation and neurodegeneration after traumatic brain injury. Journal of Neuroinflammation. 2012;**9**:43

[88] Fishman RA. Brain Edema. The New England Journal of Medicine 1975;**293**:706-711. http://www.nejm.org/doi/full/10.1056/NEJM197510022931407

[89] Available from: https://www.bruker.com/products/mr/preclinical-mri.html

[90] Available from: http://www3.gehealthcare.com/en/products/categories/magnetic_resonance_imaging

[91] Available from: https://www.usa.philips.com/healthcare/solutions/magnetic-resonance

[92] Available from: http://www.hitachimed.com/products/mri

[93] Horsman GP, Zechel DL. Phosphonate biochemistry. Chemical Reviews. 2017;**117**(8):5704

9

Age-Dependent Responses Following Traumatic Brain Injury

Thomas Brickler, Paul D. Morton, Amanda Hazy and
Michelle H. Theus

Abstract

Traumatic brain injury (TBI) is a growing health concern worldwide that affects a broad range of the population. As TBI is the leading cause of disability and mortality in children, several preclinical models have been developed using rodents at a variety of different ages; however, key brain maturation events are overlooked that leave some age groups more or less vulnerable to injury. Thus, there has been a large emphasis on producing relevant animal models to elucidate molecular pathways that could be of therapeutic potential to help limit neuronal injury and improve behavioral outcome. TBI involves a host of different biochemical events, including disruption of the cerebral vasculature and breakdown of the blood-brain barrier (BBB) that exacerbates secondary injuries. A better understanding of age-related mechanism(s) underlying brain injury will aid in establishing more effective treatment strategies aimed at improving restoration and preventing further neuronal loss. This review looks at studies that focus on modeling the adolescent population and highlights the importance of individualized aged therapeutics to TBI.

Keywords: childhood, juvenile, traumatic brain injury, brain development, functional outcome, age dependence

1. Introduction

Traumatic brain injury (TBI) is a leading cause of long-term disability among all age groups with the adolescent population having a higher incidence of TBI [1]. Males sustain TBI at a much higher rate compared to females [1], and functional outcomes vary across patient's age and severity of injury [2, 3]. Studies have shown that younger patients are more likely to demonstrate continued improvements, while older patients are more likely to decline [2, 4].

On the other hand, childhood TBI (<6 years of age) presents poorer recovery of function compared to early adolescent or adolescent-aged patients [5, 6], with severe TBI in early childhood resulting in long-term impairment. Although better neuroplasticity or adaptation to brain injury in children has once been attributed to better recovery, the effect of age on outcome depends upon the function under study and the stage of development at the time of injury. In fact, the effects of childhood TBI may take years to "grow into deficit" as the developing brain hits milestones of maturation [7, 8]. Multiple regression analyses has also identified that age-at-injury onset is a major contributor to post-injury IQ [6]. While there are distinct periods of vulnerability in the developing brain, evidence from animal models also show that metabolic and physiological alterations specific to the juvenile or early adolescent brain may induce acute protection compared to adults [9–11]. These potentially distinct age-related responses are currently understudied and require a more accurate correlation of disease outcome with the maturation stage of the brain. Moreover, both small and large animal models need to be interpreted with caution since developmental milestones are distinct between swine, mice, and rat species as well as across different strains during the postnatal stages of growth. These differences make age comparisons to human infancy, childhood, early adolescence, adolescence, and adulthood challenging. To that end, correlating age-specific TBI outcomes from rodent to human thus requires consideration of key neurobiological maturation events, rather than chronological age, to predict differential responses to TBI which may eventually help guide effective diagnostic and treatment strategies. Here, we will review key events that accompany brain development in both humans and rodents to identify temporal "benchmarks" that may positively or negatively influence age-at-injury outcome. We will also provide an overview of research findings from clinical and preclinical age-related TBI studies.

1.1. Human brain structure and development

The human brain is a remarkably complex organ which we still do not fully understand. Representing 2% of the entire body weight in adulthood, the brain requires 20% of the body's oxygen supply to accommodate its extreme metabolic demands. Human brain development is a highly dynamic process which can be broken down into orchestrated cellular and molecular epochs. The neocortex is the newest and arguably most sophisticated structure in the human brain and accounts for most of the brain size. By adulthood, the neocortex will have amassed approximately 20 billion neurons each capable of forming an average of 7000 connections with other neurons [12, 13]. The brain is considered to be immune privileged as it is isolated from the bloodstream by the blood-brain barrier (BBB). Cerebral spinal fluid (CSF) flows through the ventricles located in the center of the brain also provides a cushion. The cerebrum is described as having four lobes: frontal, parietal, temporal, and occipital. The frontal lobe is involved in higher-order executive functions such as planning, reasoning, abstract thinking, decision-making, attention, and personality. Gray and white matters represent the two broad components of the brain. Gray matter is heavily populated with neuronal cell bodies which are essential for transmitting/communicating information throughout the brain. White matter accounts for 50% of the human brain volume and is white in appearance because it is highly composed of myelin [14], a specialized membrane, densely enriched with lipids, which can accelerate neuronal communication throughout the brain.

Human brain development commences during the third week of gestation and continues through adolescence [15]. Within the first year of life, the brain doubles in volume and will grow another 15% over the following year [16]. By the age of 6, the brain will have increased in size by fourfold which is roughly 90% of the size achieved in adulthood [15]. At the beginning of the fetal period of development, the brain is smooth, and later becomes convoluted with folds and ridges. This drastic increase in cortical volume is primarily through an increase in surface area, as opposed to an increase in thickness, which is how the cortex constitutes up to 80% of the total brain mass [17]. Higher-order cognitive function requires precise connections and communication throughout the brain. For example, cortical neurons can form connections with neighboring and distant cells to enable communication and integration of sensory, cognitive, and motor modalities. The corpus callosum is the largest white matter tract in the brain and serves as a major highway of axons connecting the left and right cerebral hemispheres. These axons are wrapped in myelin to foster rapid interhemispheric communication of information. Myelination is a process that begins around the middle of the second trimester, is most appreciably robust up to the second year of life, and continues throughout adolescence, though to a much lesser degree during adulthood [18, 19]. White matter development in the human brain is an asynchronous process, commencing earlier and more rapidly in sensory than motor pathways, and is later highly prominent in the frontal and temporal lobes at 6–8 months of age [19]. The left and right cerebral hemispheres serve different functions and do not develop in a completely symmetric manner [19]. One explanation for such spatial and temporal asymmetries is a hierarchy of connections formed in an experience-dependent order, such that brain regions involved with lower-level processes need to be established earlier in life before higher-order integrative regions are required. For example, the somatosensory cortex—important for tactile information—matures earlier in development than the prefrontal cortex which is involved in higher-level executive functions such as planning [20].

Our knowledge of human brain development has primarily been gathered from noninvasive neuroimaging measurements and their functional correlates to neurological outcomes, in addition to cellular associations with histopathology. It has become increasingly clear that the brain is extremely vulnerable during key developmental epochs. During these sensitive maturation-dependent time windows, childhood TBI may increase the risk of brain dysmaturation and atypical development depending on the severity and location of the injury [21–23]. For example, generalized (frontal/extrafrontal) or extrafrontal lesion severity but not frontal lesion alone was predictive of poor performance in children who sustained a moderate to severe TBI at ages 1–9 years of age [23]. Mechanistic insights into the etiologies of the neurological deficits and age-specific regions of vulnerability are vital to the understanding and treatment of pediatric TBI. However, rodent models of childhood and adolescent TBI in the postnatal growth stage may be difficult to translate into chronological age in humans. A better understanding of the major developmental processes in the brain across species and strains at the time of injury may be more instrumental for interpreting key findings. A few of these major milestones in neurodevelopment are noted below in **Table 1**.

Embryonic day (E), postnatal day (P), months (M), years (Y)	Mouse	Rat	Human	Reference
Sexual maturation[‡]	F: P23 M: P42	F: P32-34 M: P45-48	F: 10-17Y M: 11-17Y	[1, 24]
Peak brain volume (MRI)	P20	P60	F: 10.5Y M: 14.5Y	[8, 25, 26]
Developmental processes/milestones				
Neurogenesis completed by[*,†]	P16.5	P15	7.5 M	[8]
Astrocytogenesis peak	At birth	At birth	At birth	[8, 27]
Prefrontal cortex peak synaptic density[*]	P27.5	P25	12.4 M	[28]
Corpus callosum body myelination onset[*]	P15.5	P14	2.6 M	[28]
Corpus callosum body myelination end[*]	P35.5	P32	20.4 M	[28]
Internal capsule myelination onset[*]	P13.5	P12	1.4 M	[28]
Functional blood-brain barrier	E15.5	E14	10w gestation	[29]

[*]Estimates determined across species with www.translatingtime.net, based on Workman et al. [28].

[†]Estimate based off of neurogenesis completion in rat by postnatal day 15 [8]. F, female; M, male; P, postnatal days; Y, years; M, months; E, embryonic days; na, not applicable.

[‡]Sexual maturation is strain dependent.

Table 1. Developmental processes and milestones across mammals.

1.2. Age-at-injury response to clinical TBI

The widespread conception that the young brain is more resilient in its response to TBI has been challenged as there is considerable evidence that childhood TBI results in poorer outcomes. The developing brain may actually fair much worse compared to adults in cognitive and motor functions [30–32]. *Levin and colleagues* utilized the Glasgow Coma Scale (GCS), the primary measure of functional impairment, in children at 0–4 years of age and 5–10 years of age following TBI. The 0–4-year-olds were found to suffer the worst clinical outcome, comparatively. These and other findings analyzed the long-term behavioral outcomes in children who sustained a moderate to severe head injury [33]. Moreover, given the longevity of white matter development and maturation, TBI negatively impacts white matter integrity in the chronic (13–19 post-injury) but not acute (1–5 months) phase of injury which was linked to cognitive impairments in patients at 8–19 years of age [34, 35]. Patients with a history of neurological illness, brain tumor, seizures, psychosis, ADHD, Tourette's disorder, and other developmental disabilities were excluded from the study. This study also showed that the GCS was not significantly associated with white matter tract changes, as measured by diffuse tensor imaging (DTI), suggesting that advanced imaging modalities are vital to clinical tracking of disease progression and may be a more sensitive measure of outcome compared to GCS alone. Indeed, DTI coupled with functional MRI and perhaps other imaging strategies would greatly advance our understanding of the age-related mechanisms of repair and plasticity following TBI [36–39]. White matter dysregulation after childhood TBI may also affect motor recovery and social cognitive skills which are realized once the skills reach maturity [40–43].

Therefore, given the lengthy developmental course of myelination and synaptogenesis, TBI may disrupt the maturation of functions that support higher-order cognitive outcomes later in life [39, 44, 45]. The expression of glutamate receptors NMDA and AMPA greatly changes during development [46, 47]. Typically, there is an imbalance between excitatory and inhibitory neurotransmission in the developing brain, which could heighten the sensitivity of the young brain to glutamatergic excitotoxicity after trauma that may not be amplified in a mature brain [48]. Interestingly, the younger brain has less antioxidant capacity compared to the more matured brain, which during TBI increases the amount of reactive oxygen species (ROS) that could exacerbate the injury in the younger brain [49]. Inflammation also plays a critical role in brain tissue recovery after TBI [50]. In early childhood TBI, microglial cells that have infiltrated the brain may become overactive exacerbating secondary tissue damage [51]. Taken together, improving our understanding of developmentally related differences will be vital for predicting differential, age-specific outcomes and treatment responses to TBI .

Since the adolescent population sees a disproportionate percentage of hospitalizations and deaths compared to other age groups, this population should have its own outcome category tailoring research findings and treatment outcomes [52]. While adolescents fall between the childhood and adult age groups, how to appropriately treat these patients has been particularly challenging in the hospital setting [53]. Over a 13-year study, Gross and colleagues analyzed the adolescent TBI population (15–17 years of age) treated at pediatric or adult trauma centers. Although this study found no significant differences in outcomes between the centers, it raised an important question regarding how to treat adolescent brain injury, where differences in developmental vulnerability may exist compared to early childhood [53]. While early childhood TBI is associated with deficits in memory [54, 55], attention [56], intellectual functioning [57], and language acquisition [58], few studies have compared the outcomes of adolescent aged or young adults to older adults. A multiple regression model has demonstrated that increased age negatively influences outcome, as measured by the Disability Rating Scale (DRS) [4]. This study found a greater decline in older patients (≥40 years) over 5 years post-TBI but also demonstrated that the greatest amount of improvement in disability in young adults (16–26 years) compared to adults (27–39 years) and aged (≥40 years) patients. The mechanism(s) underlying this age-specific difference may be due, in part, to a reduction in the capacity to recover or decreased synaptic plasticity and cortical volume as we age or yet undetermined protective factors present during the late adolescence. Although TBI incidence has a bimodal age distribution peaking in adolescence and again in the elderly, few age-related studies have compared acute and chronic effects across the spectrum of age ranges including early childhood, adolescence, adulthood, and elderly. One prospective study of 330 severe TBI patients showed that younger patients (0–19 years of age) had a significantly higher percentage of good outcomes, lower mortality rates, and a reduced incidence of surgical mass lesions compared to adults (20–80 years of age) [11]. Although poorer recovery of function is known to exist in early childhood compared to adolescent-aged TBI patients, it should be noted that the mean age for the abovementioned study was 15–19 years and 39 years, respectively. Taken together, these findings suggest that the greatest vulnerability in age-specific responses lies in early childhood and advanced ages. Interestingly, there may be a narrow time window during which adolescence may confer protection, the mechanism(s) of which may be fully elucidated using animal models of brain injury, discussed below.

1.3. Age-at-injury response to preclinical TBI

Rodents are the most commonly used animal models in TBI research and are therefore well characterized and cross-validated [59–62]. The following sections will comprehensively review the acute and long-term TBI responses in both mice and rats at pre-weanling (P17), post-weanling/juvenile (P21), and adult (P60-90) ages. The commonly used models of TBI are the controlled cortical impact (CCI) injury and lateral fluid percussion injuries (LFPI) which have been adapted and scaled to younger rodent animals to account for differences in animal weight and brain size. However, the initial mechanical forces to the brain depend on an array of factors that are independently determined. These factors include location, severity, focal, or diffuse injury. Similar to clinical findings, there are a spectrum of outcomes following pre-clinical TBI that are not only age dependent but species and strain specific which must be interpreted with caution. Although the importance of gyrification of the human brain, which is fully formed at birth but increases in complexity postnatally, is still under debate [63], this cross species differences should be kept in mind. Nonetheless, animal models of TBI have been instrumental in assessing the vulnerability of the developing brain to mechanical forces applied following CCI or LFP injury models.

Neurogenesis, gliogenesis, synaptogenesis, and myelination are key developmental events that may impact age-at-injury outcomes after TBI [64–66]. While neurogenesis peaks during gestational periods, by adulthood the generation of neurons is restricted to the dentate gyrus (DG) of the hippocampus and the lateral wall of the subventricular zone (SVZ) [64, 67]. Induction of post-injury neurogenesis has been suggested to play a critical role in learning and memory recovery as well as providing neurotrophic factor secretion as neuroprotective cues. While selectively ablating adult neurogenesis can dampen functional recovery [68, 69], the effects on early childhood or adolescence are unclear. Sun and colleagues analyzed the morphological changes within the subgranular zone of the DG and the SVZ following LFPI using P28 juvenile and P90 adult rats [70]. The LFPI model mimics both focal and diffuse mechanical injuries and results in histopathological changes similar to those seen in humans [60]. The study determined that LFPI enhanced proliferation within the DG of both adult and juvenile rats. However, the juvenile response in the SVZ was greater compared to adults. Furthermore, they identified twice as many neurons that were born from the juvenile SVZ compared to adults. Similarly, juvenile mice at P21 subjected to CCI injury show an increased presence of doublecortin-positive neuroblasts in the DG at 2 weeks post-injury [71]. However, a significant decline in these cells was seen at 3 months post-injury suggesting that an acute protective response may be subdued by long-term activation of yet unknown cellular programs. No comparisons to adult CCI injury were made. Unfortunately, data regarding age effects on neurogenesis are still lacking since numerous studies in mice or rats either have not performed adult comparisons [72] or have not used relevant TBI models [67, 73]. Of note, while naïve P9 mice display increased proliferation in the DG compared to P21, hypoxic-ischemic injury adversely affected neurogenesis in P9 but greatly enhanced it in P21 suggesting that early adolescence may display a critical window of regenerative potential that may be lost in adulthood. These findings would need to be confirmed using an appropriately controlled, longitudinal investigation (days, weeks, months) of neurogenesis with the inclusion of adult mice. Likewise, suitably comparable ages of rats subjected to TBI could support this hypothesis and help demonstrate a cross species phenomenon.

Synaptogenesis peaks at 2 years of age in humans and in 3 weeks in both rats and mice [65]. The number of synapses at these time points is greater, and pruning events follow to decrease the number of synapses [74–76]. In addition, myelination is an ongoing process that continues well into adulthood [66]; atypical development of these processes as a result of TBI may significantly impact synaptic reorganization and long-term neurobehavioral development [77–79]. Ajao and colleagues found that TBI in rats at P17 resulted in measurable deficits in motor performance on the rotarod and foot faults at 60 days post-injury well into adulthood [77]. Anxiety-like behaviors were also increased compared to noninjured sham controls. Sensorimotor tasks and anxiety-like behaviors are often linked to histological changes such as cell death in the brain as a consequence of childhood TBI. Neuronal loss due to focal impact can impair major electrical signaling pathways by disconnecting circuits, increasing calcium in dying cells, triggering inflammation, and blunting key trophic support. The immature rat brain is particularly sensitive to excitotoxicity in the neonatal period [80, 81]. This is regulated, in part, by developmental changes in expression of the NR2A and NR2B subunits of the NMDA receptor [82, 83] and/or GABAergic neurotransmission impairments through, for example, cortical loss of GABAergic interneurons [84, 85]. In the second and third postnatal weeks, however, this effect is reduced. In fact, minimal neuronal loss is seen following weight drop and LFPI in juvenile (P15–P19) rats [81, 86, 87] suggesting that long-term behavioral deficits following TBI are due in greater part to neuronal dysfunction rather than neuronal loss. On the other hand, a significant delay in loss of neural tissue is observed in juvenile (P21) mice after CCI injury [71, 88, 89] which correlates with progressive dysfunction. Differences in injury model, rodent species, or time of histopathological assessment after injury may account for these differences. Indeed, a gyrencephalic model of cortical impact delivered at different maturation stages to the piglet brain demonstrated increased vulnerability with age to cortical trauma, with the smallest lesions seen at 7 days post-injury in 5-day-old pigs, modest injury in 1-month-old piglets, and largest lesion volume in 4-month-olds [90, 91]. Progressive histopathological or behavioral changes over time were not evaluated.

While the maturation-dependent response of the resident neuroimmune system (microglial and astrocytes) remains under investigation, a notable difference in peripheral immune activation following TBI has been demonstrated. Bidirectional neural-immune communication exists to clear the brain of dead cellular debris from necrotic spillover of intracellular components. However, when overactivated, the immune system can mediate neurotoxicity and exacerbate secondary injury including free radical formation and oxidative damage as well as activation of microglia [92]. Although TBI increases the presence of leukocytes both in neural tissue, due to BBB disruption, and in the peripheral blood [93], the destructive phenotype of activated immune cell subpopulations is not well understood. Recent findings suggest that progressive injury in P21 mice observed months following CCI injury compared to adult may result from an age-dependent temporal patterns in leukocyte infiltration [88]. While no differences were noted for the CD4+ and CD8+ populations, CD45+ cells and GR-1+ granulocytes remained elevated for weeks in P21 mice compared to 3 days in adult. This effect may be regulated, in part, by IL-1β. Injection of IL-1β into the P21 rat brain exacerbates rapid neutrophil recruitment, CXC chemokine production, and BBB disruption compared to adult rats [94–96]. While the juvenile immune system may display increased sensitivity to neutrophil chemoattractants (CXCL1, CXCL2, CXC8) [97], extension of neutrophil life span may also translate into increased numbers [98, 99]. Indeed, adult neutrophil depletion studies appear to reduce edema, cell death, and macrophage/microglia activation while having no effect on BBB and functional outcome suggesting that neutrophils may negatively impact TBI outcome and their long-lived nature may cause progressive injury and contribute to other age-related responses [100, 101]. Findings from our laboratory have shown significant neuroprotection in P21 mice subjected to moderate CCI injury compared to adults (unpublished findings). Interestingly, we have identified numerous genes in the whole cell fractions of peripheral blood from P21 mice that are differentially regulated compared to adults (unpublished findings). Next-generation RNA sequencing and ontology analysis identified several pathways that are differentially regulated including (1) metabolic, (2) apoptotic, and (3) inflammatory processes (**Figure 1**). Peripheral blood cells isolated from P21 mice display reduced expression of several Toll-like receptors (Tlr1, Tlr6, Tlr4, Tlr2), TNF receptor (TNFRSF1A), MMP9, and upregulation of the antioxidant superoxide dismutase 2 (SOD2), autophagy-elated ATG4A, antiapoptotic Bag1, and a number of other genes that may influence their response once recruited after TBI. Enhanced survival of immune-derived cells in the brain may have long-lasting effects on tissue repair and recovery. There may be beneficial effects of early recruitment and survival in the damaged neural tissue that may be outweighed in the long run if their transient presence is extended. Differences in immune cell-type survival, gene expression, and function need to be further explored.

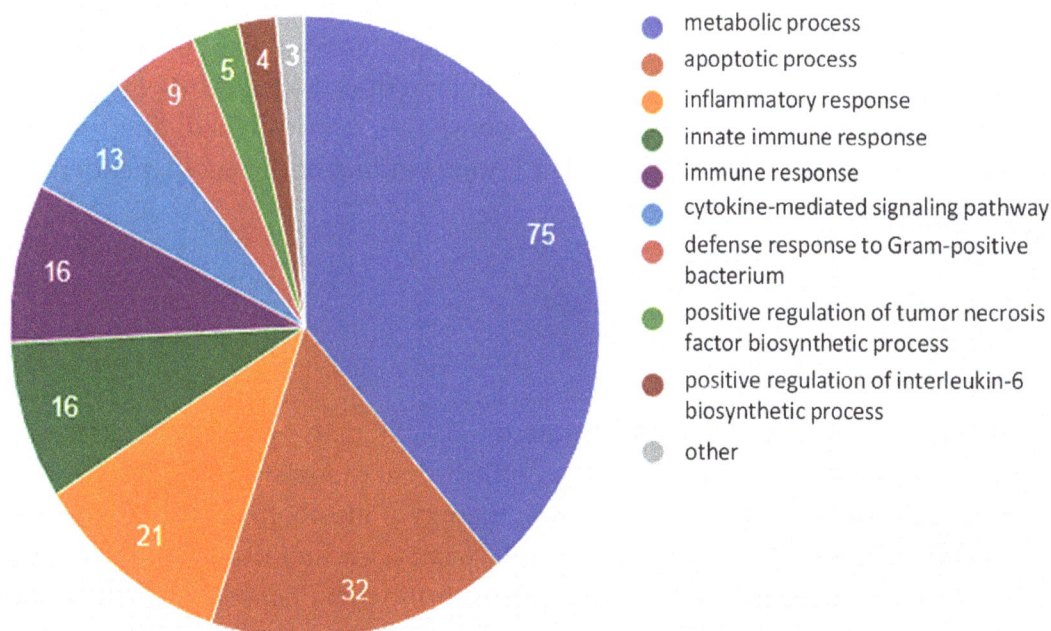

Figure 1. GO analysis of differentially expressed genes between juvenile and adult mouse peripheral blood cells. Six hundred and ten genes showed differential expression (q < 0.05) between juvenile and adults. Ontology analysis using GeneCodis (biological process) was performed using this gene list to identify differentially regulated pathways [1–3].

Lastly, subtype-specific recruitment of monocytes/macrophages (M1 vs. M2) has also been shown to play a critical role in outcome following CNS injury [102, 103]. However, age-dependent effects of these cell types in both acute and chronic TBI outcome have yet to be investigated. Further examination into the temporal–spatial recruitment of immune cell subtypes and the employment of depletion and cell-type-specific knockout studies will help address the important emerging role of the peripheral-derived immune system in responding to brain trauma across the life span.

The BBB is established during embryogenesis in rodents and humans [104, 105]; however, postnatal coverage with astrocytic end feet, which aids in the maturation and maintenance of the BBB, occurs in the first few postnatal weeks [104, 106, 107]. This maturation stage is critical with regard to changes in permeability as a result of insult. For example, systemic inflammation increases BBB permeability in P0 and P8 rats while having no effect at P20 [108, 109]. TBI induces endothelial cell dysfunction that increases the permeability of the BBB including disruption of astrocytic end feet, transporters/channels, and tight junction proteins claudin-5 and occludin-1 causing widespread vasogenic edema [110, 111]. The temporal changes in BBB permeability likely depend on the model of TBI, age-at-injury, and severity of impact. Interestingly, monocarboxylate transporter 2 (MCT2) is substantially increased in the microvessels of juvenile P35 rats following CCI injury compared to P75 adult rats [112]. This increase correlated with improved behavioral outcome and reduced cortical lesion volume in P35 rats receiving a ketogenic diet post-TBI compared to adults [113]. Pop and colleagues observed BBB disruption following CCI injury in P17 rats through high amounts of IgG staining, which is consistent with what is seen after CCI injury [114]. At 1-week after injury, a substantial reduction in BBB permeability correlated with an increase expression of tight junction protein (claudin-5). This was maintained as far out as 2 months post-injury, suggesting that tight junction proteins may modulate early disruption and subsequent repair. Likewise, administration of DHA and EPA, the main sources found in fish oil, after CCI injury in P17 juvenile rats reduces BBB permeability, behavioral deficits, and MMP9 expression [115]. The relevance of these studies to the adult response was not evaluated, and further work needs to be conducted in order to improve our understanding of the age-dependent mechanism(s) regulating the BBB following TBI.

2. Conclusions

There has been intense investigation into the brain's maturation-dependent response to TBI using numerous early childhood and juvenile rodent models. Over recent years, studies have revealed age-specific differences in the regulation of metabolism, oxidative stress, neurogenesis, innate immunity, and BBB function following acute and/or chronic injury. Further exploration into the age-specific elements of vascular function, neuroimmune regulation, and the neurovascular niche would help improve our understanding, not only of typical but also atypical developmental trajectories as a consequence of childhood TBI. The insurgence of these animal models, however, must be met with caution as key maturation stages of the brain vary considerably between murine and rat species. Studies of immature or juvenile injury must also be accompanied by appropriate comparisons to adult-aged animals, which thus far has been inadequate. The need for larger animal models that more accurately recapitulate human brain structure and maturational age is also warranted. Although predicting the age-specific response to TBI in childhood, adolescence, and young adulthood is limited based on current available animal model data, it is clear that "a window of susceptibility" exists that may deter normal growth and development. On the other hand, it is important not to underestimate the early neuroprotective findings observed in a number of studies, which may yield valuable mechanistic insight into pathways that could be utilized for neuroprotection in the adult brain.

Author details

Thomas Brickler[1], Paul D. Morton[2], Amanda Hazy[2] and Michelle H. Theus[2]*

*Address all correspondence to: mtheus@vt.edu

1 The Department of Psychiatry and Behavioral Sciences, Stanford University School of Medicine, Stanford, CA, USA

2 The Department of Biomedical Sciences and Pathobiology, Virginia-Maryland Regional College of Veterinary Medicine, Blacksburg, VA, USA

References

[1] Dewan MC, Mummareddy N, Wellons JC, 3rd CM. Bonfield, epidemiology of global pediatric traumatic brain injury: Qualitative review. World Neurosurgery. 2016;**91**:497-509 e491

[2] Mosenthal AC et al. The effect of age on functional outcome in mild traumatic brain injury: 6-month report of a prospective multicenter trial. The Journal of Trauma. 2004;**56**: 1042-1048

[3] van der Naalt J et al. Early predictors of outcome after mild traumatic brain injury (UPFRONT): An observational cohort study. Lancet Neurology. 2017;**16**:532-540

[4] Marquez de la Plata CD et al. Impact of age on long-term recovery from traumatic brain injury. Archives of Physical Medicine and Rehabilitation. 2008;**89**:896-903

[5] Catroppa C, Anderson VA, Morse SA, Haritou F, Rosenfeld JV. Outcome and predictors of functional recovery 5 years following pediatric traumatic brain injury (TBI). Journal of Pediatric Psychology. 2008;**33**:707-718

[6] Duval J et al. Brain lesions and IQ: Recovery versus decline depends on age of onset. Journal of Child Neurology. 2008;**23**:663-668

[7] Giza CC, Prins ML. Is being plastic fantastic? Mechanisms of altered plasticity after developmental traumatic brain injury. Developmental Neuroscience. 2006;**28**:364-379

[8] Semple BD, Blomgren K, Gimlin K, Ferriero DM, Noble-Haeusslein LJ. Brain development in rodents and humans: Identifying benchmarks of maturation and vulnerability to injury across species. Progress in Neurobiology. 2013;**106-107**:1-16

[9] Prins ML, Hovda DA. The effects of age and ketogenic diet on local cerebral metabolic rates of glucose after controlled cortical impact injury in rats. Journal of Neurotrauma. 2009;**26**:1083-1093

[10] Babikian T et al. Molecular and physiological responses to juvenile traumatic brain injury: Focus on growth and metabolism. Developmental Neuroscience. 2010;**32**:431-441

[11] Alberico AM, Ward JD, Choi SC, Marmarou A, Young HF. Outcome after severe head injury. Relationship to mass lesions, diffuse injury, and ICP course in pediatric and adult patients. Journal of Neurosurgery. 1987;**67**:648-656

[12] Herculano-Houzel S. The human brain in numbers: A linearly scaled-up primate brain. Frontiers in Human Neuroscience. 2009;**3**:31

[13] Pakkenberg B et al. Aging and the human neocortex. Experimental Gerontology. 2003;**38**: 95-99

[14] Filley CM. White matter dementia. Therapeutic Advances in Neurological Disorders. 2012; **5**:267-277

[15] Stiles J, Jernigan TL. The basics of brain development. Neuropsychology Review. 2010;**20**: 327-348

[16] Knickmeyer RC et al. A structural MRI study of human brain development from birth to 2 years. The Journal of Neuroscience. 2008;**28**:12176-12182

[17] Geschwind DH, Rakic P. Cortical evolution: Judge the brain by its cover. Neuron. 2013; **80**:633-647

[18] Geng X et al. Quantitative tract-based white matter development from birth to age 2years. NeuroImage. 2012;**61**:542-557

[19] Qiu A, Mori S, Miller MI. Diffusion tensor imaging for understanding brain development in early life. Annual Review of Psychology. 2015;**66**:853-876

[20] Guillery RW. Is postnatal neocortical maturation hierarchical? Trends in Neurosciences. 2005;**28**:512-517

[21] Popernack ML, Gray N, Reuter-Rice K. Moderate-to-severe traumatic brain injury in children: Complications and rehabilitation strategies. Journal of Pediatric Health Care. 2015;**29**:e1-e7

[22] Vaewpanich J, Reuter-Rice K. Continuous electroencephalography in pediatric traumatic brain injury: Seizure characteristics and outcomes. Epilepsy & Behavior. 2016;**62**:225-230

[23] Power T, Catroppa C, Coleman L, Ditchfield M, Anderson V. Do lesion site and severity predict deficits in attentional control after preschool traumatic brain injury (TBI)? Brain Injury. 2007;**21**:279-292

[24] Sengupta P. The laboratory rat: Relating its age with Human's. International Journal of Preventive Medicine. 2013;**4**:624-630

[25] Chuang N et al. An MRI-based atlas and database of the developing mouse brain. NeuroImage. 2011;**54**:80-89

[26] Mengler L et al. Brain maturation of the adolescent rat cortex and striatum: Changes in volume and myelination. NeuroImage. 2014;**84**:35-44

[27] Sauvageot CM, Stiles CD. Molecular mechanisms controlling cortical gliogenesis. Current Opinion in Neurobiology. 2002;**12**:244-249

[28] Workman AD, Charvet CJ, Clancy B, Darlington RB, Finlay BL. Modeling transformations of neurodevelopmental sequences across mammalian species. The Journal of Neuroscience. 2013;**33**:7368-7383

[29] Ben-Zvi A et al. Mfsd2a is critical for the formation and function of the blood-brain barrier. Nature. 2014;**509**:507-511

[30] Anderson VA et al. Understanding predictors of functional recovery and outcome 30 months following early childhood head injury. Neuropsychology. 2006;**20**:42-57

[31] Bruce DA, Schut L, Bruno LA, Wood JH, Sutton LN. Outcome following severe head injuries in children. Journal of Neurosurgery. 1978;**48**:679-688

[32] Taylor HG et al. Influences on first-year recovery from traumatic brain injury in children. Neuropsychology. 1999;**13**:76-89

[33] Treble-Barna A et al. Long-term neuropsychological profiles and their role as mediators of adaptive functioning after traumatic brain injury in early childhood. Journal of Neurotrauma. 2017;**34**:353-362

[34] Dennis EL et al. White matter disruption in moderate/severe pediatric traumatic brain injury: Advanced tract-based analyses. Neuroimage: Clinical. 2015;**7**:493-505

[35] Dennis EL et al. Callosal function in Pediatric traumatic brain injury linked to disrupted white matter integrity. The Journal of Neuroscience. 2015;**35**:10202-10211

[36] Mechtler LL, Shastri KK, Crutchfield KE. Advanced neuroimaging of mild traumatic brain injury. Neurologic Clinics. 2014;**32**:31-58

[37] Edlow BL, Wu O. Advanced neuroimaging in traumatic brain injury. Seminars in Neurology. 2012;**32**:374-400

[38] Ashwal S, Holshouser BA, Tong KA. Use of advanced neuroimaging techniques in the evaluation of pediatric traumatic brain injury. Developmental Neuroscience. 2006;**28**: 309-326

[39] Levin HS. Neuroplasticity following non-penetrating traumatic brain injury. Brain Injury. 2003;**17**:665-674

[40] Stephens J, Salorio C, Denckla M, Mostofsky S, Suskauer S. Subtle motor findings during recovery from Pediatric traumatic brain injury: A preliminary report. Journal of Motor Behavior. 2017;**49**:20-26

[41] Ryan NP et al. Longitudinal outcome and recovery of social problems after pediatric traumatic brain injury (TBI): Contribution of brain insult and family environment. International Journal of Developmental Neuroscience. 2016;**49**:23-30

[42] Ryan NP et al. The emergence of age-dependent social cognitive deficits after generalized insult to the developing brain: A longitudinal prospective analysis using susceptibility-weighted imaging. Human Brain Mapping. 2015;**36**:1677-1691

[43] Li L, Liu J. The effect of pediatric traumatic brain injury on behavioral outcomes: A systematic review. Developmental Medicine and Child Neurology. 2013;**55**:37-45

[44] Chapman SB, McKinnon L. Discussion of developmental plasticity: Factors affecting cognitive outcome after pediatric traumatic brain injury. Journal of Communication Disorders. 2000;**33**:333-344

[45] Cook LG, Chapman SB, Elliott AC, Evenson NN, Vinton K. Cognitive gains from gist reasoning training in adolescents with chronic-stage traumatic brain injury. Frontiers in Neurology. 2014;**5**:87

[46] Ben-Ari Y, Khazipov R, Leinekugel X, Caillard O, Gaiarsa JL. GABAA, NMDA and AMPA receptors: A developmentally regulated 'menage a trois'. Trends in Neurosciences. 1997; **20**:523-529

[47] Nunez JL, McCarthy MM. Evidence for an extended duration of GABA-mediated excitation in the developing male versus female hippocampus. Developmental Neurobiology. 2007;**67**:1879-1890

[48] McDonald JW, Trescher WH, Johnston MV. Susceptibility of brain to AMPA induced excitotoxicity transiently peaks during early postnatal development. Brain Research. 1992;**583**:54-70

[49] Bayir H, Kochanek PM, Kagan VE. Oxidative stress in immature brain after traumatic brain injury. Developmental Neuroscience. 2006;**28**:420-431

[50] Das M, Mohapatra S, Mohapatra SS. New perspectives on central and peripheral immune responses to acute traumatic brain injury. Journal of Neuroinflammation. 2012;**9**:236

[51] Hagberg H, Gressens P, Mallard C. Inflammation during fetal and neonatal life: Implications for neurologic and neuropsychiatric disease in children and adults. Annals of Neurology. 2012;**71**:444-457

[52] Coronado VG et al. Surveillance for traumatic brain injury-related deaths--United States, 1997-2007. MMWR Surveillance Summaries. 2011;**60**:1-32

[53] Gross BW et al. Big children or little adults? A statewide analysis of adolescent isolated severe traumatic brain injury outcomes at pediatric versus adult trauma centers. Journal of Trauma and Acute Care Surgery. 2017;**82**:368-373

[54] Anderson VA, Catroppa C, Morse SA, Haritou F. Functional memory skills following traumatic brain injury in young children. Pediatric Rehabilitation. 1999;**3**:159-166

[55] Anderson VA, Catroppa C, Rosenfeld J, Haritou F, Morse SA. Recovery of memory function following traumatic brain injury in pre-school children. Brain Injury. 2000;**14**:679-692

[56] Bakker K, Anderson V. Assessment of attention following pre-school traumatic brain injury: A behavioural attention measure. Pediatric Rehabilitation. 1999;**3**:149-157

[57] Anderson V, Catroppa C, Morse S, Haritou F, Rosenfeld J. Recovery of intellectual ability following traumatic brain injury in childhood: Impact of injury severity and age at injury. Pediatric Neurosurgery. 2000;**32**:282-290

[58] Morse S et al. Early effects of traumatic brain injury on young children's language performance: A preliminary linguistic analysis. Pediatric Rehabilitation. 1999;**3**:139-148

[59] Johnson VE, Meaney DF, Cullen DK, Smith DH. Animal models of traumatic brain injury. Handbook of Clinical Neurology. 2015;**127**:115-128

[60] Xiong Y, Mahmood A, Chopp M. Animal models of traumatic brain injury. Nature Reviews. Neuroscience. 2013;**14**:128-142

[61] Adelson PD. Animal models of traumatic brain injury in the immature: A review. Experimental and Toxicologic Pathology. 1999;**51**:130-136

[62] Morganti-Kossmann MC, Yan E, Bye N. Animal models of traumatic brain injury: Is there an optimal model to reproduce human brain injury in the laboratory? Injury. 2010;**41**(Suppl 1):S10-S13

[63] White T, Su S, Schmidt M, Kao CY, Sapiro G. The development of gyrification in childhood and adolescence. Brain and Cognition. 2010;**72**:36-45

[64] Rice D, Barone S Jr. Critical periods of vulnerability for the developing nervous system: Evidence from humans and animal models. Environmental Health Perspectives. 2000;**108**(Suppl 3):511-533

[65] Low LK, Cheng HJ. Axon pruning: An essential step underlying the developmental plasticity of neuronal connections. Philosophical Transactions of the Royal Society of London. Series B, Biological Sciences. 2006;**361**:1531-1544

[66] Giedd JN et al. Brain development during childhood and adolescence: A longitudinal MRI study. Nature Neuroscience. 1999;**2**:861-863

[67] Covey MV, Jiang Y, Alli VV, Yang Z, Levison SW. Defining the critical period for neocortical neurogenesis after pediatric brain injury. Developmental Neuroscience. 2010;**32**: 488-498

[68] Dixon KJ et al. Endogenous neural stem/progenitor cells stabilize the cortical microenvironment after traumatic brain injury. Journal of Neurotrauma. 2015;**32**:753-764

[69] Blaiss CA et al. Temporally specified genetic ablation of neurogenesis impairs cognitive recovery after traumatic brain injury. The Journal of Neuroscience. 2011;**31**:4906-4916

[70] Sun D et al. Cell proliferation and neuronal differentiation in the dentate gyrus in juvenile and adult rats following traumatic brain injury. Journal of Neurotrauma. 2005;**22**:95-105

[71] Pullela R et al. Traumatic injury to the immature brain results in progressive neuronal loss, hyperactivity and delayed cognitive impairments. Developmental Neuroscience. 2006;**28**:396-409

[72] Potts MB et al. Glutathione peroxidase overexpression does not rescue impaired neurogenesis in the injured immature brain. Journal of Neuroscience Research. 2009;**87**: 1848-1857

[73] Qiu L et al. Less neurogenesis and inflammation in the immature than in the juvenile brain after cerebral hypoxia-ischemia. Journal of Cerebral Blood Flow and Metabolism. 2007;**27**:785-794

[74] Herschkowitz N, Kagan J, Zilles K. Neurobiological bases of behavioral development in the first year. Neuropediatrics. 1997;**28**:296-306

[75] Huttenlocher PR. Synaptic density in human frontal cortex - developmental changes and effects of aging. Brain Research. 1979;**163**:195-205

[76] Crain B, Cotman C, Taylor D, Lynch G. A quantitative electron microscopic study of synaptogenesis in the dentate gyrus of the rat. Brain Research. 1973;**63**:195-204

[77] Ajao DO et al. Traumatic brain injury in young rats leads to progressive behavioral deficits coincident with altered tissue properties in adulthood. Journal of Neurotrauma. 2012;**29**:2060-2074

[78] Jullienne A et al. Juvenile traumatic brain injury induces long-term perivascular matrix changes alongside amyloid-beta accumulation. Journal of Cerebral Blood Flow and Metabolism. 2014;**34**:1637-1645

[79] Kamper JE et al. Juvenile traumatic brain injury evolves into a chronic brain disorder: Behavioral and histological changes over 6months. Experimental Neurology. 2013;**250**: 8-19

[80] Ikonomidou C, Qin Y, Labruyere J, Kirby C, Olney JW. Prevention of trauma-induced neurodegeneration in infant rat brain. Pediatric Research. 1996;**39**:1020-1027

[81] Bittigau P et al. Apoptotic neurodegeneration following trauma is markedly enhanced in the immature brain. Annals of Neurology. 1999;**45**:724-735

[82] Giza CC, Maria NS, Hovda DA. N-methyl-D-aspartate receptor subunit changes after traumatic injury to the developing brain. Journal of Neurotrauma. 2006;**23**:950-961

[83] Jantzie LL et al. Developmental expression of N-methyl-D-aspartate (NMDA) receptor subunits in human white and gray matter: Potential mechanism of increased vulnerability in the immature brain. Cerebral Cortex. 2015;**25**:482-495

[84] Wu C, Sun D. GABA receptors in brain development, function, and injury. Metabolic Brain Disease. 2015;**30**:367-379

[85] Robinson S, Li Q, Dechant A, Cohen ML. Neonatal loss of gamma-aminobutyric acid pathway expression after human perinatal brain injury. Journal of Neurosurgery. 2006;**104**:396-408

[86] Adelson PD et al. Histopathologic response of the immature rat to diffuse traumatic brain injury. Journal of Neurotrauma. 2001;**18**:967-976

[87] Gurkoff GG, Giza CC, Hovda DA. Lateral fluid percussion injury in the developing rat causes an acute, mild behavioral dysfunction in the absence of significant cell death. Brain Research. 2006;**1077**:24-36

[88] Claus CP et al. Age is a determinant of leukocyte infiltration and loss of cortical volume after traumatic brain injury. Developmental Neuroscience. 2010;**32**:454-465

[89] Tong W, Igarashi T, Ferriero DM, Noble LJ. Traumatic brain injury in the immature mouse brain: Characterization of regional vulnerability. Experimental Neurology. 2002;**176**:105-116

[90] Duhaime AC et al. Maturation-dependent response of the piglet brain to scaled cortical impact. Journal of Neurosurgery. 2000;**93**:455-462

[91] Grate LL, Golden JA, Hoopes PJ, Hunter JV, Duhaime AC. Traumatic brain injury in piglets of different ages: Techniques for lesion analysis using histology and magnetic resonance imaging. Journal of Neuroscience Methods. 2003;**123**:201-206

[92] Clark RS, Schiding JK, Kaczorowski SL, Marion DW, Kochanek PM. Neutrophil accumulation after traumatic brain injury in rats: Comparison of weight drop and controlled cortical impact models. Journal of Neurotrauma. 1994;**11**:499-506

[93] Furlan JC, Krassioukov AV, Fehlings MG. Hematologic abnormalities within the first week after acute isolated traumatic cervical spinal cord injury: A case-control cohort study. Spine (Phila Pa 1976). 2006;**31**:2674-2683

[94] Anthony DC, Bolton SJ, Fearn S, Perry VH. Age-related effects of interleukin-1 beta on polymorphonuclear neutrophil-dependent increases in blood-brain barrier permeability in rats. Brain. 1997;**120**(Pt 3):435-444

[95] Anthony D et al. CXC chemokines generate age-related increases in neutrophil-mediated brain inflammation and blood-brain barrier breakdown. Current Biology. 1998;**8**:923-926

[96] Campbell SJ, Carare-Nnadi RO, Losey PH, Anthony DC. Loss of the atypical inflammatory response in juvenile and aged rats. Neuropathology and Applied Neurobiology. 2007;**33**:108-120

[97]   Semple BD, Kossmann T, Morganti-Kossmann MC. Role of chemokines in CNS health and pathology: A focus on the CCL2/CCR2 and CXCL8/CXCR2 networks. Journal of Cerebral Blood Flow and Metabolism. 2010;**30**:459-473

[98]   Kigerl KA, McGaughy VM, Popovich PG. Comparative analysis of lesion development and intraspinal inflammation in four strains of mice following spinal contusion injury. The Journal of Comparative Neurology. 2006;**494**:578-594

[99]   Hazeldine J, Lord JM, Belli A. Traumatic brain injury and peripheral immune suppression: Primer and prospectus. Frontiers in Neurology. 2015;**6**:235

[100] Kenne E, Erlandsson A, Lindbom L, Hillered L, Clausen F. Neutrophil depletion reduces edema formation and tissue loss following traumatic brain injury in mice. Journal of Neuroinflammation. 2012;**9**:17

[101] Semple BD, Bye N, Ziebell JM, Morganti-Kossmann MC. Deficiency of the chemokine receptor CXCR2 attenuates neutrophil infiltration and cortical damage following closed head injury. Neurobiology of Disease. 2010;**40**:394-403

[102] Kigerl KA et al. Identification of two distinct macrophage subsets with divergent effects causing either neurotoxicity or regeneration in the injured mouse spinal cord. The Journal of Neuroscience. 2009;**29**:13435-13444

[103] Kumar A, Alvarez-Croda DM, Stoica BA, Faden AI, Loane DJ. Microglial/macrophage polarization dynamics following traumatic brain injury. Journal of Neurotrauma. 2016;**33**:1732-1750

[104] Daneman R, Zhou L, Kebede AA, Barres BA. Pericytes are required for blood-brain barrier integrity during embryogenesis. Nature. 2010;**468**:562-566

[105] Saunders NR, Liddelow SA, Dziegielewska KM. Barrier mechanisms in the developing brain. Frontiers in Pharmacology. 2012;**3**:46

[106] Cornford EM, Cornford ME. Nutrient transport and the blood-brain barrier in developing animals. Federation Proceedings. 1986;**45**:2065-2072

[107] Engelhardt B. Development of the blood-brain barrier. Cell and Tissue Research. 2003;**314**:119-129

[108] Stolp HB, Dziegielewska KM, Ek CJ, Potter AM, Saunders NR. Long-term changes in blood-brain barrier permeability and white matter following prolonged systemic inflammation in early development in the rat. The European Journal of Neuroscience. 2005;**22**:2805-2816

[109] Stolp HB et al. Breakdown of the blood-brain barrier to proteins in white matter of the developing brain following systemic inflammation. Cell and Tissue Research. 2005;**320**:369-378

[110] Price L, Wilson CG. Grant. In: Laskowitz D, Grant G, editors. Translational Research in Traumatic Brain Injury. CRC Press/Taylor and Francis Group: Boca Raton (FL); 2016

[111] Chodobski A, Zink BJ, Szmydynger-Chodobska J. Blood-brain barrier pathophysiology in traumatic brain injury. Translational Stroke Research. 2011;**2**:492-516

[112] Prins ML, Giza CC. Induction of monocarboxylate transporter 2 expression and ketone transport following traumatic brain injury in juvenile and adult rats. Developmental Neuroscience. 2006;**28**:447-456

[113] Appelberg KS, Hovda DA, Prins ML. The effects of a ketogenic diet on behavioral outcome after controlled cortical impact injury in the juvenile and adult rat. Journal of Neurotrauma. 2009;**26**:497-506

[114] Pop V, Badaut J. A neurovascular perspective for long-term changes after brain trauma. Translational Stroke Research. 2011;**2**:533-545

[115] Russell KL, Berman NE, Gregg PR, Levant B. Fish oil improves motor function, limits blood-brain barrier disruption, and reduces Mmp9 gene expression in a rat model of juvenile traumatic brain injury. Prostaglandins, Leukotrienes, and Essential Fatty Acids. 2014;**90**:5-11

10

Traumatic Penumbra: Opportunities for Neuroprotective and Neurorestorative Processes

Andrea Regner, Lindolfo da Silva Meirelles and
Daniel Simon

Abstract

Traumatic brain injury (TBI) is a major cause of morbidity and mortality worldwide. Understanding the pathophysiology of TBI is crucial for the development of more effective therapeutic strategies. At the moment of the traumatic impact, transfer of kinetic forces causes neurologic damage; this primary injury triggers a secondary wave of biochemical cascades, together with metabolic and cellular changes, called secondary neural injury. These areas of ongoing secondary injury, or areas of "traumatic penumbra," represent crucial targets for therapeutic interventions. This chapter is focused on the interplay between progression of parenchymal injury and the neuroprotective and neurorestorative processes that are emerging and developing subsequently to traumatic impact. Thus, we emphasized the role of traumatic penumbra in TBI pathogenesis and suggested a crucial contribution of the neurovascular units (NVUs) and paracrine effects of exosomes and miRNAs in promoting neurological recovery.

Keywords: traumatic brain injury, traumatic penumbra, neural injury, pericytes, neurovascular unit, neurorestoration

1. Introduction

Worldwide, injuries account for 15% of the burden of death and disability, while traumatic brain injury (TBI) accounts for up to half of all deaths from trauma [1–6], and often causes severe and long-lasting functional impairment in survivors [7]. TBI affects individuals of all age groups with a bimodal distribution in adolescents and elderly [8, 9], with a major predominance in the male population [10, 11]. Blunt trauma accounts for about 88–95% of TBI cases, whereas the remaining 5–12% of cases are the result of penetrating injuries [12]. Because of the high-impact nature of trauma-inducing accidents, patients commonly suffer concomitant injuries to multiple body regions and organs, otherwise known as multitrauma or polytrauma, that are capable of modifying the pathobiology and outcomes of TBI [13].

TBI is classified by different methods; in the 1970s, Teasdale and Jennett introduced the Glasgow Coma Scale (GCS) to objectively assess the degree of impaired consciousness [14]. Based on GCS, TBI is classified into mild (GCS score 14–15), moderate (9–13), and severe (3–8) [15]. At present, GCS is the most used method for TBI classification, however, has a number of limitations [15, 16]. A recent study reported that normal GCS did not indicate an absence of head injury, as among patients with GCS 15 in the Emergency Department, 26% had serious/critical TBI [17]. Therefore, stratification of severity and prediction of death and functional outcome is essential for determining treatment strategies and allocation of resources for patients with TBI. Among the most studied predictors of TBI outcome, age is a consistent predictor, as well as GCS scores and pupillary parameters [18]. Recent studies show a series of either tissue-specific or circulating biomarkers that are useful in the clinical status evaluation of these patients [19–22].

Intracranial hypertension is the main cause of death in patients with TBI and contributes to secondary brain injury if not managed correctly [23–25]. Therefore, the management of TBI focuses on the control of intracranial pressure (ICP) and maintenance of adequate cerebral perfusion, oxygenation, and metabolism attempting to limit secondary injury progression [26–28]. Mortality rates have decreased in the last decades, largely due to improvements in trauma systems and supportive critical care [29]. Yet, case fatality rates in severe TBI have not decreased significantly since 1990 [30], remaining with an outstanding mortality, because up to 50% of the patients will still die and nearly all survivors will present some degree of sequelae [3, 4, 6, 31–33]. To the present, regardless of over dozens of phase III clinical trials, there are no specific treatments known to improve TBI outcomes [13]. Hence, TBI is heterogeneous in terms of pathophysiology, clinical presentation, and outcome, with case fatality rates ranging from <1% in mild TBI up to 50% in severe TBI. A key issue in TBI care is the temporal progression of injury cascades and the design of therapeutic approaches to improve functional recovery after TBI.

This chapter is focused on the interplay between progression of parenchymal injury and the neuroprotective and neurorestorative processes that are emerging and developing subsequently to traumatic impact. Thus, we emphasized the role of traumatic penumbra in TBI pathogenesis and suggested a crucial contribution of the neurovascular units (NVUs) and paracrine effects of exosomes and miRNAs in promoting neurological recovery.

2. Mechanisms of neural injury in the traumatic penumbra

TBI is unique since it results from an external force, which can inflict devastating effects to brain vasculature, neighboring neural tissue, and blood-brain barrier (BBB) [34]. Together, neurons, vascular cells (endothelial cells) and perivascular components of the BBB (astrocytes and pericytes) form the neurovascular unit (NVU). NVU is at the basis of neurovascular coupling, which allows cerebral blood flow to local regulation according to neuronal activity in specific areas of the brain [34]. TBI may cause mechanical deformation and damage to the entire NVU [20, 35, 36], compromising barrier integrity and leading to dysautoregulation of brain vessels and BBB disruption. In this context, brain edema may occur and result in increased ICP and decreased cerebral perfusion [37]. In fact, compensatory mechanisms are exceeded as brain volume increases due to edema, and ICP rises exponentially and correlates with increased mortality and poor functional outcomes [20, 38–40]. The impact of trauma causes mechanical forces that engender deformation of the brain tissue, resulting in immediate neural damage, called primary injury [40]. This primary injury triggers a secondary wave of biochemical cascades, together with metabolic and cellular changes, occurring within seconds to minutes after the trauma and lasting for days, months or years [40]. The ongoing brain damage characteristic of secondary injury culminates in notable cell death [24, 40, 41]. Typically, initial neuronal death following acute brain injury occurs by necrosis, on a time scale of minutes, then, a second wave of delayed cell death occurs mostly by apoptosis [13, 42–45]. Indeed, this protracted course of cell death following TBI may represent a unique opportunity for therapeutic intervention. Following TBI, brain lesions are not limited to the site of the primary trauma, but expand progressively and centrifugally. Therefore, secondary brain injury develops and progresses in the traumatic penumbra, that is, the potentially salvageable brain tissue surrounding the primary lesion [46, 47]. Indeed, clinical studies have demonstrated that expansion of the penumbra impairs cerebral blood flow and leads to edema and compromised local metabolism, resulting in clinical deterioration [48–50].

The traumatic penumbra is characterized by metabolic changes as a consequence of neural injury progression [51–53] culminating in cell death [26, 54]. In this scenario of metabolic crisis, astrocytes may exert a neuroprotective action supplying substrates of glycogen metabolism for the survival of ischemic neurons and oligodendroglial cells [49]. Thus, astrocytes also play crucial roles in the injury site after TBI, as they exert homeostatic mechanisms critical for maintaining neural circuit function, such as buffering neurotransmitters, modulating extracellular osmolarity, and calibrating neurovascular coupling [55]. Accordingly, astrocytes are thought to exert many beneficial effects post-TBI [56] as providing neurotrophins that support and guide axons in their recovery [57], increasing cell proliferation, and promoting the long-term survival of neurons by inhibiting apoptosis [58, 59]. However, when the presence of astrocytes is too large and they become over activated, they may build a dense physical and chemical barrier surrounding the injury site (glial scar), which encapsulates and isolates the axons. This not only protects the remaining healthy brain from the neurotoxic environment of the injury site but also interferes and prevents the regeneration and repair of the damaged tissue [60, 61].

We will resume some of the phenomena involved in cellular injury in the traumatic penumbra. Particularly, excitotoxicity, oxidative stress, mitochondrial dysfunction, and neuroinflammation are processes that contribute to neurological damage and impairment of neural recovery following TBI (**Figure 1**). In the injured brain, excitotoxicity derives from an acute increase in extracellular glutamate levels due to excessive release from depolarized neurons, leakage from neuronal and glial cells exhibiting damaged membranes, or the extravasation through a disrupted BBB [53, 62–64]. TBI also involves enhanced glutamatergic activity at

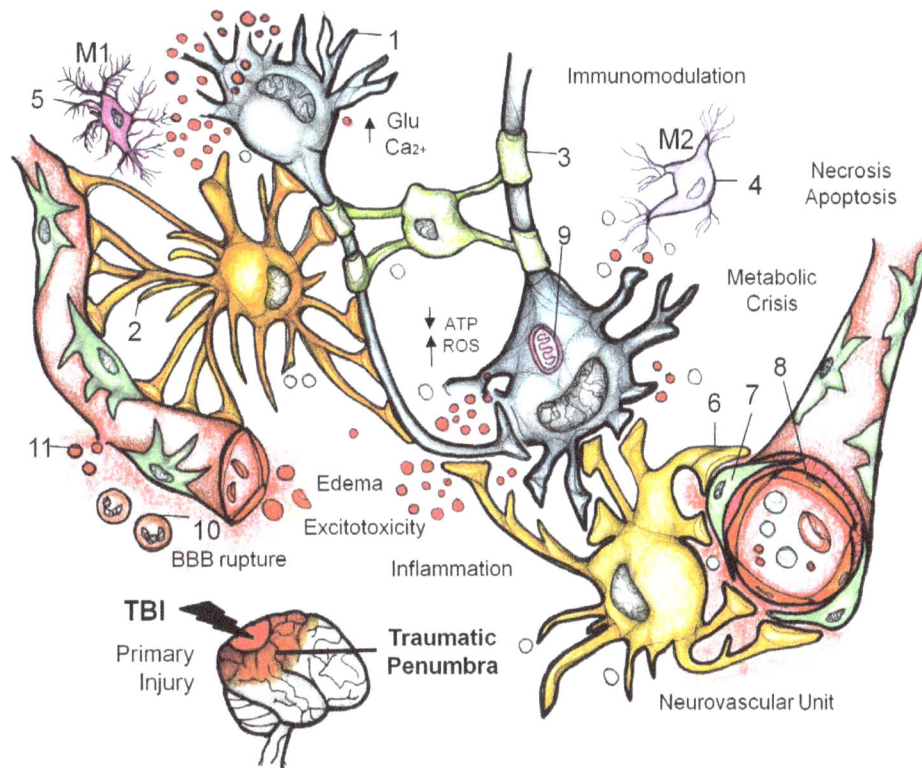

Figure 1. Schematic representation of mechanisms of neural injury in the traumatic penumbra. The neural tissue disruption of primary injury triggers a cascade of cellular events that result in areas of traumatic penumbra characteristic of secondary injury, leading to necrosis and apoptosis. Secondary injury progression can either evolve to edema that culminates in an uncontrollable increase of intracranial pressure leading to brain death or trigger mechanisms of neural tissue survival and recovery. The first 96 hours after the trauma are critical for the cellular processes involved in ongoing secondary neural injury. Various cellular components are involved in secondary injury progression in the traumatic penumbra: (1) neuron, (2) reactive astrocyte, (3) oligodendrocyte, (4) microglia M2 anti-inflammatory phenotype, (5) microglia M1 pro-inflammatory phenotype, (6) astrocyte endfoot, (7) pericyte, (8) endothelial cells, (9) mitochondria, (10) peripheral immune cells, and (11) signaling molecules. Excitotoxicity is a central mechanism of injury and triggers a cascade of events, such as increase in calcium influx, cellular damage mediated by ROS, and mitochondrial dysfunction resulting in metabolic crisis and culminating in cell death. A pro-inflammatory phase occurs in the first hours and days. In that microenvironment, microglia polarize into a M1 pro-inflammatory phenotype. Reactive astrocytosis occurs and contributes both to injury and neurorestoration. Acutely after TBI, in the neurovascular unit, swelling of perivascular astrocytes occur and the swollen endfeet constrict capillaries, leading to a reduction in oxygen availability. Also, focal microhemorrhages contribute to inflammatory processes. In this scenario, pericytes contribute to alterations in BBB permeability, angiogenesis, clearance of toxic metabolites, and hemodynamic responses. BBB rupture is evident and contributes to inflammation and edema of the neural tissue.

extrasynaptic sites due to failure of glutamate uptake, gliotransmission, reverse operation of the glutamate transporters, increase in presynaptic glutamate release or increase in the number and/or stability of glutamatergic receptors [53, 62, 65, 66]. The increase in glutamate levels occurs several minutes after the primary trauma, peaks in about 10 minutes and stays increased for several days [45, 64]. Excitotoxicity also causes calcium influx and overload [67, 68], resulting in cellular damage due to several mechanisms (i.e. activation of destructive calcium-dependent proteases, oxidative stress, mitochondrial impairment and transition pore formation, and apoptotic events) [51, 53, 62, 69–71]. Noteworthy, the massive influx of calcium causes production of reactive oxygen species (ROS) in mitochondria. The calcium overload leads to swelling and compromised function of mitochondria, instigating impaired energy metabolism [51, 72]. Conversely, the damaged tissue needs more energy for its repair than under physiological conditions, resulting in what has been termed a "flow/metabolism mismatch," a factor that aggravates injury in the traumatic penumbra [62, 73]. Furthermore, increased glutamatergic release into the extracellular milieu following injury causes marked increases in glucose use and accumulation of extracellular lactate [53, 74–79]. This deregulated cerebral metabolism leads to decreased ATP production causing the failure of ATP-dependent ion channels and proteins leading to ionic osmotic alterations that result in cell swelling and culminating in necrosis [80]. Mitochondrial dysfunction may be central to the pathophysiology of TBI through metabolic derangements, oxidative stress, and apoptosis. In fact, a recent study showed mitochondrial ultrastructural alterations at progressive distances from the center of the penumbra in tissue samples from TBI patients [81]. In the setting of TBI, the production of ROS is enhanced [82–84], and the neuroprotective systems become overwhelmed and result in oxidative cell damage. Furthermore, ROS can contribute to disruption of the BBB, edema, and neuroinflammation [34].

Importantly, neuroinflammation is known to be important for the short- and long-term consequences of TBI [85]. Various factors influence the inflammatory response of the brain to TBI. These factors include activation of resident central nervous system (CNS) immune cells and cerebral infiltration of peripheral immune cells (through a disrupted BBB); these cells mediate inflammatory processes through secretion of a variety of inflammatory cytokines, chemokines, adhesion molecules, ROS, and complement factors [86, 87]. Immediately following injury, the levels of various cytokines change drastically in the brain parenchyma and take approximately 48 hours to return to normal [45]. Accordingly, regional, intrathecal, and systemic concentrations of various inflammatory cytokines (interleukin-1, -1β, -6, -8, -10, -12, and tumor necrosis factor-alpha) are altered shortly after TBI in humans and experimental models [88–94]. Even though neuroinflammation is generally considered to have negative effects on the neural tissue, interleukins may actually exert beneficial effects on the injured brain by triggering mechanisms of response to tissue injury. Clearly, the beneficial effects of these cytokines are dependent on their concentrations and the timing/conditions of their expression following TBI [53]. The dual role of these cytokines on TBI is observable during the pro-inflammatory phase (in the first hours and days after TBI) as well as through the reparative phase, which lasts for days to months after TBI [95]. Of these cytokines, IL-1β is of special importance because its action on astrocytes makes them release of matrix metalloproteinases (MMPs) [96] that cause further BBB breakdown by promoting and prolonging neuroinflammation [97]. Modulating these inflammatory cells by changing their phenotype from pro-inflammatory to anti-inflammatory would likely promote therapeutic effects on TBI [42, 59, 98]. Additionally, peripheral injuries of the multi-injured patient may increase circulating levels of many of the inflammatory cytokines worsening TBI outcomes [13, 68].

As the major cellular component of the innate immune system in the central nervous system (CNS) and the first line of defense whenever injury or disease occurs, microglia play a critical role in neuroinflammation through the production of various cytokines, proteases, and ROS [45, 99]. In the injured brain, microglia can produce neuroprotective factors, clear cellular debris, and orchestrate neurorestorative processes that are beneficial for neurological recovery after TBI [100, 101]. Microglia can polarize into distinct phenotypes, depending on the microenvironment in which they are activated. The macrophage/microglial populations are shown to result in a mix of pro-inflammatory M1 and anti-inflammatory M2 microglia/ macrophage populations following TBI [56, 102]. It is thought that M1 microglia/macrophage populations are responsible for the production of oxidative species, increased synthesis of pro-inflammatory cytokines, low levels of anti-inflammatory cytokines, and much of the phago-cytic activity. As a result, they may contribute to injury progression. M2 populations on the other hand are believed to play a role in angiogenesis, remodeling of the extracellular matrix, and support regeneration following injury [103]. When appropriately queued, microglia can also release neurotrophins to augment neuronal growth and survival [104]. Deficits in the ability of microglia to perform these functions or to appropriately switch between M1 and M2 phenotypes detrimentally affect brain function [105]. Microglial activation within the injured area is observed within 6–48 hours post injury [99] but evidence has shown that microglia can maintain a primed or pro-inflammatory profile for weeks to months after the acute effects of injury have dissipated [106]. Recently, it was shown that extracellular vesicles may exchange pro-inflammatory molecules between brain immune cells, as well as to the systemic circula-tion, as pathways of inflammation propagation following TBI [107].

Notwithstanding the previous characterization of the pathophysiologic responses to TBI, these biologic responses occur in individuals who possess biologic differences that can modify their response to injury [53, 108]. Over the last years, evidence has showed that the brain is capa-ble of significant structural and functional repair, plasticity, and regeneration. Approaches for accomplishing this include reawakening the growth potential of the surviving neurons or antagonizing the inhibition of axonal growth and synaptogenesis. Alternatively, cellu-lar replacement is achievable in certain brain regions that possess nascent neural stem cells [25, 43, 109–111]. Thus, the discussed concept of traumatic penumbra imbues the transition between injury and repair at the NVU with profound implications for selecting the appropri-ate type and timing of neuroprotective interventions [34]. In this scenario, it is instigating to investigate which cellular pathways in the traumatic penumbra could play key roles for neu-rorestoration and, therefore, represent novel therapeutic opportunities for TBI.

2.1. The neurovascular unit in the traumatic penumbra

NVU comprises vascular cells (endothelial cells), perivascular constituents of the blood-brain barrier (pericytes and astrocytes) and their associated neurons, as well as extracellular matrix components [112]. NVU also includes microglial cells, vascular smooth muscle cells located around blood vessels, specialized cellular compartments such as the endothelial glycocalyx, the endothelial lining of cerebral capillaries, capillary tight junctions, and the capillary base-ment membrane [113]. Together, the components of NVU detect physiological needs of the neural tissue and respond accordingly to supply these demands [112]. Consequently, under normal conditions, cerebral blood flow is maintained constant despite wide changes in perfu-sion pressure [114], a phenomenon called autoregulation of cerebral blood flow [115].

Traumatic cerebral vascular injury (TCVI) is a major feature of TBI disease. While the complex molecular and cellular mechanisms responsible for functional deficits after TBI are not fully understood, substantial data indicate that TCVI underlies a significant fraction of TBI-related disability. Therefore, in view of its physiological function, the NVU plays an important role in the pathogenesis of TBI, whether responding to physical trauma or participating in the cascade of events that leads to secondary injury in the traumatic penumbra [116]. Endothelial cells, for example, respond to hemodynamic forces by releasing factors that promote constriction or dilation. Neurons associated with the neural cerebral vasculature release neurotransmitters (e.g. norepinephrine and serotonin for vasoconstriction, and acetylcholine, substance P, and vasoactive intestinal polypeptide for vasodilation) that diffuse into the tunica media and act on receptors in the smooth muscle cell layer to elicit either vasoconstriction or dilation. Based on local activity and needs, basal forebrain neurons release vasoactive mediators on cortical microvessels and supporting astrocytes to modulate microvascular tone [113]. Consequently, neuronal metabolism and activity are tightly coupled to local cerebral blood flow [117].

Microvascular injury is observed in animal models of TBI, whether the injury is caused by impact acceleration, fluid percussion or controlled cortical impact (CCI). Immediately after TBI, endothelial cells are damaged; subsequently, secondary injury extends to the other components of the NVU; decreased blood flow and focal hypoxia disturb the NVU, and various pathophysiological events, such as BBB disruption, edema, and focal ischemia, take place [118]. The NVU response to these events include the increased production of nitric oxide and consequent increase of blood flow right after TBI followed by a period of decreased production of NO and consequent decrease of blood flow [119]. Another aspect of the response of the NVU to these events is the release of damage-associated molecular patterns that trigger secretion of pro-inflammatory mediators such as tumor necrosis factor, interleukin-6, and interleukin-1β by glial cells [120]. The trade-off to this response consists of unwanted side effects such as BBB disruption, edema, hypoperfusion, and oxidative stress, all of which contribute to increase severity of the secondary injury.

Ultrastructural changes in endothelial cells at acutely injury sites are observable 3 hours after TBI and are still present 1 week later [121]. During this, time swelling of perivascular astrocytes is evident; their swollen endfeet constrict capillaries, which leads to a redistribution of capillary blood flow that can reduce oxygen availability to cerebral tissue even if ischemia is not obvious [122]. Data from experimental TBI models indicate that increased extravasation of the contents of blood vessels through microhemorrhages is evident between 3 and 12 hours after the injury [116]. Most of these focal hemorrhages occur in pericontusional tissue, while some occur within the contusion itself and diffusely throughout the ipsilateral, noncontused cerebral hemisphere; intravascular microthrombi, in turn, peak at 48 hours after TBI but persist for at least 9 days [123]. Focal microhemorrhages are accompanied by activation of microglia, reactive gliosis, and recruitment of macrophages; 3 months after the injury, these microbleed sites are surrounded by glial scars and are characterized by major loss of myelin [124].

Clearly, endothelial cells are not alone in the response to TBI. During necrotic phases, cytokines, such as TNF and IL-1, are released by astrocytes, microglia, endothelial cells, and neurons and contributed to the initiation of neuroinflammation [125]. These cytokines induce microglial activation and expression by endothelial cells of adhesion molecules, such as intercellular adhesion molecule 1, aka CD54 (ICAM-1), vascular cell adhesion protein 1, aka CD106 (VCAM-1), P-selectin (CD62P), and E-selectin (CD62E), which in turn allow attachment of leukocytes (neutrophils and monocytes) to the endothelium and their passage across the BBB. These events lead to increased production of proinflammatory factors at the injured tissue, and leukocytes start releasing MMPs [125]. These MMPs, which include MMP-2, MMP-3, and MMP-9, degrade extracellular matrix proteins and tight junction proteins that join endothelial cells with each other, which results in increased permeability of the BBB. Not surprisingly, the levels of some of these TBI-associated molecules in the blood, as is the case of MMP-9 [126], have been associated with the outcome of TBI and may become important tools for patient screening at the emergency unit in the future.

2.2. Pericytes in the traumatic penumbra

Another cell of the NVU, the pericyte, has been recognized as a component of the BBB more than a century ago [127]. Functions attributed to pericytes in the CNS include regulation of the BBB permeability, angiogenesis, clearance of toxic metabolites, and capillary hemodynamic responses [128]. Through the past two decades, pericytes have been increasingly receiving attention from researchers around the world owing to growing knowledge on their properties, which suggested they could behave as stem or progenitor cells not only in the mesodermal tissues [129–132] but also in the CNS [133]. Indeed, various types of evidence suggest that pericytes behave as mesenchymal stem cells in vivo [134], especially the fact that pericytes isolated through various techniques give rise to cultured cells with mesenchymal stem cell characteristics [135–137]. Experiments in which the progeny of cells expressing certain pericyte markers was genetically labeled indicate that pericytes give rise to differentiated progeny in situ in various tissues [138–142], while a recent fate tracing study indicates that does not happen [143]. Albeit in contrast with previous findings in this area, this latter study confirmed that isolated pericytes give rise to cultures with mesenchymal stem cell characteristics.

Most of the knowledge on mesenchymal stem cells comes from in vitro studies that used cultured cells with mesenchymal stem cell characteristics. The International Society for Cellular Therapy has proposed that these cultured cells be called mesenchymal stromal cells (MSCs) unless they are proved to be stem cells using strict criteria [144], and many studies on this cell population use this terminology, although it may be inaccurate. Even though MSCs, owing to their ability to differentiate into various mature cell types, may be used for tissue engineering, it is their ability to secrete trophic and immunomodulatory molecules [145–147] that render them so interesting for cell therapies. Therefore, the acronym "MSC" has been proposed to be used in reference to these cells, but under the designation of "medicinal signaling cells" [148] or any other that does not include "stem cells" [149].

Even though the question as to whether or not pericytes are able to give rise to mature cell types in situ warrants further experimentation, it is likely that pericytes may still be important for regenerative purposes even if they do not behave as stem cells in the body. Pericytes can give rise to cultured cells able to secrete a wide range of trophic and immunomodulatory molecules; consequently, it is possible that pericytes can secrete these types of molecules in vivo too. When tissue injury occurs, pericytes undergo a process called activation—their gene expression profile changes and they become proliferative. As MSC cultures endowed with the ability of secreting trophic molecules can be derived from prospectively isolated pericytes, it is likely that these MSCs possess characteristics of activated pericytes. An early study has shown that some pericytes detach from blood vessels and migrate toward the cerebral tissue after CCI in rats [150]. Pericytes have been shown to become activated in a CCI model and progress to a state of *reactive pericytosis* [151] in reference to the well-known reactive gliosis observed in various types of CNS injuries. In that study, the number of pericytes in the peri-contusional area decreased drastically after the injury, remained lower than normal up to 3 days after the injury, and doubled 5 days after the injury; additionally, the authors found that these activated pericytes remained limited by an area of reactive gliosis. Pericytes were shown to undergo apoptosis in a cortical organotypic slice culture subjected to hypoxia [152]. More recently, cells with characteristic pericyte markers have been detected and isolated from necrotic cerebral tissue affected by stroke; these cells were able to establish MSC cultures [153]. Human brain pericytes cultured under hypoxic conditions were shown to upregulate the expression of neurotrophin-3, which boosted NGF produced by astrocytes under hypoxia, contributing to a neuroprotective effect [154]. Whereas, noncultured pericytes isolated from human adipose tissue express message not only for neurotrophin-3 but also for other neuro-trophic factors, such as NGF, BDNF, GDNF, and persephin [155].

Another important characteristic of pericytes that can be inferred from their relationship to MSCs is the ability to secrete molecules that interfere with the action of immune system cells, blocking inflammation [156]. However, it should be noted that pericytes do not become acti-vated immediately upon TBI, and during the initial stages of the response to this injury, they may contribute to the recruitment of inflammatory cells. Some studies have presented evi-dence that pericytes may contribute to neuroinflammation owing to their ability to perceive infection-related or pro-inflammatory signals and respond through secretion of chemokines that recruit inflammatory cells [157]. In contrast, cultured pericytes have also been shown to be immunosuppressive, as they can inhibit the proliferation of T cells to the same extent as MSCs isolated through traditional methods [136]. It is likely, therefore, that pericytes display a pro-inflammatory phenotype at the onset of TBI, but become immunosuppressive as they undergo activation, thus contributing to maintenance of a balanced level of inflammation as the response to injury progresses.

Together, the information depicted above indicates that, under injury conditions such as TBI or stroke, a number of pericytes die; whereas, the surviving ones become activated, increase in number, and secrete a number of molecules that exert trophic and immunomodulatory effects on their surroundings, contributing to mitigate tissue damage caused by the insult, as previously suggested [155]. While further experimentation is warranted to gain insight into the details of this process, some questions, such as what is the mode of delivery of these soluble factors, are yet to be elucidated. Not long after the introduction of the concept that MSCs exert their reparative effects by means of paracrine factors, microvesicles were found to work as vehicles for the delivery of trophic molecules secreted by MSCs in acute tubu-lar injury [158]. The same principle could well apply to activated pericytes in TBI, but that requires validation. On the other hand, this proposed action of pericytes during the response to TBI suggests that this process could be explored for the purpose of diagnostics and inter-vention. On one hand, the detection of pericyte-related molecules in the blood could provide information on the status of the lesion in acute TBI patients. On the other hand, knowledge on the main pericyte-derived molecules involved in trophic support of the surrounding cells in the injured cerebral tissue may allow the development of novel pharmacological approaches to minimize tissue damage during the early stages of TBI. These pharmacological approaches could be further enhanced with the use of microvesicles as delivery vehicles.

3. Neuroprotective and neurorestorative processes in the traumatic penumbra

TBI triggers adaptive and maladaptive reactions to injury as damaged tissue attempts to recover [159]. The secondary injury events initiated in the traumatic penumbra lead to cellular dysfunction and death and determine the extent of brain damage. There may be overlapping signals and substrates between the initial trigger of injury and the subsequent endogenous mechanisms of neurorestoration and remodeling (**Figure 2**). The extended nature of these events and the multiplicity of targets offer opportunities for innovative therapeutic interventions [34, 160]. Undeniably, with therapeutic options centered on supportive care, trauma-related mortality and morbidity is an area with unlimited scope for advancement. Therefore, modulating endogenous repair mechanisms through enhancing neurogenesis could be an attractive approach for novel therapies for TBI [161].

Neurogenesis was once thought to be discontinued after brain development in mammals. However, certain areas of the brain retain the ability to generate neurons and glia [162, 163]. In these areas, neural stem cells (NSC) continue the developmental mechanisms to replace and replenish damaged cells. Neurogenic response includes three different phases: proliferation or generation of new cells, migration of new cells to target areas, and differentiation into proper cell types [164]. Many factors may affect adult neurogenesis, such as growth factors, exercise, enriched environment, or stress [161]. Studies have shown that TBI induces an upregulation of neurogenesis in varying types of TBI models [165]. In that sense, strategies such as supplementing varying types of trophic factors (i.e. BDNF, VEGF, S100β), manipulating transcriptional regulators, or other pharmacological approaches targeting different aspects of the endogenous neurogenic response have shown promising results improving functional recovery following experimental models of TBI [45, 155, 161, 165]. The potential use of cellular therapies to prevent secondary neural injury and promote recovery of injured tissue in trauma is an area of emerging investigation. Preclinical data indicate that restorative therapies targeting multiple parenchymal cells, including cerebral endothelial cells, neural stem/progenitor cells, and oligodendrocyte progenitor cells, enhance TBI-induced angiogenesis, neurogenesis, axonal sprouting, and oligodendrogenesis [45, 161, 166, 167].

Cellular therapies fall into two main categories of cell types: adult multipotent cells and pluripotent embryonic stem cells (ESCs). Adult multipotent cells, such as mesenchymal stem cells, multipotent adult progenitor cells (MAPCs), hematopoietic stem cells (HSCs), and bone marrow mononuclear cells (BMMNCs), have the capacity to generate a limited number of terminally differentiated cell types [168]. Cell-based therapies have been shown to improve outcomes in preclinical studies of trauma-related conditions via several mechanisms, which include: (i) production of soluble factors that regulate the exacerbated cell damage through

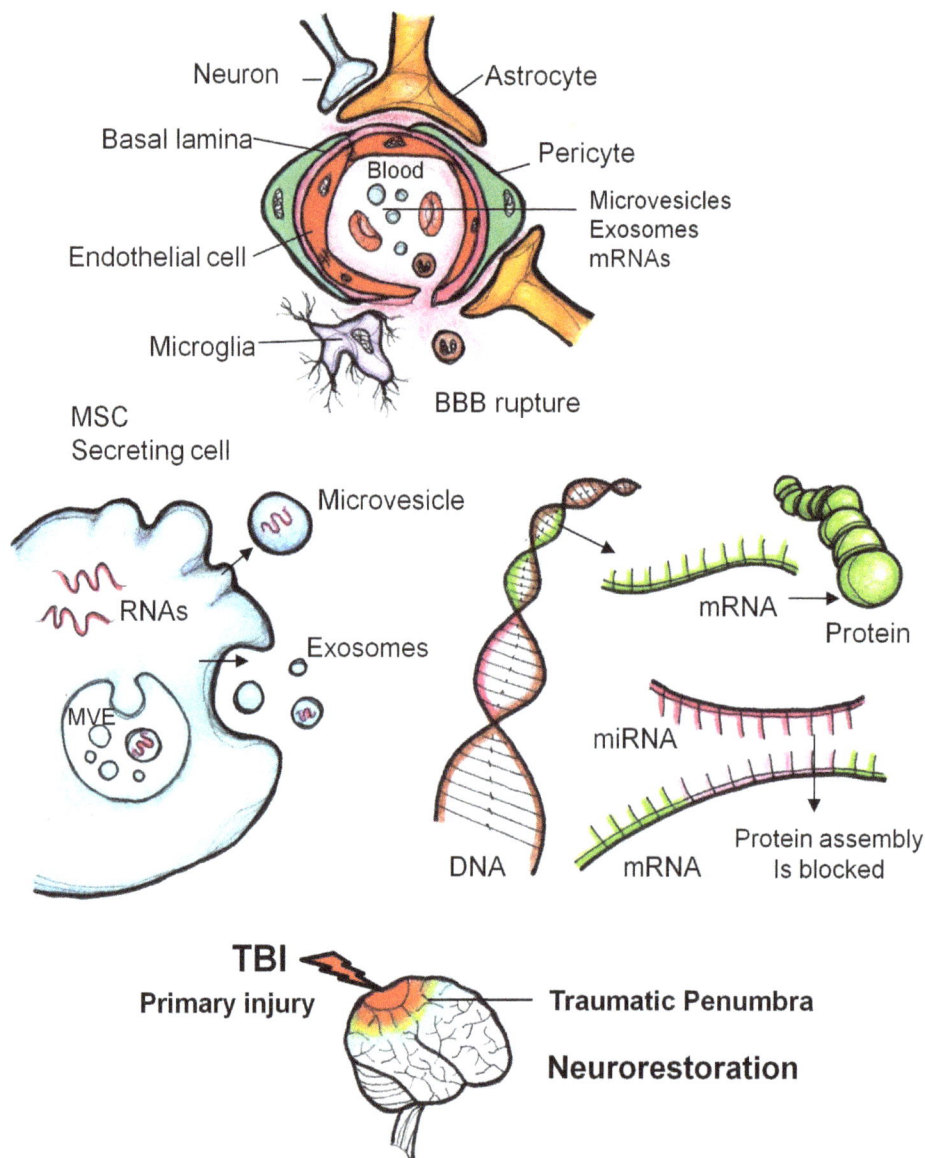

Figure 2. Schematic representation of neurorestorative mechanisms in the traumatic penumbra. Secondary injury progression in the traumatic penumbra can trigger mechanisms of neural tissue survival and recovery. After TBI, a proinflammatory phase occurs in the first hours and days and is followed by a reparative phase lasting from days to months. Secondary injury progression involves a cascade of events that results in cellular damage through diverse signaling pathways. In this scenario, components of the neurovascular unit may orchestrate several neurorestorative mechanisms in the traumatic penumbra. Of particular interest are the neurorestorative mechanisms associated to cellular therapies using mesenchymal stem cells (MSCs). MSCs may exert paracrine effects through secretion of microvesicles and exosomes, evoking endogenous reparative mechanisms, and functional recovery following TBI. Indeed, microvesicles and exosomes can deliver miRNAs to recipient cells, promoting gene regulation and enhancing neuroplasticity.

anti-inflammatory and cell-protective effects (i.e., growth factors, cytokines, microvesicles, exosomes); (ii) replacement of lost cells by differentiating and integrating into the damaged tissue microenvironment; and (iii) stimulation of endogenous regeneration of the injured tissue [167]. A multitude of cell types derived from a variety of tissues are currently under preclinical and clinical investigation for applications in trauma [167]. Multipotent MSCs have shown promise as an effective therapy for brain injuries in experimental models of acute brain injury [165, 169–172] and potentially in clinical settings [173, 174]. However, previous studies show that only a small proportion of transplanted MSCs actually survive and few MSCs differentiate into neural cells in injured brain tissues. It seems that the predominant mechanisms by which MSCs participate in brain remodeling and functional recovery are likely related to their secretion-based paracrine effect rather than a cell replacement effect [45, 175–178] (**Figure 2**).

In effect, MSCs secrete or express factors that reach neighboring parenchymal cells either via a paracrine effect or a direct cell-to-cell interaction, or MSCs may induce host cells to secrete bioactive factors, which promote survival and proliferation of the parenchymal cells (brain remodeling) and thereby improve functional recovery [178, 179]. In addition to their soluble factors, therapeutic effects of MSCs may be attributed to their generation and release of exosomes [178]. Exosomes are endosomal origin small membrane vesicles released by almost all cell types and contain not only proteins and lipids but also messenger RNAs and microRNAs (miRNAs) [180]. Recent evidence indicates that exosomes have a crucial role in cell-to-cell communication. In contrast to transplanted exogenous MSCs, nanosized exosomes derived from MSCs do not proliferate and are less immunogenic and easier to store and deliver than MSCs [181–183]. Exosomes generated from MSCs improved functional recovery in rats after TBI [45, 175]. Exosomes play an important role in intercellular communication and are promising therapeutic agents because their complex cargo of proteins and genetic materials has diverse biochemical potential to participate in multiple biochemical and cellular processes, an important attribute in the treatment of complex diseases with multiple secondary injury mechanisms involved [45]. The refinement of MSC therapy from a cell-based therapy to cell-free exosome-based therapy offers several advantages, as it eases the arduous task of preserving cell viability and function, storage, and delivery to patient [175–178]. Further exploring the mechanisms by which the secretion-based paracrine effect of MSCs participates in neurorestoration and functional recovery following TBI is an outstanding opportunity for research. The development of cell-free exosome-based therapies for TBI may allow to deliver targeted regulatory genes (miRNAs) to enhance neuroplasticity and to amplify neurological recovery in TBI.

3.1. MicroRNAs

Previous studies have demonstrated that TBI induces extensive temporal changes in the expression of brain protein, mRNA and miRNA [184–186]. There has been a growing interest on the role of miRNA in normal CNS development and function, as well as in disease, including TBI, stroke, and neurodegenerative disorders. Mature, functional miRNA sequences are single-stranded RNA molecules composed of 20–25 nucleotides, which regulate gene expression post-transcriptionally through direct effects on 3′-untranslated region (3′ UTR) of mRNA, resulting in translation repression or mRNA degradation. One miRNA usually targets more than 100 genes [187]. In turn, a gene may be regulated by multiple miRNAs [188]. It is estimated that over 2000 miRNAs have been involved in the regulation of approximately 30% of the human protein-coding genes [189].

Microarray analyses in animal models of TBI have shown a dynamic temporal regulation of miRNA expression. A report described that a peak of downregulated and upregulated miRNAs was observed after injury in rat cerebral cortex at 24 and 72 hours, respectively [190]. The research also revealed that a large number of miRNA was expressed at four different time points after injury: 136 at 6 hours, 118 at 24 hours, 149 at 48 hours, and 203 at 72 hours. In addition, only miR-21 expression was upregulated within all the four time points post injury, indicating that this miRNA may be involved in the complex process of TBI course. Another study analyzed changes in expression of 444 miRNAs within the hippocampus of rat TBI models at 3 and 24 hours after controlled cortical impact injury [184]. The results showed that 50 miRNAs had decreased expression levels and 35 miRNAs exhibited increased expression levels in the hippocampus after injury. A bioinformatic analysis of the predicted targets of a subset of the miRNAs with altered expression after TBI (miR-107, -130a, -223, -433-3p, -451, and -541) revealed that many of the target genes are involved in biological functions and processes that play a role in TBI pathophysiology, including transcription, proliferation, morphogenesis, and signal transduction. A study of microarray analyses of miRNA expression profile in rat hippocampus found that 10 of 156 reliably detected miRNAs were significantly and consistently altered from 1 hour to 7 days post injury [186]. Bioinformatic and gene ontology analyses revealed 107 putative target genes, as well as several biological processes that might be initiated by the dysregulated miRNAs, that include miR-144, miR-153, and miR-340-5p. Recently, a study analyzed the biological roles of about 600 genes that are targeted by 10 TBI-altered miRNAs [191]. Bioinformatic analysis suggested that neurodegeneration results from a global miRNA-mediated suppression of genes essential for maintaining proteostasis, the competing and integrated biological pathways that control the synthesis, folding, trafficking, and degradation of proteins. Notably, dysregulation of these essential genes would significantly impair synaptic function and functional connectivity of the brain.

MicroRNAs have emerged as novel serum diagnostic biomarkers for various diseases. The use of miRNA as biomarkers of brain injury in the serum or CSF could serve as tools for both diagnosing and stratifying TBI severity. As a biomarker of pathologic process, miRNA have several unique features, including cell-, tissue-, and disease-specific expression patterns [192, 193]. Studies of CSF in a rat model of mild blast TBI found a significant increase in levels of one miRNA, miR-let-7i, as early as 3 hours post injury [194]. Prediction analysis revealed that this miRNA targets TBI-related proteins, such as S100B and ubiquitin carboxyl-terminal hydrolase L1 (UCH-L1), suggesting a possible role for miR-let-7i in regulating TBI pathology. Studies in patients with TBI have identified other miRNAs that may serve as diagnostic biomarkers for severe (miR-16, −92a, and −765) [195] and mild brain injury (mir143-3p and mir423-3p) [196]. A recent study using a microarray platform identified 14 miRNAs differentially expressed (10 upregulated and 4 downregulated) in CFS of severe TBI patients who remained unconscious for 2 weeks compared with controls [197]. Another study using microarray analyzed the expression of 754 miRNAs in serum of TBI patients with polytrauma aiming to find biomarkers able to discriminate between mild and severe TBI [198]. The analysis revealed two miRNAs (miR-425-5p and miR-502) that were downregulated in mild TBI at early time points and two miRNAs (miR-21 and miR-335) that were upregulated in severe TBI. Moreover, miR-425-5p and miR-21 were predictors of 6-month outcome, but with differences regarding the timepoint when they were analyzed (miR-425-5p: until 1 hour and also between 4 and 12 hours from injury; miR-21: between 4 and 12 hours from injury). Overall, these studies have shown a potential role of miRNA as TBI biomarkers, but only miR21 has been identified as a candidate in more than one study [198, 199]. Given that pre-clinical optimism in finding good biomarkers in the past has not been successfully translated in clinical settings [200], further evaluation of these miRNAs with larger, multicenter patient cohorts is needed to explore their use as effective biomarkers applied to diagnosis and prognosis of TBI.

Besides the studies that evaluated miRNAs as TBI biomarkers, there was an interest about if miRNAs can be used as therapeutic targets. Hypothermia is a promising treatment for TBI patients because reducing body temperature attenuates neurological damage and improves functional outcomes [201]. A study presented an intervention on a specific miRNA-regulated pathway treating rats with an antagonist of miRNA-29c in an animal model of deep hypothermic circulatory arrest. The results showed that neurologic function, as assessed by vestibulomotor and cognitive performance tests, was improved in the pretreated animals as compared to the placebo group. Studies have shown that some miRNAs that show altered expression after TBI are also temperature sensitive and may be reduced under hypothermic conditions [202]. Since the pathways in which individual miRNAs can act are often numerous [203], further studies are needed to clarify the use of miRNAs in TBI therapy.

The analysis of miRNA in the TBI context may help in understanding the pathophysiology and possible treatments for TBI as it will provide insights into injury-related gene networks. However, the underlying molecular mechanisms of how miRNAs cause neurodegeneration or neurorestoration after TBI remains elusive. Investigating the role of miRNAs in neurological disorders is a new frontier for neurological research.

3.2. Extracellular vesicles and exosomes

MSCs have shown promise in the field of regenerative medicine, since exogenously administered MSCs target injured tissue, interact with brain parenchymal cells, and promote neurorestoration and recovery of neurological function after brain injuries [178, 191, 204, 205]. Despite the differentiation capacity of MSCs, the principal mechanism of their therapeutic action seems to be a robust paracrine capacity, related to their soluble factors as well as generation and release of microvesicles and exosomes [178, 205].

Extracellular vesicles (EVs) are membrane bound entities that transmit signals between cells via all cells and are found in all body fluids [206, 207]. The term "EV" includes microvesicles, exosomes, and oncosomes, among other vesicles that may be variously defined by origin, size, and markers [208–210]. EVs interact with target cells by binding to cell surface receptors, transfer of membrane proteins, membrane fusion, endosomal uptake, and cargo extrusion through vesicle-cell channels [206, 211, 212]. The EV protein and RNA compositions generally reflect that of progenitor cells [211]. Their ability to transport molecules and to target specific cell populations raised possibilities for their development as therapeutic tools [212–214]. MSC-EVs seem to exert positive impacts on tissue-specific stem cells, promote angiogenesis, and suppress oxidative stress and fibrosis, and, noteworthy, may suppress pro-inflammatory responses in brain injury [215, 216]. Indeed, it was shown that MSC-EVs are able to convert M1 into M2 macrophages and, therefore, by switching pro-inflammatory into tolerogenic environments, MSC-EV administration might promote regenerative processes [170, 205, 212, 215, 217–221]. These therapeutic potentials position EVs as highly competitive alternatives to stem cells, as the EVs are likely to be safer than their parental secreting stem cells [212].

Exosomes are endosome-derived small membrane nanosized vesicles (30–100 nm in diameter) generated by almost all cell types and released into extracellular fluids, playing a pivotal role in intercellular communication [178, 215]. MSC is the most prolific exosome producer among the cell types known to produce exosomes [204, 222]. Exosomes contain various molecular constituents including proteins and RNAs from maternal cells. Among these constituents are miRNAs, which play crucial roles in mediating biological function due to their prominent role in gene regulation. Via exosomes, MSCs transfer their therapeutic factors, especially miR-NAs, to recipient cells, and thereby modify gene expression [205, 208]. Although all exosomes contain the constitutive array of proteins, lipids, and RNAs, their contents vary in accordance with the cellular origin and the physiological or pathological condition of the cell and of its extracellular environment [204]. Most of the studies have demonstrated that MSC-derived exosomes contain various miRNAs, which participate in the cell-cell communication and alter the fate of recipient cells [204, 223, 224].

Overall, it has been widely accepted that the exosome secretion is an efficient adaptive mechanism since environmental challenges (such as stress conditions) can influence its composition, biogenesis, and secretion [204, 205, 225]. In fact, through preconditioning or genetic manipulation of neural cells, their exosome secretion profile can be modified [205, 215]. Of note, hypoxia and endothelial activation may be reflected in RNA and protein exosome composition [226, 227]. Furthermore, stressed cells that released exosomes conferred resistance against oxidative stress to recipient cells, suggesting that cells modulate intracellular stress situations and modify the surrounding environment via the secretion of exosomes [225, 228]. Also, the MSC exosome profile can be modified by pretreatment. When MSCs were *in vitro* exposed to brain tissue extracted from rats subjected to middle cerebral artery occlusion, the miR-133b levels in the released exosomes from MSCs were significantly increased [229]. Thus, there is a feedback between the MSC and its environment, and through which ischemic conditions will modify the exosome contents, and consequently, the secreted exosomes affect and modify the tissue environment [205, 230]. Regarding the brain, impacts of MSC-EV treatment were mainly studied in models for ischemic stroke and TBI and reduced apoptosis rates in affected brains, while promoted angiogenesis and neurogenesis [175–177, 215, 231–236]. Both systemic pro-inflammatory and neuroinflammatory cues were reduced following MSC-EV treatment [107, 215].

Administration of cell-free exosomes derived from MSCs is sufficient to exert therapeutic effects of intact MSCs after brain injury [176, 231, 232, 234]. The exosomes transfer RNAs and proteins to other cells which then act epigenetically to alter the function of the recipient cells [175, 178, 205, 215, 225]. Previous studies indicated that MSCs promised to be an effective therapy for brain injury in TBI [175–177, 215, 231–236]. Instead of brain remodeling and functional recovery by cell replacement effects, evidence suggests that the major effects of neurorestoration were due to the paracrine effects of secretion-based factors such as MSCs-derived exosomes that may reduce neuroinflammation, promote neurogenesis and angiogenesis, rescue pattern separation and spatial learning impairments, and improve functional recovery after TBI in animal models [107, 176, 178, 191, 204, 205, 215, 216, 235–237]. In addition, as exosomes contain various miRNAs, which play a key role in modifying the phenotype and/or the physiology and modulating the cellular processes of the recipient cell, and miRNAs such as miR-21 could be potential therapeutic targets for interventions after TBI, the combination of miRNAs and MSC-derived exosomes might be a novel approach for the treatment of TBI [238]. That is, MSCs-derived exosomes that carry and transfer their cargo such as miRNAs to parenchymal cells may mediate brain plasticity and improve functional recovery after TBI [204]. Furthermore, another potential application of brain endothelial-derived eMVs could be as biosignatures for monitoring the health of the BBB in CNS conditions associated with trauma and neuroinflammation [239].

Hence, MSC-derived exosomes play an important role in intercellular communication and have shown promise in the field of regenerative medicine including treatment of TBI. The refinement of MSC therapy from a cell-based therapy to cell-free exosome-based therapy offers several advantages, as it eases the arduous task of preserving cell viability, storage, and delivery to patient [178, 215]. Indeed, due to the nanosize of exosomes, they can across the BBB and present lower risk of vascular occlusion than intact stem cells [204]. Developing a cell-free exosome-based therapy for TBI may open up a variety of means to deliver targeted regulatory genes (miRNAs) to enhance multifaceted aspects of neuroplasticity and neurorestoration in TBI [178, 205].

4. Conclusions and perspectives

Despite the burden of the morbimortality of neurotrauma, currently, there are no single agent treatments known to improve TBI outcomes. Furthermore, the diverse etiology and complicated pathogenesis of TBI make it difficult for clinical diagnosis and prognosis of outcome. Since TBI acutely triggers adaptive and maladaptive reactions to injury while damaged tissue attempts to recover, understanding the mechanisms of neural injury and neurorestoration is crucial for the development of novel therapeutic approaches. The secondary injury events initiated in the traumatic penumbra lead to cellular dysfunction and death and determine the extent of brain damage. Nevertheless, recent evidence shows that response to injury may also trigger neurorestoration. In the above context, microvesicles and exosomes secreted by MSCs may induce intrinsic repair mechanisms that sustain posttraumatic recovery. Indeed, evidence shows that cell-free, exosome-based therapies for TBI may deliver molecules that regulate gene expressions to enhance neuroplasticity and neurorestoration following TBI.

Acknowledgements

The research in the authors' laboratories has been funded by Fundação de Amparo à Pesquisa do Estado do Rio Grande do Sul and Conselho Nacional de Desenvolvimento Científico e Tecnológico.

Author details

Andrea Regner[1,2]*, Lindolfo da Silva Meirelles[1,2] and Daniel Simon[1,2]

*Address all correspondence to: regner@uol.com.br

1 School of Medicine, Lutheran University of Brazil, Canoas, RS, Brazil

2 Graduate Program in Cellular and Molecular Biology Applied to Health (PPGBioSaúde), Lutheran University of Brazil, Canoas, RS, Brazil

References

[1] Manley GT, Maas AI. Traumatic brain injury: An international knowledge-based approach. Journal of the American Medical Association. 2013;**310**(5):473-474

[2] Menon DK, Schwab K, Wright DW, Maas AI. Demographics and Clinical Assessment Working Group of the International and Interagency Initiative toward common data elements for research on traumatic brain injury and psychological health. Position statement: Definition of traumatic brain injury. Archives of Physical Medicine and Rehabilitation. 2010;**91**(11):1637-1640

[3] Langlois JA, Rutland-Brown W, Wald MM. The epidemiology and impact of traumatic brain injury: A brief overview. The Journal of Head Trauma Rehabilitation. 2006;**21**(5):375-378

[4] Maas AI, Stocchetti N, Bullock R. Moderate and severe traumatic brain injury in adults. Lancet Neurology. 2008;**7**(8):728-741

[5] Masel BE, DeWitt DS. Traumatic brain injury: A disease process, not an event. Journal of Neurotrauma. 2010;**27**(8):1529-1540

[6] Faul M, Xu L, Wald MM, Coronado V. Traumatic Brain Injury in the United States: Emergency Department Visits, Hospitalizations and Deaths, 2002-2006. Atlanta, Georgia: Centers for Disease Control and Prevention, National Center for Injury Prevention and Control; 2010

[7] Finfer SR, Cohen J. Severe traumatic brain injury. Resuscitation. 2001;**48**(1):77-90

[8] Shivaji T, Lee A, Dougall N, McMillan T, Stark C. The epidemiology of hospital treated traumatic brain injury in Scotland. BMC Neurology. 2014;**14**:2

[9] Lawrence T, Helmy A, Bouamra O, Woodford M, Lecky F, Hutchinson PJ. Traumatic brain injury in England and Wales: Prospective audit of epidemiology, complications and standardised mortality. BMJ Open. 2016;**6**(11):e012197

[10] Tran TM, Fuller AT, Kiryabwire J, Mukasa J, Muhumuza M, Ssenyojo H, et al. Distribution and characteristics of severe traumatic brain injury at Mulago National Referral Hospital in Uganda. World Neurosurgery. 2015;**83**(3):269-277

[11] Song SY, Lee SK, Eom KS, Investigators K. Analysis of mortality and epidemiology in 2617 cases of traumatic brain injury: Korean Neuro-Trauma Data Bank System 2010-2014. Journal of Korean Neurosurgical Association. 2016;**59**(5):485-491

[12] Santiago LA, Oh BC, Dash PK, Holcomb JB, Wade CE. A clinical comparison of penetrating and blunt traumatic brain injuries. Brain Injury. 2012;**26**(2):107-125

[13] McDonald SJ, Sun M, Agoston DV, Shultz SR. The effect of concomitant peripheral injury on traumatic brain injury pathobiology and outcome. Journal of Neuroinflammation. 2016;**13**(1):90

[14] Teasdale G, Jennett B. Assessment of coma and impaired consciousness. A practical scale. Lancet. 1974;**2**(7872):81-84

[15] Chieregato A, Martino C, Pransani V, Nori G, Russo E, Noto A, et al. Classification of a traumatic brain injury: The Glasgow coma scale is not enough. Acta Anaesthesiologica Scandinavica. 2010;**54**(6):696-702

[16] McMillan T, Wilson L, Ponsford J, Levin H, Teasdale G, Bond M. The Glasgow outcome scale – 40 years of application and refinement. Nature Reviews. Neurology. 2016;**12**(8):477-485

[17] Savitsky B, Givon A, Rozenfeld M, Radomislensky I, Peleg K. Traumatic brain injury: It is all about definition. Brain Injury. 2016;**30**(10):1194-1200

[18] Llompart-Pou JA, Chico-Fernandez M, Sanchez-Casado M, Alberdi-Odriozola F, Guerrero-Lopez F, Mayor-Garcia MD, et al. Age-related injury patterns in Spanish trauma ICU patients. Results from the RETRAUCI. Injury. 2016;**47**(Suppl 3):S61-S5

[19] Papurica M, Rogobete AF, Sandesc D, Dumache R, Cradigati CA, Sarandan M, et al. Advances in biomarkers in critical ill polytrauma patients. Clinical Laboratory. 2016;**62**(6):977-986

[20] Kawata K, Liu CY, Merkel SF, Ramirez SH, Tierney RT, Langford D. Blood biomarkers for brain injury: What are we measuring? Neuroscience and Biobehavioral Reviews. 2016;**68**:460-473

[21] da Rocha AB, Schneider RF, de Freitas GR, Andre C, Grivicich I, Zanoni C, et al. Role of serum S100B as a predictive marker of fatal outcome following isolated severe head injury or multitrauma in males. Clinical Chemistry and Laboratory Medicine. 2006;**44**(10):1234-1242

[22] Regner A, Kaufman M, Friedman G, Chemale I. Increased serum S100beta protein concentrations following severe head injury in humans: A biochemical marker of brain death? Neuroreport. 2001;**12**(4):691-694

[23] Moscote-Salazar LR, MR A, Alvis-Miranda HR, Calderon-Miranda W, Alcala-Cerra G, Blancas Rivera MA, et al. Severe cranioencephalic trauma: Prehospital care, surgical management and multimodal monitoring. Bulletin of Emergency and Trauma. 2016;**4**(1):8-23

[24] Kinoshita K. Traumatic brain injury: Pathophysiology for neurocritical care. Journal of Intensive Care. 2016;**4**:29

[25] Hawryluk GW, Bullock MR. Past, present, and future of traumatic brain injury research. Neurosurgery Clinics of North America. 2016;**27**(4):375-396

[26] Rosenfeld JV, Maas AI, Bragge P, Morganti-Kossmann MC, Manley GT, Gruen RL. Early management of severe traumatic brain injury. Lancet. 2012;**380**(9847):1088-1098

[27] Brain Trauma F, American Association of Neurological Surgeons, Congress of Neurological Surgeons. Guidelines for the management of severe traumatic brain injury. Journal of Neurotrauma 2007;**24**(Suppl 1):S1-106

[28] Adams H, Kolias AG, Hutchinson PJ. The role of surgical intervention in traumatic brain injury. Neurosurgery Clinics of North America. 2016;**27**(4):519-528

[29] Grande PO. Critical evaluation of the Lund concept for treatment of severe traumatic head injury, 25 years after its introduction. Frontiers in Neurology. 2017;**8**:315

[30] Andriessen TM, Horn J, Franschman G, van der Naalt J, Haitsma I, Jacobs B, et al. Epidemiology, severity classification, and outcome of moderate and severe traumatic brain injury: A prospective multicenter study. Journal of Neurotrauma. 2011;**28**(10): 2019-2031

[31] Agrawal D, Ahmed S, Khan S, Gupta D, Sinha S, Satyarthee GD. Outcome in 2068 patients of head injury: Experience at a level 1 trauma centre in India. Asian Journal of Neurosurgery. 2016;**11**(2):143-145

[32] Moore L, Evans D, Hameed SM, Yanchar NL, Stelfox HT, Simons R, et al. Mortality in Canadian trauma systems: A multicenter cohort study. Annals of Surgery. 2017;**265**(1): 212-217

[33] Tagliaferri F, Compagnone C, Korsic M, Servadei F, Kraus JA. Systematic review of brain injury epidemiology in Europe. Acta Neurochirurgica. 2006;**148**(3):255-268

[34] Logsdon AF, Lucke-Wold BP, Turner RC, Huber JD, Rosen CL, Simpkins JW. Role of microvascular disruption in brain damage from traumatic brain injury. Comprehensive Physiology. 2015;**5**(3):1147-1160

[35] Rodriguez-Baeza A, Reina-de la Torre F, Poca A, Marti M, Garnacho A. Morphological features in human cortical brain microvessels after head injury: A three-dimensional and

immunocytochemical study. The Anatomical Record. Part A, Discoveries in Molecular, Cellular, and Evolutionary Biology 2003;**273**(1):583-593

[36] Vajtr D, Benada O, Kukacka J, Prusa R, Houstava L, Toupalik P, et al. Correlation of ultrastructural changes of endothelial cells and astrocytes occurring during blood brain barrier damage after traumatic brain injury with biochemical markers of BBB leakage and inflammatory response. Physiological Research. 2009;**58**(2):263-268

[37] da Fonseca AC, Matias D, Garcia C, Amaral R, Geraldo LH, Freitas C, et al. The impact of microglial activation on blood-brain barrier in brain diseases. Frontiers in Cellular Neuroscience. 2014;**8**:362

[38] Winkler EA, Minter D, Yue JK, Manley GT. Cerebral Edema in traumatic brain injury: Pathophysiology and prospective therapeutic targets. Neurosurgery Clinics of North America. 2016;**27**(4):473-488

[39] Marmarou A. A review of progress in understanding the pathophysiology and treatment of brain edema. Neurosurgical Focus. 2007;**22**(5):E1

[40] McKee AC, Daneshvar DH. The neuropathology of traumatic brain injury. Handbook of Clinical Neurology. 2015;**127**:45-66

[41] Ghajar J. Traumatic brain injury. Lancet. 2000;**356**(9233):923-929

[42] Krishnamurthy K, Laskowitz DT. Cellular and molecular mechanisms of secondary neuronal injury following traumatic brain injury. In: Laskowitz D, Grant G, editors. Translational Research in Traumatic Brain Injury. Boca Raton (FL): CRC Press/Taylor and Francis Group; 2016. Chapter 5

[43] Plummer S, Van den Heuvel C, Thornton E, Corrigan F, Cappai R. The neuroprotective properties of the amyloid precursor protein following traumatic brain injury. Aging & Disease. 2016;**7**(2):163-179

[44] Zhang X, Chen Y, Jenkins LW, Kochanek PM, Clark RS. Bench-to-bedside review: Apoptosis/programmed cell death triggered by traumatic brain injury. Critical Care. 2005;**9**(1):66-75

[45] Aertker BM, Bedi S, Cox CS Jr. Strategies for CNS repair following TBI. Experimental Neurology. 2016;**275**(Pt 3):411-426

[46] Stoffel M, Eriskat J, Plesnila M, Aggarwal N, Baethmann A. The penumbra zone of a traumatic cortical lesion: A microdialysis study of excitatory amino acid release. Acta Neurochirurgica. Supplement. 1997;**70**:91-93

[47] Harish G, Mahadevan A, Pruthi N, Sreenivasamurthy SK, Puttamallesh VN, Keshava Prasad TS, et al. Characterization of traumatic brain injury in human brains reveals distinct cellular and molecular changes in contusion and pericontusion. Journal of Neurochemistry. 2015;**134**(1):156-172

[48] Newcombe VF, Williams GB, Outtrim JG, Chatfield D, Gulia Abate M, Geeraerts T, et al. Microstructural basis of contusion expansion in traumatic brain injury: Insights from diffusion tensor imaging. Journal of Cerebral Blood Flow and Metabolism. 2013; **33**(6):855-862

[49] Wu HM, Huang SC, Vespa P, Hovda DA, Bergsneider M. Redefining the pericontusional penumbra following traumatic brain injury: Evidence of deteriorating metabolic derangements based on positron emission tomography. Journal of Neurotrauma. 2013;**30**(5):352-360

[50] Sheriff FG, Hinson HE. Pathophysiology and clinical management of moderate and severe traumatic brain injury in the ICU. Seminars in Neurology. 2015;**35**(1):42-49

[51] Algattas H, Huang JH. Traumatic brain injury pathophysiology and treatments: Early, intermediate, and late phases post-injury. International Journal of Molecular Sciences. 2013;**15**(1):309-341

[52] Buitrago Blanco MM, Prashant GN, Vespa PM. Cerebral metabolism and the role of glucose control in acute traumatic brain injury. Neurosurgery Clinics of North America. 2016;**27**(4):453-463

[53] McGinn MJ, Povlishock JT. Pathophysiology of traumatic brain injury. Neurosurgery Clinics of North America. 2016;**27**(4):397-407

[54] Ding K, Wang H, Wu Y, Zhang L, Xu J, Li T, et al. Rapamycin protects against apoptotic neuronal death and improves neurologic function after traumatic brain injury in mice via modulation of the mTOR-p53-Bax axis. The Journal of Surgical Research. 2015;**194**(1):239-247

[55] Burda JE, Bernstein AM, Sofroniew MV. Astrocyte roles in traumatic brain injury. Experimental Neurology. 2016;**275**(Pt 3):305-315

[56] Kumar A, Loane DJ. Neuroinflammation after traumatic brain injury: Opportunities for therapeutic intervention. Brain, Behavior, and Immunity. 2012;**26**(8):1191-1201

[57] Baez E, Echeverria V, Cabezas R, Avila-Rodriguez M, Garcia-Segura LM, Barreto GE. Protection by neuroglobin expression in brain pathologies. Frontiers in Neurology. 2016; **7**:146

[58] Zhao Z, Alam S, Oppenheim RW, Prevette DM, Evenson A, Parsadanian A. Overexpression of glial cell line-derived neurotrophic factor in the CNS rescues motoneurons from programmed cell death and promotes their long-term survival following axotomy. Experimental Neurology. 2004;**190**(2):356-372

[59] Lozano D, Gonzales-Portillo GS, Acosta S, de la Pena I, Tajiri N, Kaneko Y, et al. Neuroinflammatory responses to traumatic brain injury: Etiology, clinical consequences, and therapeutic opportunities. Neuropsychiatric Disease and Treatment. 2015;**11**:97-106

[60] Ziebell JM, Morganti-Kossmann MC. Involvement of pro- and anti-inflammatory cytokines and chemokines in the pathophysiology of traumatic brain injury. Neurotherapeutics. 2010;7(1):22-30

[61] Castejon OJ. Biopathology of astrocytes in human traumatic and complicated brain injuries. Review and hypothesis. Folia Neuropathologica. 2015;53(3):173-192

[62] Cheng G, Kong RH, Zhang LM, Zhang JN. Mitochondria in traumatic brain injury and mitochondrial-targeted multipotential therapeutic strategies. British Journal of Pharmacology. 2012;167(4):699-719

[63] Regner A, Alves LB, Chemale I, Costa MS, Friedman G, Achaval M, et al. Neurochemical characterization of traumatic brain injury in humans. Journal of Neurotrauma. 2001;18(8): 783-792

[64] Bullock R, Zauner A, Woodward JJ, Myseros J, Choi SC, Ward JD, et al. Factors affecting excitatory amino acid release following severe human head injury. Journal of Neurosurgery. 1998;89(4):507-518

[65] Yi JH, Pow DV, Hazell AS. Early loss of the glutamate transporter splice-variant GLT-1v in rat cerebral cortex following lateral fluid-percussion injury. Glia. 2005;49(1):121-133

[66] Parsons MP, Raymond LA, Extrasynaptic NMDA. receptor involvement in central nervous system disorders. Neuron. 2014;82(2):279-293

[67] Vink R, Nimmo AJ. Novel therapies in development for the treatment of traumatic brain injury. Expert Opinion on Investigational Drugs. 2002;11(10):1375-1386

[68] Hofman M, Koopmans G, Kobbe P, Poeze M, Andruszkow H, Brink PR, et al. Improved fracture healing in patients with concomitant traumatic brain injury: Proven or not? Mediators of Inflammation. 2015;2015:204842

[69] Saatman KE, Creed J, Raghupathi R. Calpain as a therapeutic target in traumatic brain injury. Neurotherapeutics. 2010;7(1):31-42

[70] Weber JT. Altered calcium signaling following traumatic brain injury. Frontiers in Pharmacology. 2012;3:60

[71] Lai TW, Zhang S, Wang YT. Excitotoxicity and stroke: Identifying novel targets for neuroprotection. Progress in Neurobiology. 2014;115:157-188

[72] Maciel EN, Vercesi AE, Castilho RF. Oxidative stress in Ca(2+)-induced membrane permeability transition in brain mitochondria. Journal of Neurochemistry. 2001;79(6):1237-1245

[73] Rockswold SB, Rockswold GL, Defillo A. Hyperbaric oxygen in traumatic brain injury. Neurological Research. 2007;29(2):162-172

[74] Kawamata T, Katayama Y, Hovda DA, Yoshino A, Becker DP. Administration of excitatory amino acid antagonists via microdialysis attenuates the increase in glucose utilization seen following concussive brain injury. Journal of Cerebral Blood Flow and Metabolism. 1992;12(1):12-24

[75] Bergsneider M, Hovda DA, Shalmon E, Kelly DF, Vespa PM, Martin NA, et al. Cerebral hyperglycolysis following severe traumatic brain injury in humans: A positron emission tomography study. Journal of Neurosurgery. 1997;**86**(2):241-251

[76] Bergsneider M, Hovda DA, Lee SM, Kelly DF, McArthur DL, Vespa PM, et al. Dissociation of cerebral glucose metabolism and level of consciousness during the period of metabolic depression following human traumatic brain injury. Journal of Neurotrauma. 2000;**17**(5):389-401

[77] Bergsneider M, Hovda DA, McArthur DL, Etchepare M, Huang SC, Sehati N, et al. Metabolic recovery following human traumatic brain injury based on FDG-PET: Time course and relationship to neurological disability. The Journal of Head Trauma Rehabilitation. 2001;**16**(2):135-148

[78] Wu HM, Huang SC, Hattori N, Glenn TC, Vespa PM, Hovda DA, et al. Subcortical white matter metabolic changes remote from focal hemorrhagic lesions suggest diffuse injury after human traumatic brain injury. Neurosurgery. 2004;**55**(6):1306-1315 discussion 16-7

[79] Yoshino A, Hovda DA, Kawamata T, Katayama Y, Becker DP. Dynamic changes in local cerebral glucose utilization following cerebral conclusion in rats: Evidence of a hyper- and subsequent hypometabolic state. Brain Research. 1991;**561**(1):106-119

[80] Werner C, Engelhard K. Pathophysiology of traumatic brain injury. British Journal of Anaesthesia. 2007;**99**(1):4-9

[81] Balan IS, Saladino AJ, Aarabi B, Castellani RJ, Wade C, Stein DM, et al. Cellular alterations in human traumatic brain injury: Changes in mitochondrial morphology reflect regional levels of injury severity. Journal of Neurotrauma. 2013;**30**(5):367-381

[82] Lewen A, Matz P, Chan PH. Free radical pathways in CNS injury. Journal of Neurotrauma. 2000;**17**(10):871-890

[83] Braughler JM, Hall ED. Involvement of lipid peroxidation in CNS injury. Journal of Neurotrauma. 1992;**9**(Suppl 1):S1-S7

[84] Halestrap AP, Woodfield KY, Connern CP. Oxidative stress, thiol reagents, and membrane potential modulate the mitochondrial permeability transition by affecting nucleotide binding to the adenine nucleotide translocase. The Journal of Biological Chemistry. 1997;**272**(6):3346-3354

[85] Louveau A, Smirnov I, Keyes TJ, Eccles JD, Rouhani SJ, Peske JD, et al. Structural and functional features of central nervous system lymphatic vessels. Nature. 2015;**523**(7560): 337-341

[86] Rock KL, Kono H. The inflammatory response to cell death. Annual Review of Pathology. 2008;**3**:99-126

[87] Mathew P, Graham DI, Bullock R, Maxwell W, McCulloch J, Teasdale G. Focal brain injury: Histological evidence of delayed inflammatory response in a new rodent model of focal cortical injury. Acta Neurochirurgica. Supplementum (Wien). 1994;**60**:428-430

[88] Morganti-Kossmann MC, Rancan M, Stahel PF, Kossmann T. Inflammatory response in acute traumatic brain injury: A double-edged sword. Current Opinion in Critical Care. 2002;**8**(2):101-105

[89] Csuka E, Morganti-Kossmann MC, Lenzlinger PM, Joller H, Trentz O, Kossmann T. IL-10 levels in cerebrospinal fluid and serum of patients with severe traumatic brain injury: Relationship to IL-6, TNF-alpha, TGF-beta1 and blood-brain barrier function. Journal of Neuroimmunology. 1999;**101**(2):211-221

[90] Fassbender K, Schneider S, Bertsch T, Schlueter D, Fatar M, Ragoschke A, et al. Temporal profile of release of interleukin-1beta in neurotrauma. Neuroscience Letters. 2000; **284**(3):135-138

[91] Maier B, Schwerdtfeger K, Mautes A, Holanda M, Muller M, Steudel WI, et al. Differential release of interleukines 6, 8, and 10 in cerebrospinal fluid and plasma after traumatic brain injury. Shock. 2001;**15**(6):421-426

[92] Lenzlinger PM, Morganti-Kossmann MC, Laurer HL, McIntosh TK. The duality of the inflammatory response to traumatic brain injury. Molecular Neurobiology. 2001;**24**(1-3): 169-181

[93] Ferreira LC, Regner A, Miotto KD, Moura S, Ikuta N, Vargas AE, et al. Increased levels of interleukin-6, −8 and −10 are associated with fatal outcome following severe traumatic brain injury. Brain Injury. 2014;**28**(10):1311-1316

[94] Frugier T, Morganti-Kossmann MC, O'Reilly D, McLean CA. In situ detection of inflammatory mediators in post mortem human brain tissue after traumatic injury. Journal of Neurotrauma. 2010;**27**(3):497-507

[95] Schmidt OI, Heyde CE, Ertel W, Stahel PF. Closed head injury – An inflammatory disease? Brain Research. Brain Research Reviews. 2005;**48**(2):388-399

[96] Ralay Ranaivo H, Zunich SM, Choi N, Hodge JN, Wainwright MS. Mild stretch-induced injury increases susceptibility to interleukin-1beta-induced release of matrix metalloproteinase-9 from astrocytes. Journal of Neurotrauma. 2011;**28**(9):1757-1766

[97] Roberts DJ, Jenne CN, Leger C, Kramer AH, Gallagher CN, Todd S, et al. Association between the cerebral inflammatory and matrix metalloproteinase responses after severe traumatic brain injury in humans. Journal of Neurotrauma. 2013;**30**(20):1727-1736

[98] Hanrahan F, Campbell M. Neuroinflammation. In: Laskowitz D, Grant G, editors. Translational Research in Traumatic Brain Injury. Boca Raton (FL): CRC Press/Taylor and Francis Group; 2016. Chapter 6

[99] Toklu HZ, Tumer N. Oxidative stress, brain edema, blood-brain barrier permeability, and autonomic dysfunction from traumatic brain injury. In: Kobeissy FH, editor. Brain Neurotrauma: Molecular, Neuropsychological, and Rehabilitation Aspects. Boca Raton (FL): CRC Press/Taylor & Francis; 2015. Chapter 5

[100] Loane DJ, Kumar A. Microglia in the TBI brain: The good, the bad, and the dysregulated. Experimental Neurology. 2016;**275**(Pt 3):316-327

[101] Xu H, Wang Z, Li J, Wu H, Peng Y, Fan L, et al. The polarization states of microglia in TBI: A new paradigm for pharmacological intervention. Neural Plasticity. 2017;**2017**: 5405104

[102] Hernandez-Ontiveros DG, Tajiri N, Acosta S, Giunta B, Tan J, Borlongan CV. Microglia activation as a biomarker for traumatic brain injury. Frontiers in Neurology. 2013;**4**:30

[103] Chhor V, Le Charpentier T, Lebon S, Ore MV, Celador IL, Josserand J, et al. Characterization of phenotype markers and neuronotoxic potential of polarised primary microglia in vitro. Brain, Behavior, and Immunity. 2013;**32**:70-85

[104] Parekkadan B, Berdichevsky Y, Irimia D, Leeder A, Yarmush G, Toner M, et al. Cell-cell interaction modulates neuroectodermal specification of embryonic stem cells. Neuroscience Letters. 2008;**438**(2):190-195

[105] Chiu CC, Liao YE, Yang LY, Wang JY, Tweedie D, Karnati HK, et al. Neuroinflammation in animal models of traumatic brain injury. Journal of Neuroscience Methods. 2016; **272**:38-49

[106] Witcher KG, Eiferman DS, Godbout JP. Priming the inflammatory pump of the CNS after traumatic brain injury. Trends in Neurosciences. 2015;**38**(10):609-620

[107] Kumar A, Stoica BA, Loane DJ, Yang M, Abulwerdi G, Khan N, et al. Microglial-derived microparticles mediate neuroinflammation after traumatic brain injury. Journal of Neuroinflammation. 2017;**14**(1):47

[108] Lingsma HF, Yue JK, Maas AI, Steyerberg EW, Manley GT, Investigators T-T. Outcome prediction after mild and complicated mild traumatic brain injury: External validation of existing models and identification of new predictors using the TRACK-TBI pilot study. Journal of Neurotrauma. 2015;**32**(2):83-94

[109] Hall ED. Translational principles of neuroprotective and neurorestorative therapy testing in animal models of traumatic brain injury. In: Laskowitz D, Grant G, editors. Translational Research in Traumatic Brain Injury. Boca Raton (FL): CRC Press/Taylor and Francis Group; 2016. Chapter 11

[110] Kochanek PM, Jackson TC, Ferguson NM, Carlson SW, Simon DW, Brockman EC, et al. Emerging therapies in traumatic brain injury. Seminars in Neurology. 2015;**35**(1):83-100

[111] Jablonska A, Lukomska B. Stroke induced brain changes: Implications for stem cell transplantation. Acta Neurobiologiae Experimentalis (Wars). 2011;**71**(1):74-85

[112] Muoio V, Persson PB, Sendeski MM. The neurovascular unit – Concept review. Acta Physiologica (Oxford, England). 2014;**210**(4):790-798

[113] Stanimirovic DB, Friedman A. Pathophysiology of the neurovascular unit: Disease cause or consequence? Journal of Cerebral Blood Flow and Metabolism. 2012;**32**(7):1207-1221

[114] Lassen NA. Cerebral blood flow and oxygen consumption in man. Physiological Reviews. 1959;**39**(2):183-238

[115] Harper AM. Autoregulation of cerebral blood flow: Influence of the arterial blood pressure on the blood flow through the cerebral cortex. Journal of Neurology, Neurosurgery, and Psychiatry. 1966;**29**(5):398-403

[116] Kenney K, Amyot F, Haber M, Pronger A, Bogoslovsky T, Moore C, et al. Cerebral vascular injury in traumatic brain injury. Experimental Neurology. 2016;**275**(Pt 3):353-366

[117] Villringer A, Dirnagl U. Coupling of brain activity and cerebral blood flow: Basis of functional neuroimaging. Cerebrovascular and Brain Metabolism Reviews. 1995;**7**(3): 240-276

[118] Shlosberg D, Benifla M, Kaufer D, Friedman A. Blood-brain barrier breakdown as a therapeutic target in traumatic brain injury. Nature Reviews. Neurology. 2010;**6**(7):393-403

[119] Cherian L, Hlatky R, Robertson CS. Nitric oxide in traumatic brain injury. Brain Pathology. 2004;**14**(2):195-201

[120] Simon DW, McGeachy MJ, Bayir H, Clark RSB, Loane DJ, Kochanek PM. The far-reaching scope of neuroinflammation after traumatic brain injury. Nature Reviews. Neurology. 2017;**13**(9):572

[121] Maxwell WL, Irvine A, Adams JH, Graham DI, Gennarelli TA. Response of cerebral microvasculature to brain injury. The Journal of Pathology. 1988;**155**(4):327-335

[122] Ostergaard L, Engedal TS, Aamand R, Mikkelsen R, Iversen NK, Anzabi M, et al. Capillary transit time heterogeneity and flow-metabolism coupling after traumatic brain injury. Journal of Cerebral Blood Flow and Metabolism. 2014;**34**(10):1585-1598

[123] Stein SC, Chen XH, Sinson GP, Smith DH. Intravascular coagulation: A major secondary insult in nonfatal traumatic brain injury. Journal of Neurosurgery. 2002;**97**(6):1373-1377

[124] Glushakova OY, Johnson D, Hayes RL. Delayed increases in microvascular pathology after experimental traumatic brain injury are associated with prolonged inflammation, blood-brain barrier disruption, and progressive white matter damage. Journal of Neurotrauma. 2014;**31**(13):1180-1193

[125] Jullienne A, Badaut J. Molecular contributions to neurovascular unit dysfunctions after brain injuries: Lessons for target-specific drug development. Future Neurology. 2013;**8**(6):677-689

[126] Simon D, Evaldt J, Nabinger DD, Fontana MF, Klein MG, do Amaral Gomes J, et al. Plasma matrix metalloproteinase-9 levels predict intensive care unit mortality early after severe traumatic brain injury. Brain Injury. 2017;**31**(3):390-395

[127] Sa-Pereira I, Brites D, Brito MA. Neurovascular unit: A focus on pericytes. Molecular Neurobiology. 2012;**45**(2):327-347

[128] Sweeney MD, Ayyadurai S, Zlokovic BV. Pericytes of the neurovascular unit: Key functions and signaling pathways. Nature Neuroscience. 2016;**19**(6):771-783

[129] Bianco P, Cossu G. Uno, nessuno e centomila: Searching for the identity of mesodermal progenitors. Experimental Cell Research. 1999;**251**(2):257-263

[130] Bianco P, Riminucci M, Gronthos S, Robey PG. Bone marrow stromal stem cells: Nature, biology, and potential applications. Stem Cells. 2001;**19**(3):180-192

[131] da Silva Meirelles L, Caplan AI, Nardi NB. Search of the in vivo identity of mesenchymal stem cells. Stem Cells. 2008;**26**(9):2287-2299

[132] da Silva Meirelles L, de Deus Wagatsuma VM, Malta TM, Bonini Palma PV, Araujo AG, Panepucci RA, et al. The gene expression profile of non-cultured, highly purified human adipose tissue pericytes: Transcriptomic evidence that pericytes are stem cells in human adipose tissue. Experimental Cell Research. 2016;**349**(2):239-254

[133] Dore-Duffy P, Katychev A, Wang X, Van Buren ECNS. microvascular pericytes exhibit multipotential stem cell activity. Journal of Cerebral Blood Flow and Metabolism. 2006;**26**(5):613-624

[134] da Silva Meirelles L, Bellagamba BC, Camassola M, Nardi NB. Mesenchymal stem cells and their relationship to pericytes. Front Biosci (Landmark Ed). 2016;**21**:130-156

[135] Crisan M, Yap S, Casteilla L, Chen CW, Corselli M, Park TS, et al. A perivascular origin for mesenchymal stem cells in multiple human organs. Cell Stem Cell. 2008;**3**(3): 301-313

[136] da Silva Meirelles L, Malta TM, de Deus Wagatsuma VM, Palma PV, Araujo AG, Ribeiro Malmegrim KC, et al. Cultured human adipose tissue pericytes and mesenchymal stromal cells display a very similar gene expression profile. Stem Cells and Development. 2015;**24**(23):2822-2840

[137] da Silva Meirelles L, Malta TM, Panepucci RA, da Silva Jr WA. Transcriptomic comparisons between cultured human adipose tissue-derived pericytes and mesenchymal stromal cells. Genomics Data 2016;**7**:20-25

[138] Dellavalle A, Maroli G, Covarello D, Azzoni E, Innocenzi A, Perani L, et al. Pericytes resident in postnatal skeletal muscle differentiate into muscle fibres and generate satellite cells. Nature Communications. 2011;**2**:499

[139] Feng J, Mantesso A, De Bari C, Nishiyama A, Sharpe PT. Dual origin of mesenchymal stem cells contributing to organ growth and repair. Proceedings of the National Academy of Sciences of the United States of America. 2011;**108**(16):6503-6508

[140] Humphreys BD, Lin SL, Kobayashi A, Hudson TE, Nowlin BT, Bonventre JV, et al. Fate tracing reveals the pericyte and not epithelial origin of myofibroblasts in kidney fibrosis. The American Journal of Pathology. 2010;**176**(1):85-97

[141] Maes C, Kobayashi T, Selig MK, Torrekens S, Roth SI, Mackem S, et al. Osteoblast precursors, but not mature osteoblasts, move into developing and fractured bones along with invading blood vessels. Developmental Cell. 2010;**19**(2):329-344

[142] Tang W, Zeve D, Suh JM, Bosnakovski D, Kyba M, Hammer RE, et al. White fat progenitor cells reside in the adipose vasculature. Science. 2008;**322**(5901):583-586

[143] Guimaraes-Camboa N, Cattaneo P, Sun Y, Moore-Morris T, Gu Y, Dalton ND, et al. Pericytes of multiple organs do not behave as mesenchymal stem cells in vivo. Cell Stem Cell. 2017;**20**(3):345-359

[144] Dominici M, Le Blanc K, Mueller I, Slaper-Cortenbach I, Marini F, Krause D, et al. Minimal criteria for defining multipotent mesenchymal stromal cells. The International Society for cellular therapy position statement. Cytotherapy. 2006;**8**(4):315-317

[145] Caplan AI, Dennis JE. Mesenchymal stem cells as trophic mediators. Journal of Cellular Biochemistry. 2006;**98**(5):1076-1084

[146] Meirelles Lda S, Fontes AM, Covas DT, Caplan AI. Mechanisms involved in the therapeutic properties of mesenchymal stem cells. Cytokine & Growth Factor Reviews. 2009;**20**(5-6):419-427

[147] Caplan AI. Adult mesenchymal stem cells for tissue engineering versus regenerative medicine. Journal of Cellular Physiology. 2007;**213**(2):341-347

[148] Caplan AI. What's in a name? Tissue Engineering. Part A. 2010;**16**(8):2415-2417

[149] Caplan AI. Mesenchymal stem cells: Time to change the name. Stem Cells Translational Medicine. 2017;**6**(6):1445-1451

[150] Dore-Duffy P, Owen C, Balabanov R, Murphy S, Beaumont T, Rafols JA. Pericyte migration from the vascular wall in response to traumatic brain injury. Microvascular Research. 2000;**60**(1):55-69

[151] Zehendner CM, Sebastiani A, Hugonnet A, Bischoff F, Luhmann HJ, Thal SC. Traumatic brain injury results in rapid pericyte loss followed by reactive pericytosis in the cerebral cortex. Scientific Reports. 2015;**5**:13497

[152] Zehendner CM, Wedler HE, Luhmann HJA. Novel in vitro model to study pericytes in the neurovascular unit of the developing cortex. PLoS One. 2013;**8**(11):e81637

[153] Tatebayashi K, Tanaka Y, Nakano-Doi A, Sakuma R, Kamachi S, Shirakawa M, et al. Identification of multipotent stem cells in human brain tissue following stroke. Stem Cells and Development. 2017;**26**(11):787-797

[154] Ishitsuka K, Ago T, Arimura K, Nakamura K, Tokami H, Makihara N, et al. Neurotrophin production in brain pericytes during hypoxia: A role of pericytes for neuroprotection. Microvascular Research. 2012;**83**(3):352-359

[155] da Silva Meirelles L, Simon D, Regner A. Neurotrauma: The crosstalk between neurotrophins and inflammation in the acutely injured brain. International Journal of Molecular Sciences. 2017;**18**(5):1082

[156] Caplan AI, Sorrell JM. The MSC curtain that stops the immune system. Immunology Letters. 2015;**168**(2):136-139

[157] Rustenhoven J, Jansson D, Smyth LC, Dragunow M, Brain Pericytes A. Mediators of neuroinflammation. Trends in Pharmacological Sciences. 2017;**38**(3):291-304

[158] Bruno S, Grange C, Deregibus MC, Calogero RA, Saviozzi S, Collino F, et al. Mesenchymal stem cell-derived microvesicles protect against acute tubular injury. Journal of the American Society of Nephrology. 2009;**20**(5):1053-1067

[159] Choi YK, Maki T, Mandeville ET, Koh SH, Hayakawa K, Arai K, et al. Dual effects of carbon monoxide on pericytes and neurogenesis in traumatic brain injury. Nature Medicine. 2016;**22**(11):1335-1341

[160] Tu Y, Chen C, Sun HT, Cheng SX, Liu XZ, Qu Y, et al. Combination of temperature-sensitive stem cells and mild hypothermia: A new potential therapy for severe traumatic brain injury. Journal of Neurotrauma. 2012;**29**(14):2393-2403

[161] Patel K, Sun D. Strategies targeting endogenous neurogenic cell response to improve recovery following traumatic brain injury. Brain Res. 2016;**1640**(Pt A):104-113

[162] Lois C, Alvarez-Buylla A. Proliferating subventricular zone cells in the adult mammalian forebrain can differentiate into neurons and glia. Proceedings of the National Academy of Sciences of the United States of America. 1993;**90**(5):2074-2077

[163] Gage FH, Kempermann G, Palmer TD, Peterson DA, Ray J. Multipotent progenitor cells in the adult dentate gyrus. Journal of Neurobiology. 1998;**36**(2):249-266

[164] Hallbergson AF, Gnatenco C, Peterson DA. Neurogenesis and brain injury: Managing a renewable resource for repair. The Journal of Clinical Investigation. 2003;**112**(8): 1128-1133

[165] Rolfe A, Sun D. Stem cell therapy in brain trauma: implications for repair and regeneration of injured brain in experimental TBI models. In: Kobeissy FH, editor. Brain Neurotrauma: Molecular, Neuropsychological, and Rehabilitation Aspects. Boca Raton (FL): CRC Press/Taylor & Francis; 2015. Chapter 42

[166] Xiong Y, Qu C, Mahmood A, Liu Z, Ning R, Li Y, et al. Delayed transplantation of human marrow stromal cell-seeded scaffolds increases transcallosal neural fiber length, angiogenesis, and hippocampal neuronal survival and improves functional outcome after traumatic brain injury in rats. Brain Research. 2009;**1263**:183-191

[167] Pati S, Rasmussen TE. Cellular therapies in trauma and critical care medicine: Looking towards the future. PLoS Medicine. 2017;**14**(7):e1002343

[168] Pati S, Pilia M, Grimsley JM, Karanikas AT, Oyeniyi B, Holcomb JB, et al. Cellular therapies in trauma and critical care medicine: Forging new Frontiers. Shock. 2015;**44**(6): 505-523

[169] Chen Q, Long Y, Yuan X, Zou L, Sun J, Chen S, et al. Protective effects of bone marrow stromal cell transplantation in injured rodent brain: Synthesis of neurotrophic factors. Journal of Neuroscience Research. 2005;**80**(5):611-619

[170] Chopp M, Li Y. Treatment of neural injury with marrow stromal cells. Lancet Neurology. 2002;**1**(2):92-100

[171] Mahmood A, Lu D, Chopp M. Marrow stromal cell transplantation after traumatic brain injury promotes cellular proliferation within the brain. Neurosurgery. 2004;**55**(5): 1185-1193

[172] Mahmood A, Lu D, Chopp M. Intravenous administration of marrow stromal cells (MSCs) increases the expression of growth factors in rat brain after traumatic brain injury. Journal of Neurotrauma. 2004;**21**(1):33-39

[173] Doeppner TR, Hermann DM. Stem cell-based treatments against stroke: Observations from human proof-of-concept studies and considerations regarding clinical applicability. Frontiers in Cellular Neuroscience. 2014;**8**:357

[174] Cox Jr CS, Baumgartner JE, Harting MT, Worth LL, Walker PA, Shah SK, et al. Autologous bone marrow mononuclear cell therapy for severe traumatic brain injury in children. Neurosurgery 2011;**68**(3):588-600

[175] Zhang Y, Chopp M, Meng Y, Katakowski M, Xin H, Mahmood A, et al. Effect of exosomes derived from multipluripotent mesenchymal stromal cells on functional recovery and neurovascular plasticity in rats after traumatic brain injury. Journal of Neurosurgery. 2015;**122**(4):856-867

[176] Zhang Y, Chopp M, Zhang ZG, Katakowski M, Xin H, Qu C, et al. Systemic administration of cell-free exosomes generated by human bone marrow derived mesenchymal stem cells cultured under 2D and 3D conditions improves functional recovery in rats after traumatic brain injury. Neurochemistry International. 2017;**111**:69-81

[177] Kim DK, Nishida H, An SY, Shetty AK, Bartosh TJ, Prockop DJ. Chromatographically isolated CD63+CD81+ extracellular vesicles from mesenchymal stromal cells rescue cognitive impairments after TBI. Proceedings of the National Academy of Sciences of the United States of America. 2016;**113**(1):170-175

[178] Xiong Y, Mahmood A, Chopp M. Emerging potential of exosomes for treatment of traumatic brain injury. Neural Regeneration Research. 2017;**12**(1):19-22

[179] Marsh SE, Blurton-Jones M. Neural stem cell therapy for neurodegenerative disorders: The role of neurotrophic support. Neurochemistry International. 2017;**106**:94-100

[180] Barteneva NS, Fasler-Kan E, Bernimoulin M, Stern JN, Ponomarev ED, Duckett L, et al. Circulating microparticles: Square the circle. BMC Cell Biology. 2013;**14**:23

[181] Lai RC, Arslan F, Lee MM, Sze NS, Choo A, Chen TS, et al. Exosome secreted by MSC reduces myocardial ischemia/reperfusion injury. Stem Cell Research. 2010;4(3):214-222

[182] Zhang B, Yin Y, Lai RC, Lim SK. Immunotherapeutic potential of extracellular vesicles. Frontiers in Immunology. 2014;5:518

[183] Lai RC, Yeo RW, Lim SK. Mesenchymal stem cell exosomes. Seminars in Cell & Developmental Biology. 2015;40:82-88

[184] Redell JB, Liu Y, Dash PK. Traumatic brain injury alters expression of hippocampal microRNAs: Potential regulators of multiple pathophysiological processes. Journal of Neuroscience Research. 2009;87(6):1435-1448

[185] Hu Z, Yu D, Almeida-Suhett C, Tu K, Marini AM, Eiden L, et al. Expression of miRNAs and their cooperative regulation of the pathophysiology in traumatic brain injury. PLoS One. 2012;7(6):e39357

[186] Liu L, Sun T, Liu Z, Chen X, Zhao L, Qu G, et al. Traumatic brain injury dysregulates microRNAs to modulate cell signaling in rat hippocampus. PLoS One. 2014;9(8):e103948

[187] Lu J, Clark AG. Impact of microRNA regulation on variation in human gene expression. Genome Research. 2012;22(7):1243-1254

[188] John B, Enright AJ, Aravin A, Tuschl T, Sander C, Marks DS. Human MicroRNA targets. PLoS Biology. 2004;2(11):e363

[189] Hammond SM. An overview of microRNAs. Advanced Drug Delivery Reviews. 2015;87:3-14

[190] Lei P, Li Y, Chen X, Yang S, Zhang J. Microarray based analysis of microRNA expression in rat cerebral cortex after traumatic brain injury. Brain Research. 2009;1284:191-201

[191] Boone DK, Weisz HA, Bi M, Falduto MT, Torres KEO, Willey HE, et al. Evidence linking microRNA suppression of essential prosurvival genes with hippocampal cell death after traumatic brain injury. Scientific Reports. 2017;7(1):6645

[192] Ye Y, Perez-Polo JR, Qian J, Birnbaum Y. The role of microRNA in modulating myocardial ischemia-reperfusion injury. Physiological Genomics. 2011;43(10):534-542

[193] Bartels CL, Tsongalis GJ. MicroRNAs: Novel biomarkers for human cancer. Clinical Chemistry. 2009;55(4):623-631

[194] Balakathiresan N, Bhomia M, Chandran R, Chavko M, McCarron RM, Maheshwari RK. MicroRNA let-7i is a promising serum biomarker for blast-induced traumatic brain injury. Journal of Neurotrauma. 2012;29(7):1379-1387

[195] Redell JB, Moore AN, Ward 3rd NH, Hergenroeder GW, Dash PK. Human traumatic brain injury alters plasma microRNA levels. Journal of Neurotrauma 2010;27(12):2147-2156

[196] Mitra B, Rau TF, Surendran N, Brennan JH, Thaveenthiran P, Sorich E, et al. Plasma micro-RNA biomarkers for diagnosis and prognosis after traumatic brain injury: A pilot study. Journal of Clinical Neuroscience. 2017;38:37-42

[197] You WD, Tang QL, Wang L, Lei J, Feng JF, Mao Q, et al. Alteration of microRNA expression in cerebrospinal fluid of unconscious patients after traumatic brain injury and a bioinformatic analysis of related single nucleotide polymorphisms. Chinese Journal of Traumatology. 2016;**19**(1):11-15

[198] Di Pietro V, Ragusa M, Davies D, Su Z, Hazeldine J, Lazzarino G, et al. MicroRNAs as novel biomarkers for the diagnosis and prognosis of mild and severe traumatic brain injury. Journal of Neurotrauma. 2017;**34**(11):1948-1956

[199] Redell JB, Zhao J, Dash PK. Altered expression of miRNA-21 and its targets in the hippocampus after traumatic brain injury. Journal of Neuroscience Research. 2011;**89**(2):212-221

[200] Wong VS, Langley B. Epigenetic changes following traumatic brain injury and their implications for outcome, recovery and therapy. Neuroscience Letters. 2016;**625**:26-33

[201] Choi HA, Badjatia N, Mayer SA. Hypothermia for acute brain injury--mechanisms and practical aspects. Nature Reviews. Neurology. 2012;**8**(4):214-222

[202] Truettner JS, Alonso OF, Bramlett HM, Dietrich WD. Therapeutic hypothermia alters microRNA responses to traumatic brain injury in rats. Journal of Cerebral Blood Flow and Metabolism 2011;**31**(9):1897-1907

[203] Kurlansky P. MicroRNAs: Panacea or Pandora's box? The Journal of Thoracic and Cardiovascular Surgery. 2015;**150**(2):407-408

[204] Yang Y, Ye Y, Su X, He J, Bai W, He X. MSCs-derived exosomes and neuroinflammation, neurogenesis and therapy of traumatic brain injury. Frontiers in Cellular Neuroscience. 2017;**11**:55

[205] Xin H, Li Y, Chopp M. Exosomes/miRNAs as mediating cell-based therapy of stroke. Frontiers in Cellular Neuroscience. 2014;**8**:377

[206] Yanez-Mo M, Siljander PR, Andreu Z, Zavec AB, Borras FE, Buzas EI, et al. Biological properties of extracellular vesicles and their physiological functions. Journal of Extracellular Vesicles. 2015;**4**:27066

[207] Raposo G, Stoorvogel W. Extracellular vesicles: Exosomes, microvesicles, and friends. The Journal of Cell Biology. 2013;**200**(4):373-383

[208] Cocucci E, Meldolesi J. Ectosomes. Current Biology. 2011;**21**(23):R940-R941

[209] Lener T, Gimona M, Aigner L, Borger V, Buzas E, Camussi G, et al. Applying extracellular vesicles based therapeutics in clinical trials – An ISEV position paper. Journal of Extracellular Vesicles. 2015;**4**:30087

[210] Tkach M, Thery C. Communication by extracellular vesicles: Where we are and where we need to go. Cell. 2016;**164**(6):1226-1232

[211] Kowal J, Arras G, Colombo M, Jouve M, Morath JP, Primdal-Bengtson B, et al. Proteomic comparison defines novel markers to characterize heterogeneous populations of extracellular vesicle subtypes. Proceedings of the National Academy of Sciences of the United States of America. 2016;**113**(8):E968-E977

[212] Reiner AT, Witwer KW, van Balkom BWM, de Beer J, Brodie C, Corteling RL, et al. Concise review: Developing best-practice models for the therapeutic use of extracellular vesicles. Stem Cells Translational Medicine. 2017;**6**(8):1730-1739

[213] Biancone L, Bruno S, Deregibus MC, Tetta C, Camussi G. Therapeutic potential of mesenchymal stem cell-derived microvesicles. Nephrology, Dialysis, Transplantation. 2012;**27**(8):3037-3042

[214] Fais S, O'Driscoll L, Borras FE, Buzas E, Camussi G, Cappello F, et al. Evidence-based clinical use of Nanoscale extracellular vesicles in Nanomedicine. ACS Nano. 2016;**10**(4): 3886-3899

[215] Borger V, Bremer M, Ferrer-Tur R, Gockeln L, Stambouli O, Becic A, et al. Mesenchymal stem/stromal cell-derived extracellular vesicles and their potential as novel Immunomodulatory therapeutic agents. International Journal of Molecular Sciences. 2017;**18**(7):1450

[216] Bruno S, Deregibus MC, Camussi G. The secretome of mesenchymal stromal cells: Role of extracellular vesicles in immunomodulation. Immunology Letters. 2015;**168**(2): 154-158

[217] Chen X, Li Y, Wang L, Katakowski M, Zhang L, Chen J, et al. Ischemic rat brain extracts induce human marrow stromal cell growth factor production. Neuropathology. 2002;**22**(4):275-279

[218] Zhang ZG, Chopp M. Neurorestorative therapies for stroke: Underlying mechanisms and translation to the clinic. Lancet Neurology. 2009;**8**(5):491-500

[219] Wei GJ, An G, Shi ZW, Wang KF, Guan Y, Wang YS, et al. Suppression of MicroRNA-383 enhances therapeutic potential of human bone-marrow-derived mesenchymal stem cells in treating spinal cord injury via GDNF. Cellular Physiology and Biochemistry. 2017;**41**(4):1435-1444

[220] Zhang ZG, Chopp M. Exosomes in stroke pathogenesis and therapy. The Journal of Clinical Investigation. 2016;**126**(4):1190-1197

[221] Hasan A, Deeb G, Rahal R, Atwi K, Mondello S, Marei HE, et al. Mesenchymal stem cells in the treatment of traumatic brain injury. Frontiers in Neurology. 2017;**8**:28

[222] Yeo RW, Lai RC, Zhang B, Tan SS, Yin Y, Teh BJ, et al. Mesenchymal stem cell: An efficient mass producer of exosomes for drug delivery. Advanced Drug Delivery Reviews. 2013;**65**(3):336-341

[223] Koh W, Sheng CT, Tan B, Lee QY, Kuznetsov V, Kiang LS, et al. Analysis of deep sequencing microRNA expression profile from human embryonic stem cells derived mesenchymal stem cells reveals possible role of let-7 microRNA family in downstream targeting of hepatic nuclear factor 4 alpha. BMC Genomics. 2010;**11**(Suppl 1):S6

[224] Huang JH, Yin XM, Xu Y, Xu CC, Lin X, Ye FB, et al. Systemic administration of exosomes released from mesenchymal stromal cells attenuates apoptosis, inflammation, and promotes angiogenesis after spinal cord injury in rats. Journal of Neurotrauma. 2017

[225] Kassis H, Shehadah A, Chopp M, Zhang ZG. Epigenetics in stroke recovery. Genes (Basel). 2017;**8**(3):89

[226] de Jong OG, Verhaar MC, Chen Y, Vader P, Gremmels H, Posthuma G, et al. Cellular stress conditions are reflected in the protein and RNA content of endothelial cellderived exosomes. Journal of Extracellular Vesicles. 2012;**1**. DOI: 10.3402/jev.v1i0.18396

[227] Yoon JH, Kim J, Kim KL, Kim DH, Jung SJ, Lee H, et al. Proteomic analysis of hypoxia-induced U373MG glioma secretome reveals novel hypoxia-dependent migration factors. Proteomics. 2014;**14**(12):1494-1502

[228] Eldh M, Ekstrom K, Valadi H, Sjostrand M, Olsson B, Jernas M, et al. Exosomes communicate protective messages during oxidative stress; possible role of exosomal shuttle RNA. PLoS One. 2010;**5**(12):e15353

[229] Xin H, Li Y, Buller B, Katakowski M, Zhang Y, Wang X, et al. Exosome-mediated transfer of miR-133b from multipotent mesenchymal stromal cells to neural cells contributes to neurite outgrowth. Stem Cells. 2012;**30**(7):1556-1564

[230] Feng Y, Huang W, Wani M, Yu X, Ashraf M. Ischemic preconditioning potentiates the protective effect of stem cells through secretion of exosomes by targeting Mecp2 via miR-22. PLoS One. 2014;**9**(2):e88685

[231] Doeppner TR, Herz J, Gorgens A, Schlechter J, Ludwig AK, Radtke S, et al. Extracellular vesicles improve post-stroke neuroregeneration and prevent Postischemic immunosuppression. Stem Cells Translational Medicine. 2015;**4**(10):1131-1143

[232] Chen KH, Chen CH, Wallace CG, Yuen CM, Kao GS, Chen YL, et al. Intravenous administration of xenogenic adipose-derived mesenchymal stem cells (ADMSC) and ADMSC-derived exosomes markedly reduced brain infarct volume and preserved neurological function in rat after acute ischemic stroke. Oncotarget. 2016;**7**(46):74537-74556

[233] Xin H, Katakowski M, Wang F, Qian JY, Liu XS, Ali MM, et al. MicroRNA cluster miR-17-92 cluster in exosomes enhance neuroplasticity and functional recovery after stroke in rats. Stroke. 2017;**48**(3):747-753

[234] Xin H, Li Y, Liu Z, Wang X, Shang X, Cui Y, et al. MiR-133b promotes neural plasticity and functional recovery after treatment of stroke with multipotent mesenchymal stromal cells in rats via transfer of exosome-enriched extracellular particles. Stem Cells. 2013;**31**(12):2737-2746

[235] Xin H, Wang F, Li Y, Lu QE, Cheung WL, Zhang Y, et al. Secondary release of exosomes from astrocytes contributes to the increase in neural plasticity and improvement of functional recovery after stroke in rats treated with exosomes harvested from MicroRNA 133b-overexpressing multipotent mesenchymal stromal cells. Cell Transplantation. 2017;**26**(2):243-257

[236] Drommelschmidt K, Serdar M, Bendix I, Herz J, Bertling F, Prager S, et al. Mesenchymal stem cell-derived extracellular vesicles ameliorate inflammation-induced preterm brain injury. Brain, Behavior, and Immunity. 2017;**60**:220-232

[237] Ennour-Idrissi K, Maunsell E, Diorio C. Telomere length and breast cancer prognosis: A systematic review. Cancer Epidemiology, Biomarkers & Prevention. 2017;**26**(1):3-10

[238] Sandhir R, Gregory E, Berman NE. Differential response of miRNA-21 and its targets after traumatic brain injury in aging mice. Neurochemistry International. 2014;**78**:117-121

[239] Andrews AM, Lutton EM, Merkel SF, Razmpour R, Ramirez SH. Mechanical injury induces brain endothelial-derived microvesicle release: Implications for cerebral vascular injury during traumatic brain injury. Frontiers in Cellular Neuroscience. 2016;**10**:43

11

Complementary Traditional Chinese Medicine Therapy for Traumatic Brain Injury

Ching-Chih Chen, Yu-Chiang Hung and
Wen-Long Hu

Abstract

The number of cases of traumatic brain injury (TBI) is increasing daily, predominantly because of the increasing rate of motor vehicle accidents. TBI has become one of the major causes of mortality and morbidity worldwide among individuals of all ages. TBI-inducing accidents usually occur very suddenly, leading to a heavy burden for both families and society at large. Beside conventional treatments such as surgery, medication, and rehabilitation, traditional Chinese medicine (TCM) is a promising complementary therapy that is practiced worldwide. This chapter will investigate the advances in TCM therapy for TBI.

Keywords: traumatic brain injury, traditional Chinese medicine, herbal medicine, acupuncture, Tai Chi Chuan

1. Introduction

1.1. Definition

Traumatic brain injury (TBI) is defined as an impairment of brain function that is caused by an external force [1].

1.2. Epidemiology

TBI has becoming a major health and socioeconomic problem all over the world [1]. It affects people of all ages including those living in both low-income countries and high-income countries [2]. TBI contributes largely to worldwide mortality and morbidity. According to the Centers for Disease Control and Prevention of the United States, in 2013, there were a recorded 2.8 million TBI-related emergency department visits, hospitalizations, and deaths in the United States alone; there were nearly 50,000 TBI-induced deaths and 282,000 TBI-related hospitalizations [3]. The World Health Organization (WHO) has predicted that, by 2020, TBI will be one of the main health problems and the principle cause of disability [4]. Blunt head injury caused by motor vehicle crashes is most common in young adults and children, whereas falling is the most common cause of TBI in older individuals. The incidence of TBI is twice as much for men than for women [5]. Although the average mortality rate appears to be decreasing, a review published in 2015 has indicated that there are, nonetheless, still no signs of a decreasing incidence of TBI in Europe [2].

1.3. Impact

The high incidence of TBI-associated disability and death incurs many costs and social challenges [5]. In the United States, the cost of TBI has been estimated to be greater than USD 75 billion per year, and the cost for one patient in their whole lifetime is estimated at USD 396,000 [6]. Indeed, even after emergency treatment and hospitalization, deficits persist, even in cases of mild TBI. These include both physical and neurobehavioral impairments, which result in activity limitations, a lack of social participation, and communication difficulties [7], and potentially years of rehabilitation are required after acute treatment. Therefore, it is crucial to raise concern for the recruitment of healthcare resources for TBI treatment and rehabilitation and even to consider potential alternative treatments for survivors of TBI.

2. Etiology

In the United States, the top three major etiologies of TBI are falls, motor vehicle accidents, and being struck by an object. Each of these has been reported to account for 47, 15, and 14%, respectively, of all TBI-related emergency department visits, hospitalizations, and deaths [8]. Moreover, blast-induced TBI accounted for 67–88% of all the TBIs among the casualties in warfare [9]. Falls were reportedly more common in the youngest and oldest age groups. Motor vehicle accidents have the highest fatality rate, followed by intentional self-harm [3]. Other etiologies include assault, "unknown," bicycle and other transport accidents, and suicide attempts [10].

3. Classification

TBI is classified into mild, moderate, and severe on the basis of Glasgow Coma Scale (GCS) score, which ranks functional ability from 1 to 15. Mild TBI (GCS 14–15) accounts for 80% of TBI [5]. Although it is termed "mild," the sequelae may be long lasting. Moderate TBI (GCS 9–13) accounts for 10% of TBI [5]. The mortality rate of TBI without other physical injuries is less than 20%. Among patients with moderate TBI, 40% demonstrated abnormal computed tomography (CT) findings, and 8% required neurosurgery [5]. Severe TBI (GCS 3–8) has a mortality rate approaching 40%, and less than 10% of patients are reported to experience a good recovery [5].

TBI can be categorized into primary and secondary brain injury based on whether the damage is directly or indirectly caused by the trauma.

4. Pathophysiology

4.1. Primary brain injuries

Primary brain injuries are those caused by direct mechanical forces to the brain, which contribute to deformation of brain tissue and disruption of normal brain function. When encountering a force against the head, the soft brain hits the intracranial surface of the skull, resulting in brain damage at the area of contact and at the area opposite to the point of contact. The location and severity of such an impact directly influence the patient's outcome. Penetration to the brain can tear axons and damage neuron conduction, and vascular damage could lead to blood and leukocyte migration into the normally immune-privileged brain [11]. Primary brain injuries include contusions, intracranial hematomas, diffuse axonal injuries, direct cellular damage, loss of electrochemical function, and blood-brain-barrier (BBB) dysfunction.

4.2. Secondary brain injuries

Secondary brain injuries are caused by a cascade of secondary events after primary injuries of the brain. One common example is secondary neurotoxic cascade, which leads to progressive brain damage and eventually results in poor outcomes. The process of secondary neurotoxic cascade involves a massive release of neurotransmitters into synaptic clefts; this ultimately induces mitochondrial damage and leads to cell death and necrosis [12, 13]. The inflammatory response can also cause secondary damage in TBI, especially around the locations of contusions and hemorrhages. Neurotransmitter release and inflammatory responses can last days after TBI, leading to BBB dysfunction and immune-mediated activation of cell death and apoptosis.

5. Conventional treatment and rehabilitation

5.1. Conventional treatment

Emergent treatment for TBI, including surgery and intensive care, is crucial because cerebral edema can lead to several pathologies associated with primary and secondary injuries [14]. Initially, prehospital care is primarily aimed at preventing hypoxia and hypotension, which can lead to secondary brain injury; hence, fluid resuscitation with crystalloids and colloids and oxygen supplementation are implemented. Osmotherapy with rapid infusion of mannitol, which creates an osmolality gradient to maintain fluid in vessels, therefore, improves focal cerebral blood flow. Decompressive craniectomy has also been practiced on TBI patients to lower intracranial pressure and treat brain edema for decades [1].

5.2. Rehabilitation treatment

Further rehabilitation strategies include hyperbaric oxygen therapy, noninvasive brain stimulation, and limb or organ function reconstruction [4]. Hyperbaric oxygen therapy has been shown to inhibit apoptosis, suppress inflammation, protect the integrity of the BBB, and promote angiogenesis and neurogenesis [15, 16]. Several studies have revealed that noninvasive brain stimulation, including transcranial magnetic stimulation and transcranial direct current stimulation, can reduce TBI-associated depression, tinnitus, neglect, memory deficits, and attention disorders [4]. Another study demonstrated that electrical stimulation enhanced energy and glucose metabolism in patients who could not voluntarily exercise [17].

5.3. Outcomes and prognosis

Experience has shown that about 85% of recovery occurs within 6 months after head injury [1]. The most frequently used scale for outcome prediction is the GCS scale; however, further detailed functional and neuropsychological assessment is required during rehabilitation to fully assess outcomes. Early and intensive rehabilitation is recommended in order to obtain the best possible functional outcome and social reintegration [1].

6. Traditional Chinese medicine in the treatment of TBI

Traditional Chinese medicine (TCM), which has been practiced in China for thousands of years, has attracted increasing attention in recent years. There is sufficient evidence supporting the clinical benefits of TCM in the treatment of TBI, including Chinese herbal medicine compounds, acupuncture, and electroacupuncture [18–20]. This chapter will thus discuss the complementary treatment of TBI with TCM.

6.1. Chinese herbal medicine for TBI

Chinese herbal medicine treatment comes in different forms, including decoctions, pills, and powders. Numerous studies have suggested that Chinese medicine has multiple neuroprotective effects, including improvement of brain edema, anti-inflammatory responses, and antioxidative effects. Reviews of several studies have concluded that TCM plays an important role in the prevention and treatment of neural diseases and is potentially effective in neural regeneration and CNS functional recovery [21, 22].

6.1.1. Single Chinese herb for TBI

Ginseng, the root of *Panax ginseng C.A. Meyer* (Araliaceae), has been widely used for treating qi depletion patterns. Generally, qi represents the energy flow in the meridian that maintains the proper function of the organs, and therefore, qi depletion represents a decrease of function of the organs. The biologically active substance in Ginseng is ginsenoside, which has been reported to have neuroprotective effects, regulate nerve-regulating factors, and improve the proliferation of neural stem cells. This suggests that ginsenoside might improve the recovery of neurological functions, such as memory and learning [23, 24]. Rhein (the active part of *Rheum rhabarbarum*) also has the potential to be utilized as a neuroprotective drug in TBI because of its anti-oxidative effects and its ability to cross the BBB and it increases permeability the BBB [25, 26] (**Table 1**).

6.1.2. Traditional Chinese herbal formulae for TBI

TCM formulae are potentially neuroprotective and beneficial in cases of brain edema through a reduction of brain water content, improvement of the permeability of the BBB, and reduction of tumor necrosis factor-alpha (TNF-α)/nitric oxide (NO) levels after TBI [27]. One study has demonstrated that the Sheng-Nao-Kang decoction, which contains 15 different traditional Chinese medicines, has a protective effect against ischemia and reperfusion injuries [28]. The Shen-Nao-Kang decoction was developed to activate blood circulation, dissipate blood stasis, and dredge meridians and collaterals [28]. The Xuefu-Zhuyu (XFZY) decoction is also documented to have multiple benefits for TBI, including improving neurological recovery after TBI, reducing TBI-induced elevation of arachidonic acid (a precursor of prostaglandins and leukotrienes) levels in the brain, restraining the TBI-induced increase of pro-inflammatory factors in the brain, and inhibiting the inflammatory pathways mediated by Akt/mammalian target of rapamycin (mTOR)/p70S6 kinase [29]. NeuroAid is a TCM compound that contains 14 different herb components and has been found to have neuroprotective and neurorestorative actions in animal models and, hence, leads to improved cognitive function following TBI [30, 31] (**Table 2**).

Study	N	Design	Herb extracts	Conclusion
Hu et al. [23]	48	(1) Animal model (2) RCT	GTS	GTS alleviates secondary brain injury and improves neurological function through regulation of the expression of nerve growth related factors
Ji et al. [24]	24	(1) Animal model (2) RCT	GTS	GTS has a neuroprotective effect after TBI
Xu et al. [25]	36	(1) Animal model (2) RCT	Rhein	Rhubarb (and its component rhein) has anti-oxidative properties and decreases the overproduction of free radicals after oxidative stress in TBI
Tang et al. [26]	6:6:6	(1) Animal model (2) RCT	Rhein	Rhubarb could ameliorate cerebral edema; rhein may inhibit the transcription and translation of the aquaporin-4 gene

GTS, ginseng total saponins; TBI, traumatic brain injury; RCT, randomized controlled trial

Table 1. Studies on the effects of single herbal medicines on brain injury.

6.2. Acupuncture and electroacupuncture for TBI

6.2.1. The benefit of treating patients with TBI through acupuncture and electroacupuncture

In TCM theory, acupuncture regulates the function of qi, blood, and organs through the stimulation of acupoints and eliminates pathogenic factors [32]. Acupuncture plays an important role in treating TBI, and its popularity as a supplementary treatment continues to increase. In the first year after TBI, patients in one study that received acupuncture treatment experienced a decreased risk of hospitalization and lower use of emergency medical care compared to patients who did not receive acupuncture treatment [33]. In an animal study, early, low-frequency electroacupuncture treatment after TBI was shown to be beneficial, decreasing TNF-α expression in activated microglia and astrocytes and reducing neural apoptosis and, therefore, improving functional outcome after TBI [34]. Neural stem cell proliferation and differentiation could also be affected by acupuncture, by upregulating gene expression, shortening the time for recovery, and regulating astrocyte proliferation and differentiation [35, 36]. Despite these aspects of neural recovery, some sequelae after TBI have also been shown to be benefited by acupuncture. Insomnia after TBI is a common complaint; one study has found that acupuncture has beneficial effect on the perception of sleep or sleep quality as well as benefiting cognition in 24 adult patients with TBI [37]. In patients with spastic muscle hyperactivity and chronic disorders of consciousness following TBI, evidence has shown that acupuncture can immediately reduce the excitability of spinal motor neurons [38]. However, another study has shown that acupuncture could increase the excitability of the corticospinal system; this suggests that acupuncture might accelerate the recovery of motor function in patients with disorders of consciousness following TBI [20]. Moreover, a cohort study has demonstrated that patients with TBI who received acupuncture had a lower risk of new-onset stroke than those who did not receive acupuncture [39] (**Table 3**).

Study	N	Design	TCM compound	Conclusion
Yang et al. [27]	25	(1) Systematic review (2) Animal model		TCM compound recipes may improve brain edema via increasing BBB permeability and decreasing TNF-α/NO expression after TBI
Chen et al. [28]	36	(1) RCT (2) Animal model	Sheng-Nao-Kang	Sheng-Nao-Kang demonstrates a protective effect against cerebral ischemia/reperfusion injury
Xing et al. [29]	64	(1) RCT (2) Animal model	XFZY decoction	XFZY decoction reduces mNSS, AA, TNF-α, and IL-1β levels and downregulates AKT/mTOR/p70S6K proteins in the brain; XFZY decoction may reduce TBI-associated inflammation
Quitard et al. [30]	6:6:6	(1) RCT (2) Animal model	NeuroAid (MLC901)	MLC901 has neuroprotective and neurorestorative effects in TBI animal models

TNF-α, tumor necrosis factor α; NO, nitric oxide; TBI, traumatic brain injury; RCT, randomized controlled trial; mNSS, modified neurologic severity score; AA, arachidonic acid; mTOR, mechanistic target of rapamycin; XFZY, Xuefu-Zhuyu

Table 2. Studies on the effects of traditional Chinese medicine compounds in the treatment of brain injury.

Study	N	Design	Test group	Control group	Acupoints	Conclusion
Tang et al. [34]	6:6:6	RCT animal study	EA	(1) Control (2) Sham	DU20, DU26, LI4, and KI1	EA ameliorates TBI neuroinflammation in the acute stage by attenuating TNF-α expression
Zhang et al. [35]	36:36:16:16	RCT animal model	Acupuncture	(1) Model (2) Normal (3) Sham	DU20, DU26, DU16, DU15, and LI4	Acupuncture promotes *notch1*, *hes1*, and *hes5* expression in brain tissue, which are important for stem cell proliferation
Jiang et al. [36]	32:36:36	RCT animal model	Acupuncture	(1) Normal (2) TBI	DU20, DU26, DU16, DU15, and LI4	Acupuncture induces endogenous neural stem cell proliferation and differentiation
Zollman et al. [37]	12:12	Pilot RCT	Acupuncture	WCM	KI3, HR3, BL60, LR3, LI4, PC7, DU20, ear point Tranquilizer, and Shen Men	Acupuncture is beneficial for treatment of insomnia and improving cognitive function after TBI
Matsumoto-Miyazaki et al. [20]	12	Crossover study	Acupuncture first	Control first	DU26, Ex-HN3, LI4, and ST36	Acupuncture could improve corticospinal tract excitability and, therefore, improve spastic muscle hypertonia in patients with TBI
Matsu moto-Miyazaki et al. [36]	11	Crossover study	Acupuncture first	Control first	DU26, Ex-HN3, LI4, and ST36	Acupuncture could reduce the excitability of spinal motor neurons and improve spastic muscle hypertonia in patients with TBI
Shih et al. [37]	29,636	Cohort study	Acupuncture treatment	Non-acupuncture treatment		Compared to patients with TBI not receiving acupuncture, those with acupuncture have a lower risk of new-onset stroke

EA, electroacupuncture; TBI, traumatic brain injury; RCT, randomized controlled trial; TNF-α, tumor necrosis factor-α; WCM, Western conventional medicine

Table 3. Studies on the effects of acupuncture and electroacupuncture in the treatment of brain injury.

6.2.2. Zusanli (ST36)

Zusanli (ST36) is an acupoint on the stomach meridian that is rich in blood and qi. Stimulation of this point has several effects in TCM theory, including supplementing the qi and blood, fortification of the spleen, and harmonizing the stomach. Several neuroprotective effects of ST36 have been noted in recent studies, including enhancing neural plasticity, suppressing neuron apoptosis, increasing cerebral blood flow, and improving microcirculation [40]. One study found that acupuncture performed at certain acupoints, including Baihui (DU20), Renzhong (DU26), Hegu (LI4), and Zusanli (ST36), improved neurological recovery after TBI through the brain-derived neurotrophic factor (BDNF)/tropomyosin receptor kinase B (TrkB) pathway; not only was this effect immediate, but it persisted for 168 hours after acupuncture [32]. Electroacupuncture at ST36 might also encourage neurological recovery through upregulation of angiopoietin-1 and angiopoietin-2 [40]. Moreover, electroacupuncture at ST36 could enhance endothelial cell proliferation and, consequently, upregulate the level of hypoxia-inducible factor-1α (HIF-1α) protein, which accelerates angiogenesis [41] (**Table 4**).

6.2.3. Baihui (DU20)

DU20, also named GV20, when the ears are folded, DU20 is located at the midpoint of the connecting line between the auricular apices [42]. According to TCM theory, DU20 belongs

Study	N	Design	Test group	Control group	Acupoints	Conclusion
Zhou et al. [40]	30:30:30	RCT animal model	Stroke-EA group	(1) Sham (2) Stroke-no acupuncture	ST36	EA in ICH rats remarkably increases Angiopoietin-1 and −2 levels
Li et al. [32]	20:20:20:20	RCT animal model	(1) TBI + Acupuncture group (2) TBI + Acupuncture + K252α group	(1) TBI (2) TBI-placebo-acupuncture group	DU20, DU26, LI4, ST36	Acupuncture aids neurological recovery through activation of the BDNF/TrkB pathway
Luo et al. [41].	24:24:24:24	RCT animal model	(1) ICH + Acupuncture	(1) Sham (2) ICH group (3) ICH non-acupoint acupuncture	ST36	EA at ST36 increases the number of cerebral endothelial cells and increases the expression of HIF-1 and may, therefore, accelerate ICH-induced angiogenesis

EA, electroacupuncture; ICH, intracranial hemorrhage; TBI, traumatic brain injury; BDNF, brain-derived neurotrophic factor; TrkB, tropomyosin receptor kinase B; HIF-1, hypoxia-induced factor-1; RCT, randomized controlled trial

Table 4. Studies on the effects of acupuncture at ST36 for the treatment of brain injury.

to the governor vessel, which governs the yang qi all over the body. The function of DU20 is to wake the brain and open the orifices, lift the spirit, tonify yang, strengthen the ascending function of the spleen, dredge qi and the blood, and lift up yang qi [43]. Therefore, researchers have targeted a combination of DU20 and ST36 for the treatment of cerebral injury; results revealed that rats with cerebral ischemia reperfusion injuries had better neurological scores and reduced volumes of brain infarction than those who did not receive postoperative treatment [44]. Another study found that acupuncture and electroacupuncture at DU20 and ST36 could decrease the infiltration of inflammatory cells and pro-inflammatory enzymes [45]. More importantly, acupuncture and electroacupuncture significantly attenuate the expression of aquaporins in the ischemic brain, including aquaporin 4 and aquaporin 9, indicating that protective mechanisms are partially dependent on the reduction of inflammation-related brain edema [46]. One study of electroacupuncture at DU20 demonstrated improvements in the microenvironment via neural regeneration and neuroprotection in newborn rats with TBI [47] (**Table 5**).

6.3. Tai Chi Chuan for TBI

Tai Chi Chuan (also known as "Tai Chi"), as a traditional Chinese aerobic exercise, has been popular in both the Western and Eastern worlds for years. Tai Chi Chuan was used as a novel supplementation to a comprehensive rehabilitation program [48]. Many studies have demonstrated the physiological and psychological benefits of Tai Chi Chuan in chronic conditions, including benefits in cardiovascular function, musculoskeletal condition, and reduction of anxiety [49]. In one randomized pilot study, patients with TBI were allocated to either a Tai Chi group (n = 20) that received supervised Tai Chi instruction for 8 weeks (1 h per week) or

Study	N	Design	Test group	Control group	Acupoints	Conclusion
Chen et al. [44]	24:24:24	RCT animal model	Acupuncture group	(1) Sham-operated group (2) Model group	DU20, ST36	Acupuncture at DU20 and ST 36 in rats could upregulate miRNA 124 and reduce the expression of laminin and integrin β1
Xu et al. [45]	48:48:48:8	RCT animal model	Acupuncture group	(1) Sham operated (2) Model (3) Normal	DU20, ST36	Acupuncture at DU20 and ST36 could reduce or delay the expression of HSP70 and TNF-α, which are related to neuroprotection
Chen et al. [47]	6:6:6:6	RCT animal model	20-min fetal distress + DU20 group	(1) Blank control group (2) 20-min fetal distress group (3) 20-min fetal distress-non-acupoint group	DU20	EA regulates NeuroD expression by affecting the brain's microenvironment

RCT, randomized controlled trial; miRNA, micro ribonucleic acid; HSP-70, heat-shock protein 70; TNF-α, tumor necrosis factor-α; EA, electroacupuncture

Table 5. Studies on the effect of acupuncture at DU20 on brain injury.

a control group (n = 20) that performed a non-exercise leisure activity for the same amount of time. The results revealed that the Tai Chi group had a better mood and higher self-esteem scores [50]. Another study investigated the effects of a 6-week Tai Chi practice in patients with TBI and revealed increased happiness and energy, with significant improvements in sadness, confusion, anger, tension, and fear compared to a control group [51]. However, there was no significant difference in fatigue between the intervention group and control group. Although our knowledge of the mechanisms underlying such effects of Tai Chi Chuan is still lacking, evidence suggests that smooth exercise can improve mood and self-esteem and might, therefore, help patients with TBI become more involved in social activities.

7. Conclusions

The use of TCM as a complementary treatment for TBI is becoming increasingly popular. Although more evidence on the effects and mechanisms of TCM therapy is certainly required, previous results are encouraging. Chinese herbal medicine, acupuncture, and Tai Chi Chuan were found to have beneficial effects in patients with TBI. The possible mechanisms and effects of TCM for the treatment of TBI have been shown and proven to be effective based on animal studies mostly. Nevertheless, we are optimistic regarding the results of further TCM studies and look forward to more evidence confirming the TCM theory, as this would be beneficial for all patients.

Author details

Ching-Chih Chen[1], Yu-Chiang Hung[1,2] and Wen-Long Hu[1,3,4]*

*Address all correspondence to: oolonghu@gmail.com

1 Department of Chinese Medicine, Kaohsiung Chang Gung Memorial Hospital and School of Traditional Chinese Medicine, Chang Gung University College of Medicine, Kaohsiung, Taiwan

2 School of Chinese Medicine for Post Baccalaureate, I-Shou University, Kaohsiung, Taiwan

3 Fooyin University College of Nursing, Kaohsiung, Taiwan

4 Kaohsiung Medical University College of Medicine, Kaohsiung, Taiwan

References

[1] Maas AI, Stocchetti N, Bullock R. Moderate and severe traumatic brain injury in adults. The Lancet Neurology. 2008;**7**:728-741

[2] Peeters W, van den Brande R, Polinder S, Brazinova A, Steyerberg EW, Lingsma HF, et al. Epidemiology of traumatic brain injury in Europe. Acta Neurochirurgica. 2015;**157** (10):1683-1696

[3] Larson K. Centers for Disease Control and Prevention (CDC). 1600 Clifton Rd. Atlanta, GA 30333. Retrieved 24-02-2012, from http://www.cdc.gov. Gov Inf Q.2012;29:304-5

[4] Dang B, Chen W, He W, Chen G. Rehabilitation treatment and progress of traumatic brain injury dysfunction. Neural plasticity. 2017;**2017**:6. Article ID 1582182 DOI: 10.1155/2017/1582182

[5] Tintinalli JE. Emergency medicine. In: JAMA [Internet]. 1996. p. 1804. Available from: http://ezproxy.library.dal.ca/login?url=http://search.proquest.com/docview/211352415?accountid=10406%5Cnhttp://sfxhosted.exlibrisgroup.com/dal?url_ver=Z39.88-2004&rft_val_fmt=info:ofi/fmt:kev:mtx:journal&genre=article&sid=ProQ:ProQ%3Anursing&atitle=Emerge

[6] Peeters W, Majdan M, Brazinova A, Nieboer D, Maas AIR. Changing epidemiological patterns in traumatic brain injury: A longitudinal hospital-based study in Belgium. Neuroepidemiology. 2017;**48**(1-2):63-70. Available from: https://www.karger.com/?doi=10.1159/000471877%0Ahttp://www.ncbi.nlm.nih.gov/pubmed/28448968

[7] DeLisa Joel A. Frontera WR, editor. DeLisa's Physical Medicine & Rehabilitation Principles and Practice. 5th ed. 2010. pp. 575-624

[8] Larson K. Centers for Disease Control and Prevention (CDC). [Internet]. 2012. Available from https://www.cdc.gov/traumaticbraininjury/get_the_facts.html. [Accessed: 08-07-2017]

[9] Jones E, Fear NT, Wessely S. Shell shock and mild traumatic brain injury: A historical review. The American Journal of Psychiatry. 2007;**164**:1641-1645

[10] Langlois JA, Rutland-Brown W, Wald MM. The epidemiology and impact of traumatic brain injury. The Journal of Head Trauma Rehabilitation. 2006;**21**(5):375-378. Available from: http://content.wkhealth.com/linkback/openurl?sid=WKPTLP:landingpage&an=00001199-200609000-00001

[11] Dixon KJ. Pathophysiology of traumatic brain injury. Physical Medicine and Rehabilitation Clinics of North America. 2017;**28**(2):215-225. Available from: http://dx.doi.org/10.1016/j.pmr.2016.12.001

[12] McIntosh TK, Smith DH, Meaney DF, Kotapka MJ, Gennarelli TA, Graham DI. Neuropathological sequelae of traumatic brain injury: Relationship to neurochemical and biomechanical mechanisms. Laboratory Investigation. 1996;**74**(2):315-342

[13] Goodman JC, Van M, Gopinath SP, Robertson CS. Pro-inflammatory and pro-apoptotic elements of the neuroinflammatory response are activated in traumatic brain injury. Acta Neurochirurgica. Supplement. 2008;**102**:437-439

[14] Xi G, Keep RF, Hoff JT. Pathophysiology of brain edema formation. Neurosurgery Clinics of North America. 2002;**13**:371-383

[15] Braswell C. Hyperbaric oxygen therapy. Compendium: Continuing Education for Veterinarians. 2012;**34**(3):E1-E6

[16] Sánchez EC. Mechanisms of action of hyperbaric oxygenation in stroke: A review. Critical Care Nursing Quarterly. 2013;**36**(3):290-298. Available from: http://www.ncbi. nlm.nih.gov/pubmed/23736668

[17] Hamada T. Electrical stimulation of human lower extremities enhances energy consumption, carbohydrate oxidation, and whole body glucose uptake. Journal of Applied Physiology. 2003;**96**(3):911-916. Available from: http://jap.physiology.org/cgi/ doi/10.1152/japplphysiol.00664.2003

[18] Saito S, Kobayashi T, Osawa T, Kato S. Effectiveness of Japanese herbal medicine yokukan-san for alleviating psychiatric symptoms after traumatic brain injury. Psychogeriatrics. 2010;**10**(1):45-48

[19] JW G, Zhang X, Fei Z, Wen AD, Qin SY, Yi SY, et al. Rhubarb extracts in treating complications of severe cerebral injury. Chinese Medical Journal (England). 2000;**113**(6):529-531

[20] Matsumoto-Miyazaki J, Asano Y, Yonezawa S, Nomura Y, Ikegame Y, Aki T, et al. Acupuncture increases the excitability of the cortico-spinal system in patients with chronic disorders of consciousness following traumatic brain injury. Journal of Alternative and Complementary Medicine. 2016;**22**(11):887-894. Available from: http:// online.liebertpub.com/doi/10.1089/acm.2014.0356

[21] De Qin X, Kang LY, Liu Y, Huang Y, Wang S, Zhu JQ. Chinese medicine's intervention effect on Nogo-a/NgR. Evidence-based Complementary and Alternative Medicine. 2012;**2012**

[22] Li L, Fan X, Zhang X-T, Yue S-Q, Sun Z-Y, Zhu J-Q, et al. The effects of Chinese medicines on cAMP/PKA signaling in central nervous system dysfunction. Brain Research Bulletin. 2017;**132**(November 2016):109-117. Available from: http://linkinghub.elsevier. com/retrieve/pii/S0361923016304336

[23] Hu BY, Liu XJ, Qiang R, Jiang ZL, Xu LH, Wang GH, et al. Treatment with ginseng total saponins improves the neurorestoration of rat after traumatic brain injury. Journal of Ethnopharmacology. 2014;**155**(2):1243-1255

[24] Yong CJ, Young BK, Seung WP, Sung NH, Byung KM, Hyun JH, et al. Neuroprotective effect of ginseng total saponins in experimental traumatic brain injury. Journal of Korean Medical Science. 2005;**20**(2):291-296

[25] Xu X, Lv H, Xia Z, Fan R, Zhang C, Wang Y, et al. Rhein exhibits antioxidative effects similar to rhubarb in a rat model of traumatic brain injury. BMC Complementary and Alternative Medicine. 2017;**17**(1):140. Available from: http://bmccomplementalternmed. biomedcentral.com/articles/10.1186/s12906-017-1655-x

[26] Tang YP, Cai DFLJ. Research on acting mechanism of rhubarb on aquaporin-4 in rats with blood-brain barrier injury after acute cerebral hemorrhage. Zhingguo Zhong Xi Yi Jie He Za Zhi. 2006;**26**(2):152-156

[27] Yang B, Wang Z, Sheng C, Wang Y, Zhou J, Xiong G-X, Peng WJ, et al. Evidence-based review of oral traditional Chinese medicine compound recipe administration for treating weight drop- induced experimental traumatic brain injury. BMC Complementary and Alternative Medicine. 2016;**2016**:1695. Available from: https://www.ncbi.nlm.nih.gov/pmc/articles/PMC4784383/

[28] Chen L, Zhao Y, Zhang T, Dang X, Xie R, Li Z, et al. Protective effect of sheng-Nao-Kang decoction on focal cerebral ischemia-reperfusion injury in rats. Journal of Ethnopharmacology. 2014;**151**(1):228-236. Available from: http://dx.doi.org/10.1016/j.jep.2013.10.015

[29] Xing Z, Xia Z, Peng W, Li J, Zhang C, Fu C, et al. Xuefu Zhuyu decoction, a traditional Chinese medicine, provides neuroprotection in a rat model of traumatic brain injury via an anti-inflammatory pathway. Scientific Reports. 2016;**6**(1):20040. Available from: http://www.nature.com/articles/srep20040

[30] Quintard H, Lorivel T, Gandin C, Lazdunski M, Heurteaux C. MLC901, a traditional Chinese medicine induces neuroprotective and neuroregenerative benefits after traumatic brain injury in rats. Neuroscience. 2014;**277**:72-86. Available from: http://dx.doi.org/10.1016/j.neuroscience.2014.06.047

[31] Tsai MC, Chang CP, Peng SW, Jhuang KS, Fang YH, Lin MT, et al. Therapeutic efficacy of Neuro AiDTM (MLC 601), a traditional Chinese medicine, in experimental traumatic brain injury. Journal of Neuroimmune Pharmacology. 2015;**10**(1):45-54

[32] Li X, Chen C, Yang X, Wang J, Zhao ML, Sun H, et al. Acupuncture improved neurological recovery after traumatic brain injury by activating BDNF/TrkB pathway. Evidence-based Complementary and Alternative Medicine. 2017;9. Article ID 8460145, http://dx.doi.org/10.1155/2017/8460145

[33] Shih C-C, Lee H-H, Chen T-L, Tsai C-C, Lane H-L, Chiu W-T, et al. Reduced use of emergency care and hospitalization in patients with traumatic brain injury receiving acupuncture treatment. Evidence-based Complementary and Alternative Medicine. 2013;**2013**:1-7. Available from: http://www.hindawi.com/journals/ecam/2013/262039/

[34] Tang W-C, Hsu Y-C, Wang C-C, C-Y H, Chio C-C, Kuo J-R. Early electroacupuncture treatment ameliorates neuroinflammation in rats with traumatic brain injury. BMC Complementary and Alternative Medicine. 2016;**16**(1):470. Available from: http://bmc-complementalternmed.biomedcentral.com/articles/10.1186/s12906-016-1457-6

[35] Zhang Y, Chen S, Dai Q, Jiang S, Chen A, Tang C, et al. Effect of acupuncture on the notch signaling pathway in rats with brain injury. Chinese Journal of Integrative Medicine. 2015;**510632**. Available from: http://link.springer.com/10.1007/s11655-015-1969-9

[36] Jiang S, Chen W, Zhang Y, Zhang Y, Chen A, Dai Q, et al. Acupuncture induces the proliferation and differentiation of endogenous neural stem cells in rats with traumatic brain injury. Evidence-based Complementary and Alternative Medicine. 2016;**2016**(20150114205420):1-8

[37] Zollman F, Larson E, Wasek-Throm L, Cyborski C, Bode R. Acupuncture for treatment of insomnia in patients with traumatic brain injury: A pilot intervention study. The Journal of Head Trauma Rehabilitation. 2012;27:135-142. Available from: http://ovidsp.ovid.com/ovid-web.cgi?T=JS&PAGE=reference&D=ovftm&NEWS=N&AN=00001199-201203000-00007

[38] Matsumoto-Miyazaki J, Asano Y, Ikegame Y, Kawasaki T, Nomura Y, Shinoda J. Acupuncture reduces excitability of spinal motor neurons in patients with spastic muscle overactivity and chronic disorder of consciousness following traumatic brain injury. Journal of Alternative and Complementary Medicine. 2016;22(11):895-902 Available from: http://online.liebertpub.com/doi/10.1089/acm.2016.0180

[39] Shih C-C, Hsu Y-T, Wang H-H, Chen T-L, Tsai C-C, Lane H-L, et al. Decreased risk of stroke in patients with traumatic brain injury receiving acupuncture treatment: A population-based retrospective cohort study. PLoS One. 2014;9(2):e89208. Available from: http://dx.plos.org/10.1371/journal.pone.0089208

[40] Zhou HJ, Tang T, Zhong JH, Luo JK, Cui HJ, Zhang QM, et al. Electroacupuncture improves recovery after hemorrhagic brain injury by inducing the expression of angiopoietin-1 and -2 in rats. BMC Complementary and Alternative Medicine. 2014;14:2-7

[41] Luo JK, Zhou HJ, Wu J, Tang T, Liang QH. Electroacupuncture at Zusanli (ST36) accelerates intracerebral hemorrhage-induced angiogenesis in rats. Chinese Journal of Integrative Medicine. 2013;19(5):367-373

[42] World Health Organization Regional Office for the Western Pacific (WPRO). WHO Standard Acupuncture Point Locations in the Western Pacific Region. WPRO: Manila, Philippines; 2009. pp. 213. ISBN: 978-92-9061-248-7

[43] Wang W, Xie C, Lu L, Zheng GA. Systematic review and meta-analysis of Baihui (GV20)-based scalp acupuncture in experimental ischemic stroke. Scientific Reports. 2014;4:1-16. Available from: http://www.nature.com/articles/srep03981

[44] Chen SH, Sun H, Zhang YM, Xu H, Yang Y, Wang FM. Effects of acupuncture at Baihui (GV 20) and Zusanli (ST 36) on peripheral serum expression of microRNA 124, laminin and integrin β1 in rats with cerebral ischemia reperfusion injury. Chinese Journal of Integrative Medicine. 2016;22(1):49-55

[45] Xu H, Sun H, Chen SH, Zhang YM, Piao YL, Gao Y. Effects of acupuncture at Baihui (DU20) and Zusanli (ST36) on the expression of heat shock protein 70 and tumor necrosis factor α in the peripheral serum of cerebral ischemia-reperfusion-injured rats. Chinese Journal of Integrative Medicine. 2014;20(5):369-374

[46] Xu H, Zhang Y, Sun H, Chen S, Wang F. Effects of acupuncture at GV20 and ST36 on the expression of matrix metalloproteinase 2, aquaporin 4, and aquaporin 9 in rats subjected to cerebral ischemia/reperfusion injury. PLoS One. 2014;9(5):e97488. Available from: http://journals.plos.org/plosone/article?id=10.1371/journal.pone.0097488

[47] Chen L, Liu Y, Lin Q, Xue L, Wang W, Electroacupuncture XJ. At Baihui (DU20) acupoint up- regulates mRNA expression of NeuroD molecules in the brains of newborn rats suffering in utero fetal distress. 2016 Apr;11(4):604-609. DOI: 10.4103/1673-5374.180745

[48] Wang C, Collet JP, Lau J. The effect of tai chi on health outcomes in patients with chronic conditions. Archives of Internal Medicine. 2004;**164**(5):493. Available from: http://archinte. jamanetwork.com/article.aspx?doi=10.1001/archinte.164.5.493

[49] Blake H, Batson M. Exercise intervention in brain injury: A pilot randomized study of Tai Chi Qigong. Clinical Rehabilitation. 2009;**23**(7):589-598. Available from: http://cre.sage-pub.com/cgi/doi/10.1177/0269215508101736

[50] Gemmell C, Leathem JM. A study investigating the effects of tai chi Chuan: Individuals with traumatic brain injury compared to controls. Brain Injury. 2006;**20**(2):151-156. Available from: http://www.ncbi.nlm.nih.gov/pubmed/164210

[51] Tomaszewski W, Manko G, Pachalska M, et al. Improvement of the quality of life of persons with degenerative joint disease in the process of a comprehensive rehabilitation program enhanced by tai chi: The perspective of increasing therapeutic and rehabilitative effects through the applying of eastern techniques combining healthenhancing exercises and martial arts. Archives of Budo. 2012;**8**:169-177

12

Head Injury Mechanisms

Esmaeil Fakharian, Saeed Banaee,
Hamed Yazdanpanah and Mahmood Momeny

Abstract

Head injury is a major cause of death and disability in young, active population. It may introduce energy through the skin to the deepest structures of the brain. The entered energy may cause direct or primary injury, or result in other, secondary, events to the tissues. These are mechanical loads and are classified as static when the duration of loading is more than 200 ms and dynamic when less than this. The dynamic loads are further classified as impact if the injurious agent has contact with the head or impulsive when the load exerted to other body part/s results in damage to the brain by the change in speed of the head motion. Impact loads can either exert their effect with direct contact to the tissue or may cause inertial loads. The direct contact can cause deformation of the skull or induce energy stress waves to the head and brain. All of these events will result in tissue strain due to compression, tension, or shear. The strain will culminate in injury, which may be a scalp abrasion, laceration, skull fracture, or different kinds of intracranial traumatic lesions.

Keywords: TBI, biomechanics, acceleration, primary events, secondary events

1. Introduction

Trauma defined as a physical harm from an external source is probably one of the earliest experiences of the man on the earth. The first evidence of head injury in human was found in Tanzania. It is due to a crocodile bite about 2,000,000–1,800,000 years BC [1]. On the base of Holy Quran and Genesis, the first death is that of Abel happened by a heavy object struck on head by his brother Cain [2]. Along the history these lesions have included all kinds of blunt and penetrating injuries to the head, more commonly in occupational activities such as those reported in Edwin-Smith papyrus in workers of the Egyptian pyramids [1, 3] or conflicts and quarrels as in Goliath and David confrontation or those gladiators managed by Galen [4]. By the development of the human society and increasing speeds particularly in transportation after industrial revolution, new injurious events appeared so that gradually traffic accidents became one of the most important causes of morbidity and mortality in all parts of the world [2].

Management of head injury has significantly changed in the past few decades with better understanding of the mechanisms of load transfer to the tissues and biophysical, biochemical, and physiological consequences which result in many different clinical presentations from a simple scalp laceration to brief periods of loss of consciousness and extending to persistent vegetative state [5–11].

Considering the mechanisms of load transfer to the head, different kinds of traumatic pathologies, including skull fracture; epidural, subdural, intracerebral, and intraventricular hematoma; as well as different kinds of contusion and finally diffuse brain injuries, could be identified and their behavior and injurious effects on the brain and clinical consequences defined [10].

In this chapter, we are going to discuss about different kinds of head trauma, their classification, and some aspects of biomechanics of these events.

2. Head injury biomechanics

The consequences of trauma as an energy transmitted to the head is dependent on physical characters of the invading substance, including the density of the invading substance, its size, speed, and duration of loading [12].

By the entrance of a damaging energy load or mechanical input to the head, the first delineating factor for the evolving injury will be the duration of the energy loading [13]. This time interval has defined in a range of 50 to 200 ms. Those lasting more than 200 ms are labeled as static loads, and those less than this, and most frequently less than 50 ms, are considered as dynamic loads [14, 15].

The static causes of injury are very rare and are usually seen when the head is entrapped between hard objects, e.g., the ground and the ruined elements of a building in an earthquake. These heavy loads may cause deformation of the skin or bone and their damage (usually a focal injury).

3. Dynamic injuries

The dynamic causes of injury include a wide variety of mechanisms. The first of these is produced by the transmission of energy to the brain tissue through the changes in speed (as either of acceleration or deceleration) which are known as impulsive loads. Impulsive loading occurs when the head is not directly struck, but set into motion as a result of a force applied to another part of the body [16]. In such instances, usually, there is no direct and gross evidence of injury to head, i.e., the injury is produced by the inertial changes of the head. In the next group, which is known as impact loads, the offending object when strikes the head may result in injury to tissues from the skin level downwardly depending to the surface area, density, size, and speed of object, directly. On the other hand, it may change the speed of the head and cause its acceleration or deceleration. So, there are inertial changes in the head, and the final result may include those produced by the impulsions.

The inertial loads produced by either impulsions or impactions are exerted by different kinds of acceleration/deceleration. These include translational, rotational, and angular ones, which are defined on the base of the changes on the center of gravity of the skull, the pineal gland. In translation, the changes should be along one of the X, Y, or Z planes. In rotation, the process should be around the axes. These two kinds of acceleration/decelerations are not very common due to the articulation of the skull to the spine; however, the former when happened usually is not associated with severe events, while the latter is highly injurious. The most common kind of event is the angular change, which may be a combination of the abovementioned accelerations.

The impaction of an object to the head can result in change in the configuration of the tissue, either the skin, bone, or deep structures. If this change is above the elasticity of the tissue, it

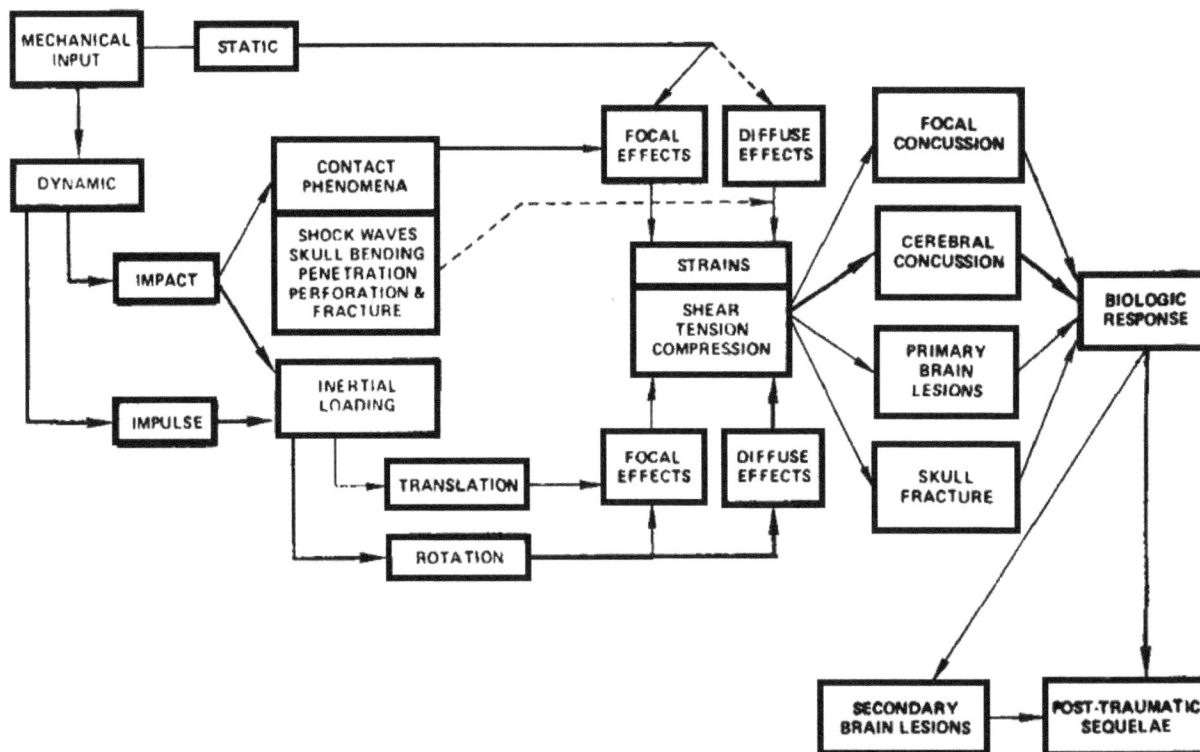

Figure 1. A diagram of head injury mechanisms (from Ommaya and Gennarlli [14]).

will result in its permanent deformity, laceration of the skin, or fracture in the bone. With the greater loads, the offending agent may cause depression of the bone into the intracranial space, namely, depressed skull fracture and laceration of deeper tissues, i.e., dura, brain, and vessels, causing epidural hematoma (EDH), subdural hematoma (SDH), contusion, and intra-cerebral hematoma (ICH). In more severe cases, especially when the speed is high and the size of the agent is small, perforation and penetration may also happen, e.g., in gunshot wounds. Instead, the impaction may be associated with the passage of a load of energy through the skull and the brain. This energy load causes deformation of the brain and its friction to the surrounding structures including skull base and dural membranes or distortion of the cerebral fiber tracts around each other and finally contusion of the brain tissue (**Figure 1**) [17, 18].

4. Tissue strain and tissue injury

All of these elements, tissue deformation, shock wave, and acceleration/deceleration, will exert energy to the tissue and result in tissue strain as compression, tension, or shear. These may result in injury to the tissues, which in the skull are either neural components, vessels, or bone. It must be reiterated that tissue injury will appear when the load entered to the tissue is above the tolerance and elasticity of the tissue so that the changes appeared on that result in an irreversible event. The tolerance of tissues is dependent on their physical characteristics, the amount of energy, duration of energy loading, and the size of the load, and so it is different for different tissues and even different ages for the same tissue. Most of our experiences in usual daily activity are within the physiological tolerance of our tissues and so are harmless, while more aggressive activities such as some of the professional sports, although still within the range, are at the upper limit of physiologic tolerance and if happened repeatedly will result in gradual or even acute appearance of brain dysfunction. What is happening in different accidents, either vehicles or falling from heights, is above the physical tolerance of the tissues and results in different sequels depending on the involved component.

5. Primary and secondary injuries

These are the mechanisms involved in the condition known as primary injury [19, 20], i.e., the direct result of the entered energy to the head. They may in themselves result in other consequences with further injurious effects either as complications of the first phenomenon or exaggerating it. These are known as secondary injuries, the most common of which are hypoxia and hypotension. Secondary injury may also involve mitochondrial dysfunction, excitotoxicity, free radical production, activation of injurious intracellular enzymes, and other mechanisms within the injured nervous tissues which may result in further dysfunctions of the system [13, 20]. Some of the secondary events are similar to the primary phenomenon which will be dealt here, soon. There are also tertiary injuries, which are usually later effects of the energy loading of the head resulting in other system dysfunctions such as electrolyte imbalance due to kidney problems, different kinds of heart disturbances, liver insufficiency, and so on, which are not under the scope of this section.

Considering the abovementioned components in production of an injury to the head, different kinds of the clinical cases can be identified. It can be started with the injury to the bone. In a static loading, the long duration of the time of the entered load results in change in the normal configuration of the skull. When this is above the elasticity of the bone for toleration of the entering energy which is usually a compression at the entrance point (outer table of the skull) and tension in either just below the load inner table or the periphery of the entered load, it will result in tissue failure as fracture of the skull. The severity of fracture is dependent on the amount of load and timing. If it is not so big and lasts for brief periods, there will be no further damage to the deeper structures, and usually the victim will be conscious with a single line or stellate pattern of fracture. On occasions with a great load, the whole skull is severely broken into fragments and the brain tissue disrupted, so that it may ooze from the lacerated scalp or nose and ear canals. In such instances, the victim is in deep coma with severe impairment of the brain and brain stem function, resulting in death.

Skull fracture may result from impaction of the head by an object and its contact resulting in change in configuration of the skull. The consequence of this contact if the surface area of the object is more than five square centimeters may be fracture in the skull. If the surface area is smaller, the object denser with a higher speed, it may penetrate the skull or even perforate it and pass through the brain tissue, as mentioned previously. If the event is in an eloquent region, there may be neurological deficit dependent on the brain function. These are the direct or primary sequel of the injury. There are other events which may appear as a complication of the mentioned events, secondary traumatic effects. Different kinds of intracranial hematomas, including EDH, SDH, ICH, and even intraventricular hematoma (IVH), as well as contusion of the brain tissue (admixture of vascular and brain tissue injury), may result from injury to the vessels in the related places. These lesions may result in mass effect in intracranial space, increase in intracranial pressure, and herniation of the brain. Brain laceration as a primary lesion may predispose the patient to convulsion and epilepsy. Another important complication of this kind of injury is infection of the bone and intracranial content, if the overlying skin is lacerated and prepares access for the microorganisms to the deeper structures. These latter events are other examples of secondary effects, although except EDH, which is always a complication of skull deformation (with or without fracture) and always a secondary phenomenon; all other events may happen as a primary event, as discussed in Section 3.

An important point regarding static and impact contact loads to the head is that they usually cause focal lesions in the brain, and these kinds of lesions are not accompanied by change in level of consciousness, primarily. This can be used as a hallmark for those injuries which are not produced by the inertial loads to the brain. It should be reiterated that changing level of consciousness in the above discussed lesions may happen as a complication of either enlargement of the produced hematoma or contusion or the mass effect produced by other secondary effects of injury like edema around the lesions. However, the mechanism of disturbed consciousness in these lesions, usually, is not injury to the brain as the main source of consciousness, because it is a wholistic function and focal damages cannot produce it, but it is mainly produced by the displacement of the brain tissue from its connecting hiatuses and compression/ischemia of the brain stem sources of the condition. These are well known as cerebral herniations, as another example of secondary injury.

Concussion, diffuse axonal injury (DAI), SDH, ICH, and IVH as primary lesions should be discussed with the mechanism of change in speed of movement of tissues in the head or inertial loads [21]. These can be viewed as a wide spectrum of injuries with very mild cases as brief period of confusion and memory disturbance to short interval of loss of consciousness or concussion [16], to long-standing deep coma or persistent vegetative state (PVS) due to diffuse injury to neurons and axons of the brain or DAI. In normal circumstances, axons are compliant and readily return to their original length after loading. However, with rapid application of tissue strain, such as at the time of head impact, with the anisotropic and complex arrangement, axons behave differently, essentially becoming brittle and vulnerable to injury [22].

In between there are injury to vascular components either in the surface of the brain (SDH), due to the difference in the elasticity and ability of the brain movement and the bridging veins connecting the brain to the venous sinuses placed in the dural layers, or in deeper parts from the cortex and subcortical layers (ICH) to the ventricle (IVH). As was stated previously, the common presentation of all of these events is loss of consciousness (LOC) of the patient from the time of event. The duration of LOC is dependent on the energy load, its effect on the specific parts of the brain, and severity of the injury in the brain.

A key clinical point is that when these lesions are produced by non-inertial loads, as discussed in previous paragraphs, and cause disturbance of level of consciousness due to their secondary effects, appropriate and in time decompression may result in recovery of the consciousness, while in those with inertial loads, decompression may not be followed by recovery of consciousness just after operation or even in longer durations. So, restrict consideration on the clinical course of the patient at the time of admission and focusing on the possible unconsciousness will help the surgeon to predict probable surgical findings and the early post-op outcome.

6. Conclusion

We suggest that application of the discussed algorithm for assessment of the injured patients may help clinicians for predictions of the sequelae outcomes. If used appropriately it even can be used for clinical evaluation of the injured patients and decision-making for a rational paraclinical study. Although increasing availability of computed tomographic (CT) scanners in most hospitals has supplanted the need for skull X-ray study as one of the primary steps in patients with head injury, however whenever inertial loads are considered as the main mechanism of trauma, even in the absence of CT scanners, the use of skull X-ray will not be helpful for the diagnosis of the probable injuries.

Finally, it must be kept in mind that classifications and delineations are used for better understanding of the events on the base of current knowledge and so may occasionally not comply with all of the events in reality. While managing head injury patients, one of these pitfalls is the definition of dynamic and static loadings of the brain on the base of duration of the event which is a small fraction of a second for both. This means that it is always possible to have a spectrum of different mechanisms and lesions due to both of the mechanisms. The algorithm should be used for better prediction, understanding, and explanation of the events on the base of detailed clinical evaluation and not as a restrict rule.

Author details

Esmaeil Fakharian[1,2]*, Saeed Banaee[1], Hamed Yazdanpanah[1] and Mahmood Momeny[1]

*Address all correspondence to: efakharian@gmail.com

1 Department of Neurosurgery, Kashan University of Medical Sciences (KAUMS), Kashan, IR Iran

2 Trauma Research Center, KAUMS, Kashan, IR Iran

References

[1] Bertullo G. History of traumatic brain injury (TBI). African Journal of Business Management. 2015;**3**(7):381-409. DOI: 10.18081/2333-5106/015-07/381-409

[2] Fakharian E. Trauma research and its importance. Archives of Trauma Research. 2012;**1** (1):1-2. DOI: 10.5812/atr.5287

[3] Ghannaee Arani M, Fakharian E, Sarbandi F. Ancient legacy of cranial surgery. Archives of Trauma Research. 2012;**1**(2):72-74. DOI: 10.5812/atr.6556

[4] Ghannaee Arani M, Fakharian E, Ardjmand A, Mohammadian H, Mohammadzadeh M, Sarbandi F. Ibn Sina's (Avicenna) contributions in the treatment of traumatic injuries. Trauma Monthly. 2012;**17**(2):301-304. DOI: 10.5812/traumamon.4695

[5] Cloots RJH, Gervaise HMT, van Dommelen JAW, Geers MGD. Biomechanics of traumatic brain injury: Influences of the morphologic heterogeneities of the cerebral cortex. Annals of Biomedical Engineering. 2008;**36**(7):1203-1215. DOI: 10.1007/s10439-008-9510-3

[6] Gaetz M. The neurophysiology of brain injury. Clinical Neurophysiology. 2004;**115**:4-18

[7] Cloots RJH, van Dommelen JAW, Kleiven S, Geers MGD. Multi-scale mechanics of traumatic brain injury: Predicting axonal strains from head loads. Biomechanics and Modeling in Mechanobiology. 2013;**12**:137-150. DOI: 10.1007/s10237-012-0387-6

[8] Greve MW, Zink BJ. Pathophysiology of traumatic brain injury. Mount Sinai Journal of Medicine. 2009;**76**:97-104. DOI: 10.1002/msj.20104

[9] Post A et al. The dynamic response characteristics of traumatic brain injury. Accident Analysis and Prevention. 2015;**79**:33-40. DOI: 10.1016/j.aap.2015.03.017

[10] Saatman KE et al. Classification of traumatic brain injury for targeted therapies. Journal of Neurotrauma. 2008;**25**:719-738. DOI: 10.1089/neu.2008.0586

[11] Stein SC. Patrick G, Meghan S, Mizra K, Seema SS. 150 years of treating severe traumatic brain injury: A systematic review of progress in mortality. Journal of Neurotrauma. 2010;**27**:1343-1353. DOI: 10.1089/neu.2009.1206

[12] McLean AJ, Anderson RWG: Biomechanics of closed head injury. In: Reilly P, Bullock R, editors. Head Injury. London: Chapman & Hall; 1997. ISBN 0 412 58540 5

[13] Meythaler JM, Peduzzi JD, Eleftheriou E, Novack TA. Current concepts: Diffuse axonal injury-associated traumatic brain injury. Archives of Physical Medicine and Rehabilitation. 2001;**82**:1461-1471. DOI: 10.1053/apmr.2001.25137

[14] Ommaya AK, Gennarelli TA. Cerebral concussion and traumatic unconsciousness. Brain. 1974;**97**:633-654

[15] Smith DH, Meaney DF, Shull WH. Diffuse axonal injury in head trauma. The Journal of Head Trauma Rehabilitation. 2003;**18**(4):307-316

[16] Poirier MP. Concussions: Assessment, management, and recommendations for return to activity. Clinical Pediatric Emergency Medicine. 2003;**4**:179-185. DOI: 10.1016/S1522-8401 (03)00061-2

[17] Bayly PV, Cohen TS, Leister EP, Ajo D, Leuthardt EC, GM: Deformation of the human brain induced by mild acceleration. Journal of Neurotrauma. 2005;**22**(8):845-856. DOI: doi.org/10.1089/neu.2005.22.845

[18] Feng Y, Abney TM, Okamoto RJ, Pless RB, Genin GM, Bayly PV. Relative brain displacement and deformation during constrained mild frontal head impact. Journal of The Royal Society Interface. 2010;**7**:1677-1688. DOI: 10.1098/rsif.2010.0210

[19] Hawryluk GWJ, Manley GT. Classification of traumatic brain injury: past, present, and future. In: Grafman J, Salazar AM, editors. Handbook of Clinical Neurology. Vol. 127 (3rd series). Traumatic Brain Injury, Part I. Waltham, USA: Elsevier B.V.; 2015. pp. 15-21

[20] Werner C, Engelhard K. Pathophysiology of traumatic brain injury. British Journal of Anaesthesia. 2007;**99**(1):4-9. DOI: 10.1093/bja/aem131

[21] Post A, Hoshizaki TB. Mechanisms of brain impact injuries and their prediction: A review. Trauma. 2012;**14**(4):327-349. DOI: 10.1177/1460408612446573

[22] Johnson VE, Stewart W, Smith DH. Axonal pathology in traumatic brain injury. Experimental Neurology. August 2013;**246**:35-43. DOI: 10.1016/j.expneurol.2012.01.013

Permissions

All chapters in this book were first published in TBI, by InTech Open; hereby published with permission under the Creative Commons Attribution License or equivalent. Every chapter published in this book has been scrutinized by our experts. Their significance has been extensively debated. The topics covered herein carry significant findings which will fuel the growth of the discipline. They may even be implemented as practical applications or may be referred to as a beginning point for another development.

The contributors of this book come from diverse backgrounds, making this book a truly international effort. This book will bring forth new frontiers with its revolutionizing research information and detailed analysis of the nascent developments around the world.

We would like to thank all the contributing authors for lending their expertise to make the book truly unique. They have played a crucial role in the development of this book. Without their invaluable contributions this book wouldn't have been possible. They have made vital efforts to compile up to date information on the varied aspects of this subject to make this book a valuable addition to the collection of many professionals and students.

This book was conceptualized with the vision of imparting up-to-date information and advanced data in this field. To ensure the same, a matchless editorial board was set up. Every individual on the board went through rigorous rounds of assessment to prove their worth. After which they invested a large part of their time researching and compiling the most relevant data for our readers.

The editorial board has been involved in producing this book since its inception. They have spent rigorous hours researching and exploring the diverse topics which have resulted in the successful publishing of this book. They have passed on their knowledge of decades through this book. To expedite this challenging task, the publisher supported the team at every step. A small team of assistant editors was also appointed to further simplify the editing procedure and attain best results for the readers.

Apart from the editorial board, the designing team has also invested a significant amount of their time in understanding the subject and creating the most relevant covers. They scrutinized every image to scout for the most suitable representation of the subject and create an appropriate cover for the book.

The publishing team has been an ardent support to the editorial, designing and production team. Their endless efforts to recruit the best for this project, has resulted in the accomplishment of this book. They are a veteran in the field of academics and their pool of knowledge is as vast as their experience in printing. Their expertise and guidance has proved useful at every step. Their uncompromising quality standards have made this book an exceptional effort. Their encouragement from time to time has been an inspiration for everyone.

The publisher and the editorial board hope that this book will prove to be a valuable piece of knowledge for researchers, students, practitioners and scholars across the globe.

List of Contributors

Sombat Muengtaweepongsa
Division of Neurology, Department of Medicine, Thammasat University, Pathum Thani, Thailand

Pornchai Yodwisithsak
Division of Neurosurgery, Department of Surgery, Thammasat University, Pathum Thani, Thailand

Christ Ordookhanian, Katherine Tsai and Paul E. Kaloostian
Riverside School of Medicine, University of California, Riverside, CA, USA

Sean W. Kaloostian
Irvine Medical Center, University of California, Irvine, CA, USA

Sung Ho Jang
Department of Physical Medicine and Rehabilitation, College of Medicine, Yeungnam University and Daemyungdong, Namku, Taegu, Republic of Korea

Nino Muradashvili, Suresh C. Tyagi and David Lominadze
Department of Physiology, University of Louisville, School of Medicine, Louisville, KY, USA

Christ Ordookhanian, Dina Elias and Paul E. Kaloostian
University of California, Riverside School of Medicine, Riverside, CA, United States

Meena Nagappan
St. Georges School of Medicine, True Blue, Grenada

John Magnuson and Geoffrey Ling
Department of Neurology, Uniformed Services University of the Health Sciences, Bethesda, MD, United States

Geoffrey Ling
Inova Neuroscience and Spine Institute, Inova Fairfax Hospital, Fairfax, VA, United States
Department of Neurology, Johns Hopkins Medical Institutions, Baltimore, MD, United States

Cino Bendinelli, Shannon Cooper, Christian Abel and Zsolt J. Balogh
John Hunter Hospital, University of Newcastle, Newcastle, NSW, AU

Andrew Bivard
Hunter Medical Research Institute, University of Newcastle, Newcastle, NSW, AU

Noam Naphatali Tal
Independent Scientist and Former student, Department of Medical Device Technology, Maltash College, Tel Aviv, Israel

Tesla Yudhistira, Woo Hyun Lee, Youngsam Kim and David G. Churchill
Molecular Logic Gate Laboratory, Department of Chemistry, Korea Advanced Institute of Science and Technology (KAIST), Daejeon, Republic of Korea

Youngsam Kim and David G. Churchill
Center for Catalytic Hydrocarbon Functionalizations, Institute for Basic Science (IBS), Daejeon, Republic of Korea

Tesla Yudhistira
Lembaga Pengelola Dana Pendidikan (LPDP), Indonesia Endowment Fund for Education, Kementrian Keuangan Republik Indonesia, Jakarta, Indonesia

David G. Churchill
Schulich Faculty of Chemistry at T echnion, Israel Institute of Technology, Haifa, Israel

Thomas Brickler
The Department of Psychiatry and Behavioral Sciences, Stanford University School of Medicine, Stanford, CA, USA

Paul D. Morton, Amanda Hazy and Michelle H. Theus
The Department of Biomedical Sciences and Pathobiology, Virginia-Maryland Regional College of Veterinary Medicine, Blacksburg, VA, USA

Andrea Regner, Lindolfo da Silva Meirelles and Daniel Simon
School of Medicine, Lutheran University of Brazil, Canoas, RS, Brazil
Graduate Program in Cellular and Molecular Biology Applied to Health (PPGBioSaúde), Lutheran University of Brazil, Canoas, RS, Brazil

Ching-Chih Chen, Yu-Chiang Hung and Wen-Long Hu
Department of Chinese Medicine, Kaohsiung Chang Gung Memorial Hospital and School of Traditional Chinese Medicine, Chang Gung University College of Medicine, Kaohsiung, Taiwan

Yu-Chiang Hung
School of Chinese Medicine for Post Baccalaureate, I-Shou University, Kaohsiung, Taiwan

Wen-Long Hu
Fooyin University College of Nursing, Kaohsiung, Taiwan

Kaohsiung Medical University College of Medicine, Kaohsiung, Taiwan

Esmaeil Fakharian, Saeed Banaee, Hamed Yazdanpanah and Mahmood Momeny
Department of Neurosurgery, Kashan University of Medical Sciences (KAUMS), Kashan, IR Iran

Esmaeil Fakharian
Trauma Research Center, KAUMS, Kashan, IR Iran

Index

www.ingramcontent.com/pod-product-compliance
Lightning Source LLC
Chambersburg PA
CBHW080631200326
41458CB00013B/4589